Pocket
ImmunoFacts™

vaccines &
immunologics

Pocket ImmunoFacts
Vaccines and Immunologics

John D. Grabenstein, MSPharm, EdM, FASHP
Laurie A. Grabenstein, RN, BSN

Pocket ImmunoFacts™ - Vaccines and Immunologics, 1997 Edition

ISBN 1-57439-018-X

Printed in the United States of America

Pocket
ImmunoFacts™

vaccines & immunologics

John D. Grabenstein, MSPharm, EdM, FASHP

Laurie A. Grabenstein, RN, BSN

Facts and Comparisons Staff

President	C. Sue Sewester
Publisher	Paul S. Heirendt
Director of Drug Information	Bernie R. Olin, PharmD
Business Development	Heidi L. Meredith
Editorial Development	Cathy H. Reilly
Print Products Manager	Noël A. Shamleffer
Assistant Editors	Stephanie Hug
	Bridget Sinclair

To Emily, to Andrea, and to Erica,
with hope, and to all our families,
with love and thanks.

Table of Contents

Introduction

Pocket *ImmunoFacts* is designed with the busy vaccine administrator in mind. Whether you see one person or a thousand people a day who need immunizations, this book helps you give each one just the right immunologic and preventive care needed.

For the first time, *Pocket ImmunoFacts* brings together, in summary form, information about vaccines, antibodies and other immunologic drugs. The format allows quick, reliable access to information. It also helps readers compare and contrast information for similar products or uses.

We assembled this book from the work of national and international experts. Pocket *ImmunoFacts* is based on *ImmunoFacts: Vaccines and Immunologic Drugs*. *ImmunoFacts* is the premier reference book reviewed by experts in immunology therapeutics, vaccinology, and drug information. Other authorities from government, universities and the pharmaceutical industry also contributed, ensuring information of the highest quality and reliability.

To keep *Pocket ImmunoFacts* concise and convenient, we have limited this book to the immunologic and vaccine data you need every day. For comprehensive discussions of all there is to know about vaccines and immunologic drugs read the primary book, *ImmunoFacts: Vaccines and Immunologic Drugs*.

How to Use This Book

You can use *Pocket ImmunoFacts* in several ways. The detailed table of contents and index will help you find the information you want, fast. Take a glance at them to learn your way around.

If you are interested in a particular vaccine or antibody, go directly to that monograph. Monographs are grouped according to type of agent (eg, viral vaccines). Monographs include:

Name
Manufacturer
Viability
Antigenic Form
Antigenic Type
Indications
Contraindications, including
   absolute and relative
Elderly
Adults
Pregnancy
Lactation
Children
Adverse Reactions
Dosage
Route and Site
Documentation Requirements
Efficacy
Onset
Duration
Drug Interactions
Concentration
Packaging
Dose Form
Diluent for Reconstitution
Storage/Stability
Handling

The appendices include a variety of information regarding the use of vaccines and immunologics. "Immunization Needs" explains the various vaccines required based on age, personal factors, occupation and travel. A section about weakened immune systems and immune suppressive drugs also is included.

Bacterial Vaccines and Toxoids

Bacillus Calmette Guérin (BCG) Vaccine

Cholera Vaccine

Diphtheria, Tetanus & Pertussis Overview

Diphtheria & Tetanus Toxoids & Whole-Cell
Pertussis Vaccine (DTwP)

DTwP-HIB

Diphtheria & Tetanus Toxoids & Acellular
Pertussis Vaccine (DTaP)

Diphtheria & Tetanus Toxoids Adsorbed,
for Pediatric Use (DT)

Tetanus and Diphtheria Toxoids Adsorbed,
for Adult Use (Td)

Tetanus Toxoid Adsorbed

Pertussis Vaccine Adsorbed

Haemophilus Influenzae Type B
Conjugate Vaccine

Meningococcal Polysaccharide,
Groups A, C, Y, and W-135

Pneumococcal Vaccine, 23-Valent

Typhoid Vaccine (Parenteral)

Typhoid Vaccine (Oral)

NAME:

Tice BCG for intravesical or per-cutaneous use, ♣ Generic

MANUFACTURERS:

Tice BCG, Organon Teknika Cor-poration; ♣ Generic, Connaught, IAF Biovac

Synonyms: Bacille or Bacillus Cal-mette-Guérin, BCG. BCG is not synonymous with tuberculosis. The disease tuberculosis has been called by various names, including consump-tion, phthisis, the "white plague" (Oliver Wendell Holmes, Sr.) and the "captain of all these men of death" (John Bunyan).

Comparison: *Tice BCG* and other BCG products are not generically equiva-lent, due to differences in potency, route of administration and indica-tions. The various strains of BCG are microbiologically distinct.

Viability: Live, attenuated

Antigenic Form: Whole bacterium

Antigenic Type: Protein

Use Characteristics

Indications: Induction of active immunity against *Mycobacterium tuberculosis* variant *hominus*, to lower the risk of serious complications of tuberculosis. BCG vaccination is rec-ommended for skin-test negative infants and children with repeated exposure to persistently untreated or ineffectively treated sputum and pul-monary tuberculosis. BCG probably confers protection against serious forms of disease (eg, miliary and meningeal tuberculosis), but data on pulmonary disease are unclear. BCG does not appear to prevent infection, but may reduce transmission (Gheo-rghiu, 1990).

BCG vaccination will protect well-defined communities against tubercu-losis in which the rate of new infection exceeds 1% per year. It will also protect those for whom the usual surveillance and treatment programs

have been attempted but are not oper-ationally feasible. These groups include persons without regular access to health care, those for whom usual health care is culturally or socially unacceptable, or groups who have demonstrated an inability to effective-ly use existing accessible care.

Induction of active immunity against tuberculosis in certain international travelers is recommended. CDC sug-gests, however, that BCG vaccination be considered only for travelers with insignificant reaction to tuberculin skin test who will be in a high-risk environment for prolonged periods of time without access to tuberculin skin-test surveillance.

Treatment of carcinoma in situ of the urinary bladder: (1) primary treatment in the absence of an associated inva-sive cancer without papillary tumors or with papillary tumors after transurethral resection (TUR); (2) sec-ondary treatment in the absence of an associated invasive cancer in patients failing to respond or relapsing after intravesical chemotherapy with other agents; or (3) primary or secondary treatment in the absence of invasive cancer for patients with medical contraindications to radical surgery.

Unlabeled Uses: BCG vaccine induces antibodies that bind to *Mycobacterium leprae* and may be effective in the prevention of leprosy. ACIP no longer recommends BCG vaccination of healthcare workers at risk of repeated exposure to tuberculosis, but recommends that these individuals receive periodic tuberculin skin tests and receive isoniazid prophylaxis in case of tuberculin skin-test conversion. Greenberg et al (1991), on the other hand, published a decision analysis suggesting that house-staff physicians may benefit from routine BCG vaccination over a 10 year period, given that the prevalence of tuberculosis among physicians is twice the age-specific rate in the general population. CDC does not recommend routine BCG vaccination of health-care workers, but urges increased compliance with existing screening programs and antituberculous prophylaxis.

Contraindications:

STOP *Absolute:* Immunodeficient patients and patients with a history of hypersensitivity or other serious adverse reactions. Avoid BCG use in asymptomatic carriers with a positive HIV serology and in patients receiving corticosteroids at immunosuppressive doses or other immunosuppressive therapies because of the possibility of systemic BCG infection.

A positive ID tuberculin skin test to 5-TU of PPD is an absolute contraindication to immunization against tuberculosis, but a contraindication to use for treatment of bladder cancer only if an active tuberculosis infection is in progress or suspected. If the patient exhibits a significant reaction to a 5-TU PPD test, use a physical examination including chest radiograph to assess tuberculosis infection.

Bladder cancer—Postpone treatment until resolution of a concurrent febrile illness, urinary tract infection or gross hematuria. Seven to 14 days should elapse between biopsy, TUR or traumatic catheterization and BCG instillation. Administration of BCG onto bleeding mucosa may result in a life-threatening disseminated infection.

Elderly: The mean age of subjects in clinical trials that established safety and efficacy for treatment of bladder cancer was 68.8 years of age (range, 38 to 97 years).

Pregnancy: *Category* C. Avoid use. Use only if clearly needed. It is not known if BCG vaccine or corresponding antibodies cross the placenta. Generally, most IgG passage across the placenta occurs during the third trimester.

Lactation: It is not known if BCG vaccine or corresponding antibodies are excreted in breast milk. Problems in humans have not been documented. A recent Canadian study (Pabst et al, 1989) suggests that breast-feeding enhanced cell-mediated immune response to BCG given at birth, but had no significant effect if vaccine was given 1 month or more after birth.

Children: Safety and efficacy have not been established in children with regard to bladder cancer. BCG is an effective vaccine against tuberculosis in children. Give children 1 month of age one-half the adult immunizing dose.

Adverse Reactions:

Reactions to Vaccination: Mild reactions include fever, anorexia, myalgia and neuralgia lasting a few days. Severe or prolonged ulceration occurs (1% to 10%). Anaphylaxis, lymphadenitis, osteomyelitis (1 case per million doses), disseminated BCG infection (1 to 10 cases per 10 million doses) self-inoculation of BCG bacteria to other body sites, and death have followed vaccination.

Reactions to Bladder Instillation: Reactions localized to the bladder—Bladder irritability (60%, beginning 3 to 4 hours after instillation, lasting 24 to 72 hours), dysuria, urinary frequency, hematuria, cystitis, urgency, nocturia, cramps or pain, urinary incontinence, urinary debris, genital inflammation or abscess, urinary tract infection, urethritis, pyuria, epididymitis or prostatitis, urinary obstruction, contracted bladder, orchitis.

Systemic Reactions: "Flu"-like syndrome, fever, malaise or fatigue, shaking chills, nausea or vomiting, arthritis or myalgia, headache or dizziness, anorexia or weight loss, abdominal pain, anemia, diarrhea, pneumonitis, GI and neurologic effects, rash, BCG sepsis, coagulopathy, leukopenia, thrombocytopenia, hepatic granuloma, hepatitis, allergic, cardiac, respiratory effects.

Febrile episodes with "flu"-like symptoms lasting longer than 48 hours, fever >38.3°C (101°F), symptoms resistant to standard antipyretic treatment, systemic manifestations increasing in intensity with repeated instillations or persistent abnormalities of liver function tests, suggest systemic BCG infection and require antitubercular therapy. Persons with small bladder capacity are at increased risk of severe local irritation.

Occupational Exposure: PPD-negative healthcare personnel who routinely handle BCG vaccine should record annual PPD skin-test results. In case BCG vaccine splashes into an eye, flush the affected eye(s) with large volumes of water for 15 minutes while holding the eyelid(s) open. In case of accidental self-inoculation, give a PPD skin test at the time of the accident and 6 weeks later to detect any skin-test conversion. Asymptomatic skin-test conversion attributable to BCG exposure is equivalent to BCG vaccination and does not require antituberculous medication.

Pharmacologic & Dosing Characteristics

Dose Preparation: Draw diluent into syringe and expel into ampule 3 times for thorough mixing; do not filter.

Dosage: *Tuberculosis:* Drop 0.2 to 0.3 ml onto the cleansed surface of the skin and use a sterile multiple-puncture disc to percutaneously penetrate the tensed skin. Give children <1 month of age one-half the adult immunizing dose.

In a successful procedure, the points penetrate the skin. Remove the disc and spread the vaccine into the puncture sites and allow to dry. No dressing is required, but keep the site dry for 24 hours. Normal reactions to tuberculosis immunization consist of skin lesions of small red papules, appearing within 10 to 14 days. The papules may reach a maximum diameter of about 3 mm after 4 to 6 weeks, after which they may scale and then slowly subside.

Keep the vaccination site clean until the local reaction disappears. Usually, no visible sign of vaccination persists 6 months later, although a discernible pattern of puncture points may remain in persons prone to keloid formation. Such marks are typically a permanent, very slightly excavated, round scar 4 to 8 mm in diameter.

Bladder Cancer: Suspend the contents of one 50 mg ampule suspended in 50 ml of preservative free 0.9% sodium chloride, delivered by gravity through a urethral catheter. Administer 1 instillation per week for 6 weeks. The patient refrains from drinking liquids for 4 hours before treatment and empties the bladder before BCG instillation. The patient retains the product in the bladder for 2 hours and then voids while seated.

Route & Site:

Tuberculosis: Percutaneous. Order multiple-puncture discs with attached magnet for tuberculosis immunization from the manufacturer. The disc is a wafer-like stainless-steel plate, $\frac{7}{8}$ inch wide and $1\frac{1}{8}$ inch long, from which 36 points protrude, to which a magnetic holder attaches. The anatomic site of vaccination is not standardized and may appear at various locations on the body, although the product labeling suggests the upper arm.

In some nations, including Canada, other BCG products are administered by ID injection for prevention of tuberculosis.

Bladder Cancer: Intravesical, by bladder instillation. Do not administer this product intradermally, SC or IV.

Additional Doses:

Tuberculosis: Repeat vaccination against tuberculosis after 2 to 3 months for those persons who remain negative to a 5-TU tuberculin skin test. If a vaccinated infant remains tuberculin negative to 5-TU PPD, and if indications for vaccination persist, give the infant a full dose after 1 year of age. Immunity to tuberculosis is considered generally long-lasting and routine booster immunizations are not recommended. Tuberculin reactivity after BCG exposure diminishes in probability as time since BCG exposure increases.

Bladder Cancer: Give 1 treatment monthly for at least 6 to 12 months after initial treatment.

Efficacy: *Tuberculosis* Clinical trials have yielded inconsistent results, with vaccine-efficacy estimates ranging from near zero in trials in India, to 14% in the southern US, or 80% in Europe and Canada. Likely explanations of these discrepancies include differences in BCG strains, regional mycobacterial ecology, trial methods, stages of mycobacterial infection and disease, and other factors (Fine and Rodrigues, 1990). Ironically, BCG may be the most widely used vaccine in the world, yet has the least scientific evidence of efficacy, mechanism of action and utility. BCG probably confers protection against serious forms of disease (eg, miliary and meningeal tuberculosis), but data on pulmonary disease is unclear. BCG does not appear to prevent infection, but may reduce transmission (Gheorghiu, 1990).

Bladder Cancer: During clinical trials, an overall response rate of 75.6% was reported in 119 evaluable patients with carcinoma in situ of the bladder.

Leprosy: Estimates range from 20% to 80% reduction in disease incidence among contacts of leprosy patients.

Onset: Vaccinated persons typically become skin-test positive to PPD within 8 to 14 weeks.

Duration:

Tuberculosis: Induced immunity to tuberculosis is generally considered long-lasting and routine booster immunizations are not recommended. Tuberculin reactivity after BCG exposure diminishes in probability as time since BCG exposure increases.

Bladder Cancer: Estimated median duration of response is ≥48 months after BCG treatment. The median time to cystectomy in patients who achieved a complete response was >74 months, whereas the median time to cystectomy for nonresponders was 31 months.

Drug Interactions: Like all live bacterial vaccines, administration of BCG to patients receiving immunosuppressant drugs, including high-dose corticosteroids, or radiation therapy may predispose patients to disseminated infection or insufficient response to immunization. They may remain susceptible despite immunization. BCG vaccine does not interfere with oral poliovirus vaccine.

BCG immunization or therapy usually induces hypersensitivity to tuberculin skin tests. This false-positive effect diminishes in probability as time since BCG exposure increases. It may be useful to determine tuberculin sensitivity prior to BCG therapy of bladder cancer.

Antitubercular therapy (eg, isoniazid) will antagonize disseminated BCG infections. Antitubercular or other antimicrobial therapy can interfere with the effectiveness of BCG therapy of bladder cancer. Some BCG strains available in other countries (eg, Evans Medical Ltd., England) are resistant to isoniazid.

BCG vaccination can decrease the elimination of theophylline, increasing its biological half-life. Observe theophylline patients who receive BCG vaccine for theophylline toxicity and advise them to seek assistance if symptoms of toxicity appear (eg, nausea, vomiting, palpitations).

Pharmaceutical Characteristics

Concentration: *Organon*: 1 to 8 x 10^8 colony-forming units per 50 mg wet weight per ampule

Connaught: 8 to 32 x 10^5 CFU per 0.1 ml dose

IAF Biovac: 75 mcg per 0.1 ml dose (750 mcg per vial)

Packaging: 2 ml single-dose ampule

Dose Form: Powder for suspension

Diluent for Reconstitution: 1 ml sterile water for injection, when injected percutaneously, or 1 ml preservative free 0.9% sodium chloride, when administered by bladder instillation.

In either case, store diluent at a temperature ranging from 4° to 25°C (39° to 77°F).

Storage/Stability: Store at 2° to 8°C (35° to 46°F). Protect from light. Lyophilized product can be stored frozen, and then reconstituted and used effectively. After reconstitution, refrigerate product until used. There is no data to support freezing and thawing of reconstituted product. Shipped in insulated containers with dry ice.

Discard 2 hours after reconstitution.

Comparison of BCG Products

	Tice BCG	TheraCys[1]
Manufacturer	Organon Teknika	Connaught
Concentration	1 to 8 x 10^8 CFU or 50 mg per ampule	1.7 to 19.2 x 10^8 CFU or 81 mg per vial
Packaging	2 ml amp (no diluent)	1 vial of powder, 1 vial of diluent
Indications	Tuberculosis prevention, treatment of bladder carcinoma in situ	Treatment of bladder carcinoma in situ only
Diluent	1 ml sterile water per amp for vaccination; 1 ml preservative free 0.9% sodium chloride per amp for bladder cancer	3 ml phosphate-buffered saline per vial
Dose and route	0.2 to 0.3 ml percutaneously as tuberculosis vaccine; 1 amp diluted in 50 ml preservative free 0.9% sodium chloride given through urinary catheter for bladder carcinoma	1 vial diluted in 50 ml 0.9% sodium chloride given through urinary catheter for baldder carcinoma

[1]For complete prescribing information for *TheraCys* refer to *ImmunoFacts™: Vaccines and Immunologic Drugs.*

Cholera Vaccine
BACTERIAL VACCINES & TOXOIDS

NAME:
Generic

MANUFACTURERS:
Wyeth-Lederle Vaccines & Pediatrics, ❦ Connaught

Viability: Inactivated
Antigenic Form: Whole bacterium

Antigenic Type: Protein toxin and lipopolysaccharide

Use Characteristics

Indications: Induction of active immunity against cholera, such as in individuals traveling to or residing in endemic or epidemic areas.

Contraindications:
Absolute: Patients with a history of a severe systemic or allergic response following a prior dose of cholera vaccine.

Relative: Defer immunization during the course of any acute illness.

Elderly: No specific information is available about geriatric use of cholera vaccine.

Pregnancy: *Category* C. Use only if clearly needed. It is not known if cholera vaccine or corresponding antibodies cross the placenta. Generally, most IgG passage across the placenta occurs during the third trimester.

Lactation: It is not known if cholera vaccine or corresponding antibodies are excreted into human breast milk. Problems in humans have not been documented.

Children: Give children a varying dose, based on age. Do not inject ID in children <5 years of age. No studies have been conducted in populations <6 months old.

Adverse Reactions:
Local reactions occur in most recipients and consist of erythema, induration, pain and tenderness at the injection site. These reactions may persist for a few days. Recipients frequently develop malaise, headache and mild to moderate temperature elevations for 1 to 2 days. Anaphylactic and other systemic reactions occur rarely.

Pharmacologic & Dosing Characteristics

Dosage: Primary immunizing series: 2 doses 1 week to 1 month or more apart, followed by booster doses every 6 months. Shake well before withdrawing each dose. Persons ≥5 years of age may receive 0.2 ml of vaccine ID for each dose. By SC or IM injection, give persons 6 months to 4 years of age 0.2 ml each dose, those 5 to 10 years of age 0.3 ml, and those >10 years 0.5 ml each dose. In areas where cholera occurs in a 2 to 3 month season, maximize protection by giving the booster dose at the beginning of the season.

Route and Site: ID, SC or IM. The volume varies according to the route of administration chosen.

Efficacy: About 50% effective in reducing disease incidence for 3 to 6 months. Protection in humans corre-

Dosage of Cholera Vaccine			
Route	Age	Dose (ml)	Regimen
ID	≥5 years	0.2	Two doses given 1 week to ≥1 month apart. Repeat every 6 months if risk persists.
SC or IM	6 months to 4 years	0.2	
	5 to 10 years	0.3	
	>10 years	0.5	

lates to acquisition of circulating vibriocidal antibody.

Onset: Data not provided. Induction of protective antibody titers probably occurs by 2 weeks after the second dose.

Duration: 3 to 6 months

Drug Interactions: Like all inactivated vaccines, administration of cholera vaccine to persons receiving immunosuppressant drugs, including high-dose corticosteroids, or radiation therapy may result in an insufficient response to immunization. They may remain susceptible despite immunization. Yellow-fever vaccination within 3 weeks before or after cholera vaccine results in reduced response to each vaccine. Cholera vaccine has reduced seroconversion to poliovirus type 1 vaccine when given simultaneously. Separate doses of these vaccines by 1 month, if possible. Avoid concurrent administration of cholera vaccine with other reactogenic vaccines (eg, SC typhoid, plague) if possible, to avoid the theoretical risk of increased reactogenicity.

As with other drugs administered by IM injection, give cholera vaccine with caution to persons receiving anticoagulant therapy.

Pharmaceutical Characteristics

Concentration: 8 units (4 billion vibrios) of each type per ml

Packaging: 1.5 ml multidose vial and 20 ml multidose vial

Dose Form: Suspension

Solvent: Phosphate-buffered saline 0.02 molar

Storage/Stability: Store at 2° to 8°C (35° to 46°F). Discard frozen vaccine. Product can tolerate 10 days at 45°C (113°F). Shipping data not provided.

Diphtheria, Tetanus & Pertussis Overview
BACTERIAL VACCINES & TOXOIDS

The following tables summarize the various formulations of diphtheria, tetanus and pertussis and related information. Detailed discussions of these formulations can be found in the individual monographs that follow the Overview section.

Diphtheria, Tetanus & Pertussis—Combination Summary					
	Diphtheria, tetanus toxoids & whole-cell pertussis vaccine	Diphtheria, tetanus toxoids & acellular pertussis vaccine	Diphtheria & tetanus toxoids (pediatric)	Tetanus & diphtheria toxoids (adult)	Diphtheria & tetanus toxoids and Hib conjugate & whole cell pertussis vaccines
Synonyms	DTP, DTwP	DTP, DTaP	DT	Td	DTwP-Hib
Manufacturer	several	Connaught, Wyeth-Lederle	several	several	Wyeth-Lederle
Concentration (per 0.5 ml) Diphtheria Tetanus Pertussis Hib	6.5-12.5 Lf u 5-5.5 Lf u 4 u none	6.7-7.5 Lf u 5 Lf u either 46.8 mcg or 300 HA u none	6.6-12.5 Lf u 5-7.6 Lf u none none	2 Lf u 2-5 Lf u none none	6.7 or 12.5 Lf u 5 Lf u 4 u 10 mcg
Packaging	5 or 7.5 ml vials	5 or 7.5 ml vials	5 ml vial, 0.5 ml syringe	5 or 30 ml vials, 0.5 ml syringe	5 ml vial
Appropriate age range	2 months to <7 years	18 months to <7 years	2 months to <7 years	7 years to adult	typically 2 to 15 months
Standard schedule[1]	five 0.5 ml doses: at 2, 4, 6 and 18 months and 4-6 years of age	for doses 4 and 5: at 18 months and at 4-6 years of age	three 0.5 ml doses: at 2, 4 and 10-16 months of age	three 0.5 ml doses: the second 4-8 weeks after the first and the third 6-12 months after the second	four 0.5 ml doses: at 2, 4, 6 and 15 months of age
Routine additional doses	none	none	none	every 10 years	none
Route	IM	IM	IM	IM, jet	IM

[1]See monographs for alternate schedules

CDC Wound-Management Guidelines

History of adsorbed tetanus toxoid	Clean, minor wounds		All other wounds[1]	
	Td [2]	TIG	Td [2]	TIG
Unknown or <3 doses	Yes	No	Yes	Yes
≥3 doses[3]	No[4]	No	No[5]	No

[1]Including, but not limited to, wounds contaminated with dirt, feces, soil or saliva; puncture sounds; avulsions; or wounds resulting from missles, crushing, burns or frostbite.

[2]For children <7 years of age, trivalent DTP (diphtheria and tetanus toxoids with pertussis vaccine) is preferred to tetanus toxoid alone. Use DT (pediatric-strength diphtheria and tetanus toxoids) if pertussis vaccine is validly contraindiacted. For persons ≥7 years of age, Td (adult-strength tetanus and diphtheria toxoids) is preferred to tetanus toxoid alone.

[3]If the patient has received only 3 doses of fluid toxoid, then give a fourth dose of toxoid, preferably an adsorbed toxoid.

[4]Yes, if >10 years have elapsed since the last dose of tetanus toxoid.

[5]Yes, if >5 years have elapsed since the last dose of tetanus toxoid. More frequent booster doses are not needed and may increase the incidence and severity of adverse effects.

Diphtheria & Tetanus Toxoids & Whole-Cell Pertussis Vaccine (DTwP)

BACTERIAL VACCINES & TOXOIDS

NAME:

Generic, *Tri-Immunol*

MANUFACTURERS:

Generic, Connaught Laboratories; Massachusetts Public Health Biologic Laboratories, distributed free of charge within the State of Massachusetts. Manufactured and distributed by Michigan Department of Public Health. Also distributed by SmithKline Beecham Pharmaceuticals, *Tri-Immunol*, Wyeth-Lederle Vaccines & Pediatrics; ❧ *Tri-Immunol*, Wyeth-Ayerst

Synonyms: DTP, DPT, DTwP

Comparison: The various whole-cell DTP products have traditionally been considered generically equivalent, but one study found the Lederle vaccine to induce higher pertussis-toxoid antibody titers than the Connaught vaccine (Edwards et al, 1991), although no significant differences in filamentous hemagglutinin (FHA) antibodies were seen.

The whole-cell and acellular DTP (DTwP and DTaP) products are not generically equivalent, due to differences in composition and side-effect incidence. DTaP results in fewer common side effects. The degree of protection from DTaP and DTwP are comparable. Clinical trials of the relative protection from disease provided by DTaP and DTwP have yielded inconsistent results. Refer to that monograph for details.

Connaught's DTwP may be used as the diluent for *ActHIB* and *OmniHIB* brands of *Haemophilus influenzae* type b conjugate vaccine.

Viability: Inactivated

Antigenic Form: Toxoid mixture with whole-cell pertussis bacteria

Antigenic Type: Protein

> **Note:** Trivalent DTaP is the preferred immunizing agent for most children. Trivalent vaccines against diphtheria, tetanus and pertussis are the preferred immunizing agent for most children. Tetanus and diphtheria toxoids for adult use (Td) is the preferred immunizing agent for adults and older children.
> Specific information about the individual components of this drug appears in the individual monographs on diphtheria toxoid, tetanus toxoid and pertussis vaccine.

Use Characteristics

Indications: Induction of active immunity against diphtheria, tetanus and pertussis in infants and children from age 6 weeks up to the seventh birthday.

Refer to CDC's wound-management guidelines in the DTP Overview.

Contraindications:

Absolute: Do not give further doses of a vaccine containing pertussis antigens to children who have recovered from culture-confirmed pertussis. Do not vaccinate patients with a history of serious adverse reactions to a previous dose of a pertussis-containing vaccine. Do not vaccinate patients hypersensitive to any component of the vaccine, including thimerosal.

Data on the use of DTaP in children for whom whole-cell pertussis vaccine is contraindicated are not available. Until such data are available, consider contraindications to whole-cell pertussis vaccine administration adopted by ACIP and AAP to be contraindications to DTaP also. These contraindications include an immediate anaphylactic reaction or encephalopathy occurring within 7 days following DTwP or DTaP vaccination. Such encephalopathies may include major alterations in consciousness, unresponsiveness, generalized or focal seizures that persist more than a few hours and failure to recover within 24 hours or other generalized or focal neurological signs.

Relative: Until safety, immunogenicity and efficacy data are evaluated, administration of DTaP to children <15 months of age is not recommended. Defer immunization during the course of any febrile illness or acute infection. A minor respiratory illness such as a mild upper respiratory infection is not usually reason to defer immunization. Give DTwP or DTaP with caution to children with thrombocytopenia or any coagulation disorder that would contraindicate IM injection.

If a contraindiaction to the pertussis-vaccine component occurs, substitute diphtheria and tetanus toxoids for pediatric use (DT) for each of the remaining doses.

Several events were previously listed as contraindications, but are now listed simply as precautions, warranting careful consideration: Temperature 40.5°C (105°F) within 48 hours after DTP administration not due to another identifiable cause, collapse or shock-like state (hypotonic-hyporesponsive episode) within 48 hours, persistent inconsolable crying lasting ≥3 hours within 48 hours, or convulsions with or without fever within 3 days. There may be circumstances, such as a high local incidence of pertussis, in which the potential benefits outweigh possible risks, particularly because these events are not associated with permanent sequelae.

The occurrence of any type of neurological symptoms or signs, including one or more convulsions, following DTwP or DTaP administration is generally a contraindication to further use. The presence of any evolving or changing disorder affecting the CNS contraindicates administration of pertussis vaccine regardless of whether the suspected neurological disorder is associated with occurrence of seizure activity of any type.

ACIP and AAP recognize certain circumstances in which children with stable CNS disorders, including well controlled seizures or satisfactorily explained single seizures, may receive pertussis vaccine. ACIP and AAP do not consider a family history of seizures to be a contraindication to pertussis vaccine. Studies suggesting that infants and children with a history of convulsions in first-degree family members (ie, siblings and parents) have an increased risk for neurologic events, compared with those without such histories (Noble et al, 1987; Livengood et al, 1989) may be flawed by selection bias or genetic confounding.

Elderly: DTwP amd DTaP are generally contraindicated after the seventh birthday.

Adults: Since the incidence of, and mortality due to, pertussis decreases with advancing age, while some local and systemic reactions to DTP may increase, routine immunization of persons ≥7 years of age is not recommended. The benefit of routine pertussis immunization of adults to reduce their role as community disease reservoirs is being investigated. Tetanus and diphtheria toxoids for adult use (Td) is the preferred immunizing agent for adults and older children.

Pregnancy: Category C. DTwP and DTaP are generally contraindicated after the seventh birthday. It is not known if DTP antigens or corresponding antibodies cross the placenta. Generally, most IgG passage across the placenta occurs during the third trimester.

Lactation: It is not known if DTP antigens or corresponding antibodies are excreted into breast milk. Problems in humans have not been documented.

Children: Do not reduce or divide the DTwP or DTaP dose for preterm infants or any other children. DTwP and DTaP are contraindicated in children <6 weeks of age, because the product may not be immunogenic. DTwP and DTaP are also contraindicated in children >7 years of age, because of their decreased risk of pertussis and increased likelihood of adverse effects. Trivalent DTwP or DTaP is the preferred immunizing agent for most children up to their seventh birthday. Tetanus and diphtheria toxoids for adult use (Td) is the preferred immunizing agent for adults and older children.

Adverse Reactions:

Not all adverse events following administration of DTwP are causally related to DTwP vaccine.

Mild local and constitutional reactions (40% to 60%): Pain, induration and redness at the injection site, usually beginning within 72 hours after vaccination. Occasionally a nodule is induced at the injection site that can persist for several weeks. These reactions are self-limiting and usually require no treatment. Rarely, an abscess develops at the injection site, with an incidence of 6 to 10 cases per million doses. Mild constitutional reactions consist chiefly of febrile reactions (38.2° to 40.4°C; 101° to 104.7°F). Constitutional reactions usually begin within 12 hours after vaccination, persist for 1 to 7 days, and may be accompanied by irritability, malaise, sleepiness or vomiting.

Severe Reactions: Several severe postimmunization illnesses have occurred following administration of both pertussis and DTwP vaccines. These ill nesses are usually considered reactions to the vaccine because of the temporal association between administration of DTwP vaccine and the onset of symptoms, and most of the reactions are usually ascribed to the pertussis component. Reactions that constitute absolute contraindications to further vaccination with the pertussis component: Convulsions, encephalopathy, focal neurological disease, collapse, shock or altered consciousness. Reactions such as thrombocytopenic purpura and demonstrable hypersensitivity reactions such as anaphylaxis, generalized urticarial eruptions, or Arthus-type reactions after administration of either pertussis or DTwP vaccines also constitute an absolute contraindication to additional immunization with these vaccines.

Other Reactions: Excessive somnolence, excessive screaming (persistent crying or screaming for ≥3 hours), temperature >40.5°C (105°F). Peripheral neuropathy can follow DTwP vaccination, possibly due in some cases to injection of vaccine too close to a peripheral nerve. An expert panel assembled by the Institute of Medicine has concluded that no causal association exists between pertussis vaccination and autism, infantile spasms, hypsarrhythmia, Reye's syndrome, SIDS, aseptic meningitis, chronic neurologic damage, erythema multiforme or other rash, Guillain-Barré syndrome, hemolytic anemia, juvenile diabetes, learning disabilities, attention deficit disorder, peripheral mononeuropathy or thrombocytopenia.

The panel found evidence consistent with a causal association between DTwP and acute encephalopathy, shock and "unusual shock-like state," anaphylaxis and protracted, inconsolable crying.

When a child returns for the next dose in a series of either pertussis or DTwP or DTaP vaccine injections, question the adult accompanying the child about possible side effects following the prior dose. If any of the effects that contraindicate additional pertussis vaccine doses occur, continue childhood immunization with bivalent diphtheria and tetanus toxoids for pediatric use (DT).

Pharmacologic & Dosing Characteristics

 Dosage: Shake vial well. Do not use if resuspension is not possible.

Primary Immunizing Series: 0.5 ml at 6 weeks of age, then a second 0.5 ml dose 4 to 8 weeks later, then a third 0.5 ml dose 4 to 8 weeks later, then a fourth reinforcing 0.5 ml dose 1 year after the third dose. But if the fourth primary dose (ie, the reinforcing dose) is given after the fourth birthday, omit the booster dose. The standard schedule is to give 5 doses at 2, 4, 6 and 12 to 18 months of age, and 4 to 6 years or age.

Do not use partial or fractional doses of DTwP or DTaP because the immunogenicity and clinical efficacy of such practices have not been adequately studied. Give preterm infants a full 0.5 ml dose at the normal chronologic age after birth.

Do not dilute.

Refer to CDC's wound-management guidelines in the DTP Overview.

Route & Site: IM, preferably into the midlateral muscles of the thigh or the deltoid muscle of the upper arm. Preferably, do not inject the same muscle group for successive injections. Using a 1 inch needle, insert at a 45 degree angle to the long axis of the leg.

Documentation Requirements: Federal law requires that (1) the manufacturer and lot number of this vaccine, (2) the date of its administration, and (3) the name, address and title of the person administering the vaccine be documented in the recipient's permanent medical record or in a permanent office log. Certain adverse events must be reported to the VAERS system, 1-800-822-7967.

Efficacy: 80% to 90% or greater reduction in disease incidence

Onset: After third dose

Duration: Greater than 4 to 6 years

Drug Interactions: Like all inactivated vaccines, administration of DTwP to persons receiving immunosuppressant drugs, including high-dose corticosteroids, or radiation therapy may result in an insufficient response to immunization. They may remain susceptible despite immunization. Several routine pediatric vaccines may safely and effectively be administered simultaneously at separate injection sites (eg, DTP, MMR, e-IPV, Hib, hepatitis B, influenza). National authorities recommend simultaneous immunization at separate sites as indicated by age or health risk, if return of a vaccine recipient for a subsequent visit is doubtful. Delay diphtheria toxoid administration until 3 to 4 weeks after diphtheria antitoxin use to avoid the hypothetical possibility of antitoxin-toxoid interference. As with other drugs administered by IM injection, give DTwP or DTaP with caution to persons on anticoagulent therapy.

Concurrent administration of tetanus toxoid and tetanus immune globulin may delay development of active immunity by several days through partial antigen-antibody antagonism, but this interaction is not clinically significant and does not preclude concurrent administration of both drugs if both are needed.

A Canadian DTwP vaccine evoked a higher pertussis antibody response given with e-IPV or OPV than did a tetravalent, parenteral DTwP-IPV vaccine from the same manufacturer or DTwP and IPV given as separate injections (Baker et al, 1992).

Systemic chloramphenicol therapy may impair anamnestic response to tetanus toxoid. Avoid concurrent use of these two drugs.

As with other drugs administered by IM injection, give DTP with caution to persons on anticoagulant therapy.

Pharmaceutical Characteristics

Concentration:

Connaught-US: 6.5 Lf units diphtheria toxoid, 5 Lf units tetanus toxoid and 4 units pertussis vaccine per 0.5 ml

Wyeth-Lederle: 12.5 Lf units diphtheria toxoid, 5 Lf units tetanus toxoid and 4 units pertussis vaccine per 0.5 ml

Massachusetts: 10 Lf units diphtheria toxoid, 5.5 Lf units tetanus toxoid and 4 units pertussis vaccine per 0.5 ml

Michigan/SKB: 10 Lf units diphtheria toxoid, 5.5 Lf units tetanus toxoid and 4 units pertussis vaccine per 0.5 ml

Connaught-Canada: 25 Lf units diphtheria toxoid, 5 Lf units tetanus toxoid and 4 units pertussis vaccine per 0.5 ml (adsorbed) or 40 Lf units diphtheria toxoid, 8 Lf units tetanus toxoid and 4 units pertussis vaccine per 0.5 ml (fluid)

Packaging:

Connaught: 5 doses per 2.5 ml multidose vial, 10 doses per 5 ml multidose vial, 15 doses per 7.5 ml multidose vial

Wyeth-Lederle: 15 doses per 7.5 ml multidose vial

Massachusetts: 10 doses per 5 ml multidose vial. Distributed free of charge, but only within the state of Massachusetts.

Michigan/SKB: 10 doses per 5 ml multidose vial. Supplied as single vials and packages of 10 vials.

Dose Form: Suspension

Solvent: Variously formulated with sodium chloride, with or without phosphate buffers.

Storage/Stability: Store at 2° to 8°C (35° to 46°F). Discard frozen vaccine. Contact manufacturers regarding exposures to prolonged room temperature or elevated temperatures. Temperature extremes can adversely affect ability to resuspend this product. Shipped in insulated containers with coolant packs.

Diphtheria & Tetanus Toxoids with *Haemophilus influenza* Type B Conjugate & Whole-cell Pertussis Vaccines (DTwP-HIB)

BACTERIAL VACCINES & TOXOIDS

Names:
Tetramune, ActHIB/DTP

Manufacturers:
Wyeth-Lederle Vaccines & Pediatrics (*Tetramune*)
Pasteur-Merieux Serums et Vaccins and Connaught Laboratories (*ActHIB/DTP*)

Synonym: DTwP-Hib, DTwP-HbOC (Wyeth-Lederle), DTwP-PRP-T (Connaught)

Comparison: *Tetramune* is a simple combination of *Tri-Immunol* and *HibTITER* in liquid form. *ActHIB*/DTP uses Connaught's DTP vaccine as the diluent for *ActHIB* powder. *ActHIB* powder is equivalent to SmithKline's *OmniHIB* powder. See those specific monographs for details.

Tetramune and *ActHIB*/DTP are not generically equivalent, based on immunogenicity and antigenic content. Each Hib conjugate vaccine is immunogenically unique. *ActHIB* plain and *OmniHIB*, both in powder form, are the same vaccine.

Whole-cell and acellular DTP (DTwP and DTaP) products are not generically equivalent, due to differences in composition and side-effect incidence. DTaP results in fewer common side effects. The degree of protection from DTaP and DTwP are comparable. Clinical trials of the relative protection from disease provided by DTaP and DTwP have yielded inconsistent results.

Viability: Inactivated

Antigenic Form: Mixture of two toxoids and two forms of bacterial vaccine

Antigenic Type: Proteins with capsular polysaccharide fragments conjugated to a protein carrier

Note: Products containing diphtheria, tetanus and pertussis antigens are the preferred immunizing agents for most children. Tetanus & diphtheria toxoids for adult use (Td) is the preferred immunizing agent for adults and other children.

Specific information about the individual components of this drug appears in the individual monographs on diphtheria toxoid, tetanus toxoid, pertussis vaccine and Hib vaccine.

Use Characteristics

Indications: Induction of active immunity against diphtheria, tetanus and pertussis and against invasive diseases caused by encapsulated Haemophilus influenzae type b in infants and children from age 2 months up to the fifth birthday. Refer to CDC's wound-management guidelines in the DTP Overview.

Contraindications:

STOP

Absolute: Do not give further doses of a vaccine containing pertussis antigens to children who have recovered from culture-confirmed pertussis. Do not vaccinate patients with a history of serious adverse reactions to a previous dose of a pertussis-containing vaccine. Do not vaccinate patients hypersensitive to any component of the vaccine, including thimerosal.

Data on the use of DTaP in children for whom whole-cell pertussis vaccine is contraindicated are not available. Until such data are available, consider contraindications to whole-cell pertussis vaccine administration adopted by ACIP and AAP to be contraindications to DTaP also. These contraindications include an immediate anaphylactic reaction or encephalopathy occurring within 7 days following DTwP or DTaP vaccination. Such encephalopathies may include major alterations in consciousness, unresponsiveness, generalized or focal seizures that persist more than a few hours and failure to recover within 24 hours or other generalized or focal neurological signs.

Relative: Patients with a history of a hypersensitivity reaction to any component. Any febrile illness or acute infection is reason for delaying immunization with this vaccine. A mild afebrile illness such as a mild upper respiratory infection is not usually reason to defer immunization.

Several events were previously listed as contraindications, but are now listed simply as precautions, warranting careful consideration: Temperature >40.5°C (105°F) within 48 hours after DTwP or DTaP administration not due to another identifiable cause, collapse or shock-like state (hypotonic-hyporesponsive episode) within 48 hours, persistent inconsolable crying lasting ≥3 hours occurring within 48 hours, or convulsions with or without fever within 3 days. There may be circumstances, such as a high local incidence of pertussis, in which the potential benefits outweigh possible risks, particularly because these events are not associated with permanent sequelae.

The occurrence of any type of neurological symptoms or signs, including one or more convulsions, following DTwP or DTaP administration is generally a contraindication to further use. The presence of any evolving or changing disorder affecting the CNS contraindicates administration of pertussis vaccine regardless of whether the suspected neurological disorder is associated with occurrence of seizure activity of any type.

ACIP and AAP recognize certain circumstances in which children with stable CNS disorders, including well-controlled seizures or satisfactorily explained single seizures, may receive pertussis vaccine. ACIP and AAP do not consider a family history of seizures to be a contraindication to pertussis vaccine.

Studies suggesting that infants and children with a history of convulsions in first-degree family members (ie, siblings and parents) have an increased risk for neurologic events, compared with those without such histories (Noble et al, 1987; Livengood et al, 1989) may be flawed by selection bias or genetic confounding. Give DTwP-Hib with caution to children with thrombocytopenia or any coagulation disorder that would contraindicate IM injection.

If a contraindication to the pertussis--

vaccine component occurs, substitute diphtheria & tetanus toxoids for pediatric use (DT) and a monovalent Hib vaccine for each of the remaining doses.

Elderly: DTwP and DTaP are generally contraindicated after the seventh birthday.

Adults: Since the incidence of and mortality due to pertussis decreases with advancing age, while some local and systemic reactions to DTP may increase, routine immunization of persons ≥7 years of age is not recommended. Tetanus and diphtheria toxoids for adult use (Td) is the preferred immunizing agent for adults and older children. Hib vaccination is not generally recommended after the fifth birthday. The benefit of routine pertussis immunization of adults to reduce their role as community disease reservoirs is being investigated.

Pregnancy: Category C. Products containing DTP are generally contraindicated after the seventh birthday. It is not known if DTP or Hib antigens or corresponding antibodies cross the placenta. Generally, most IgG passage across the placenta occurs during the third trimester.

Lactation: It is not known if DTP or Hib antigens or corresponding antibodies are excreted in breast milk. Problems in humans have not been documented.

Children: Routine immunization of all infants beginning at 2 months of age is recommended in the US. Do not reduce or divide the dose for preterm infants or any other children. Children who have recovered from culture-confirmed pertussis do not need further doses of a pertussis-containing vaccine. DTwP and DTaP are contraindicated in children 6 weeks of age, because the product may not be immunogenic. DTwP and DTaP are also contraindicated in children 7 years of age, because of their decreased risk of pertussis and increased likelihood of adverse effects. Trivalent DTwP or DTaP is the preferred immunizing agent for most children up to their seventh birthday. Tetanus & diphtheria toxoids for adult use (Td) is the preferred immunizing agent for adults and older children.

Adverse Reactions: Not all adverse events following administration of DTwP are causally related to DTwP vaccine.

Mild local and constitutional reactions (40% to 60%): Pain, induration, and redness at the injection site, usually beginning within 72 hours after vaccination. Occasionally a nodule is induced at the injection site that can persist for several weeks. These reactions are self-limiting and usually require no treatment.

Rarely, an abscess develops at the injection site, with an incidence of 6 to 10 cases per million dose. Mild constitutional reactions consist chiefly of febrile reactions (38.2° to 40.4°C; 101° to 104.7°F). Constitutional reactions usually begin within 12 hours after vaccination, persist for 1 to 7 days, and may be accompanied by irritability, malaise, sleepiness, or vomiting.

Severe Reactions: Several severe postimmunization illnesses have occurred following administration of both pertussis and DTwP vaccines. These illnesses are usually considered reactions to the vaccine because of the temporal association between administration of DTwP vaccine and the onset of symptoms and most of the reactions are usually ascribed to the pertussis component. Reactions that constitute absolute contraindications to further vaccination with the pertussis component: Convulsions, encephalopathy, focal neurological disease, collapse, shock, or altered consciousness. Reactions such as thrombocytopenic purpura and demonstrable hypersentivity reactions such as anaphylaxis, generalized urticarial eruptions, or Arthus-type reactions after administration of either pertussis or DTwP vaccines also constitute an absolute contraindication to additional immunization with these vaccines.

Other Reactions: Excessive somnolence, excessive screaming (persistent crying or screaming for ≥3 hours), temperature 40.5°C (105°F). Peripheral neuropathy can follow DTwP vaccination, possibly due in some cases to injection of vaccine too close to a peripheral nerve.

An expert panel assembled by the Institute of Medicine has concluded that no causal association exists between pertussis vaccination and autism, infantile spasms, hypsarrhythmia, Reye's syndrome, SIDS, aseptic meningitis, chronic neurologic damage, erythema multiforme or other rash, Guillain-Barré syndrome, hemolytic anemia, juvenile diabetes, learning disabilities, attention deficit disorder, peripheral mononeuropathy, or thrombocytopenia. The panel found evidence consistent with a causal association between DTwP and acute encephalopathy, shock and "unusual shock-like state," anaphylaxis, and protracted, inconsolable crying.

When a child returns for the next dose in a series of either pertussis or DTP vaccine injections, question the adult accompanying the child about possible side effects following the prior dose. If any of the effects that contraindicate additional pertussis vaccine doses occur, continue childhood immunization with bivalent diphtheria and tetanus toxoids for pediatric use (DT).

A fever >38.3°C (101°F) occurred at least once in 2% of recipients during HibTITER vaccine clinical trials. Other possible reactions include erythema, swelling, or tenderness, which are generally infrequent, mild, transient, with no serious sequelae. A cause-effect relationship between Hib vaccine and observed postvaccinal irritability, restless sleep, diarrhea, vomiting, loss of appetite, rash, hives, thrombocytopenia, convulsions, renal failure, or Guillain-Barré syndrome has not been established.

Pharmacologic & Dosing Characteristics

Dosage: 0.5 ml per dose. Typically, four doses would be given, at 2, 4, 6 and 12 to 18 months of age. Shake vial well. Do not use if resuspension is not possible.

Do not use partial or fractional doses of DTwP or DTaP since the immunogenicity and clinical efficacy of such practices have not been adequately studied. Give preterm infants a full 0.5 ml dose at the normal chronologic age after birth. Do not dilute. Refer to CDC's wound-management guidelines in the DTP Overview.

Route & Site: IM, preferably in the outer aspect of the vastus lateralis, mid-thigh muscle or the outer aspect of the upper arm. Do not administer IV or ID. Do not inject in the gluteal area or other areas where there may be a major nerve trunk. Preferably, do not inject the same muscle group for successive injections.

Documentation Requirements: Federal law requires that (1) the manufacturer and lot number of this vaccine, (2) the date of its administration, and (3) the name, address, and title of the person administering the vaccine be documented in the recipient's permanent medical record or in a permanent office log. Certain adverse events must be reported to the VAERS system, 1-800-822-7967. Refer to Immunization Documents in the resources section for complete information.

Efficacy: DTP: 80% to 90% or greater reduction in disease incidence. Two months after the second dose of Hib vaccine, 95% of infants' sera had bactericidal activity and 99.5% of infants vaccinated at 7 to 11 months of age responded with anti-Haemophilus polysaccharide antibody levels of at least 1 mcg/ml. One month after the third dose, 98% had bactericidal activity.

Onset: After multiple doses in infants

Duration: Adequate immunization against diphtheria and tetanus generally persists for 10 years. Protection against pertussis persists about 4 to 6 years. Hib antibody titers 1 mcg/ml correlate with prolonged protection from disease, generally implying several years of protection.

Drug Interactions: Like all inactivated vaccines, administration of DTwP-Hib vaccine to persons receiving immunosuppressant drugs, including high-dose corticosteroids, or radiation therapy may result in an insufficient response to immunization. They may remain susceptible despite immunization.

Several routine pediatric vaccines may safely and effectively be administered simultaneously at separate injection sites (eg, DTP, MMR, OPV or e-IPV, Hib, hepatitis B, influenza). National authorities recommend simultaneous immunization at separate sites as indicated by age or healthrisk, if return of a vaccine recipient for a subsequent visit is doubtful. Delay diphtheria toxoid administration until 3 to 4 weeks after diphtheria antitoxin use, to avoid the hypothetical possibility of antitoxin-toxoid interference.

A Canadian DTwP vaccine evoked a higher pertussis antibody response given with e-IPV or OPV than did a tetravalent, parental DTwP-IPV vaccine from the same manufacturer or DTwP and IPV given as separate injections (Baker et al, 1992).

Concurrent administration of tetanus toxoid and tetanus immune globulin may delay development of active immunity by several days through partial antigen-antibody antagonism. But this interaction is not clinically significant and does not preclude concurrent administration of both drugs if both are needed.

Systemic chloramphenicol therapy may impair anamnestic response to tetanus toxoid. Avoid concurrent use of these two drugs.

Hib, meningococcal, and penumococcal vaccines may safely and effectively be administered simultaneously at separate injection sites.

As with other drugs administered by IM injection, give with caution to persons receiving anticoagulant therapy.

Laboratory Interferences: Antigenuria has been detected following receipt of Hib vaccines and therefore antigen detection (eg, with latex agglutination kits) may have no diagnostic value in suspected Hib disease within a short period (eg, 2 weeks) after immunization. (Connaught: 3 days; Wyeth-Lederle: 2 weeks). False-positive latex agglutination tests of cerebrospinal fluid have also been reported 1 to 21 days following Hib vaccination (Perkins, 1993).

Pharmaceutical Characteristics

Concentration:

Connaught: 6.7 Lf units of diphtheria toxoid, 5 Lf units of tetanus toxoid, 4 units of pertussis vaccine, and 10 mcg Haemophilus influenzae type b polysaccharide, each per 0.5 ml

Wyeth-Lederle: 12.5 Lf units of diphtheria toxoid, 5 Lf units of tetanus toxoid, 4 units of pertussis vaccine, and 10 mcg Haemophilus influenzae type b oligosaccharide, each per 0.5 ml

Packaging:

Connaught: One package containing one 7.5 ml of Connaught's DTwP vaccine and 10 single-dose vials of *ActHIB* vaccine

Wyeth-Lederle: 10 doses per 5 ml multi-dose vial

Doseform:

Connaught: Powder for reconstitution with suspension

Wyeth-Lederle: Suspension

Solvent:

Wyeth-Lederle: Sodium chloride added for isotonicity. Contains a trace quantity of glycine.

Diluent for Reconstitution:

Connaught: 0.6 ml per dose. Connaught's DTwP vaccine suspension is the only form of DTP to be used to reconstitute *ActHIB* or *OmniHIB* brands of Hib vaccine. Use no other form of DTP. Alternately, 0.6 ml of 0.4% sodium chloride, the diluent accompanying *OmniHIB*, may be used.

Storage/Stability: Store at 2° to 8°C (35° to 46°F). Discard frozen vaccine. Contact manufacturer regarding exposures to prolonged room temperature or elevated temperatures. Temperature extremes can adversely affect ability to resuspend this product. Shipped in insulated containers with coolant packs.

Connaught: Administer vaccine within 30 minutes of reconstitution.

Diphtheria & Tetanus Toxoids & Acellular Pertussis Vaccine (DTaP)

BACTERIAL VACCINES AND TOXOIDS

Tripedia, Acel-Immune,
🍁 *Tripacel*

MANUFACTURERS:

Tripedia, Connaught Laboratories. The pertussis component is produced by The Research Foundation for Microbial Disease of Osaka University (*Biken*), and combined with diphtheria and tetanus toxoids manufactured by Connaught. *Acel-Immune,* Wyeth-Lederle Vaccines & Pediatrics. The pertussis component is produced by Takeda Chemical Industries, Osaka, Japan, and combined with diphtheria and tetanus toxoids manufactured by Wyeth-Lederle. 🍁 *Acel-Imune,* Wyeth-Ayerst;
🍁 *Tripacel,* Connaught

Synonyms: DTP, DPT, DTaP, APDT

Comparison: The various acellular DTaP products are not generically equivalent, given their differences in contents and methods of standardization. Whole-cell and acellular DTP (DTwP and DTaP) products are not generically equivalent, due to differences in composition and side-effect incidence. DTaP results in fewer common side effects than DTwP vaccines. The degree of protection from DTaP and DTwP are comparable. Clinical trials of the relative protection form disease provided by DTaP and DTwP have yielded inconsistent results, but DTaP may be effective more in preventing pertussis.

Viability: Inactivated

Antigenic Form: Toxoid mixture with acellular pertussis bacterial vaccine

Connaught: The acellular pertussis component contains equal parts of pertussis toxin (PT) and filamentous hemagglutinin (FHA), treated with formaldehyde to inactivate the toxin into a toxoid.

Wyeth-Lederle: The acellular pertussis component contains approximately 40 mcg, but not >60 mcg, of pertussis antigens per 0.5 ml dose. The pertussis component consists of approximately 86% filamentous hemagglutinin (FHA), 8% lymphocytosis-promoting factor (LPF, also known as pertussis toxin, PT), 4% 69-kilodalton (69-kd) outer membrane protein and 2% type-2 fimbriae (pertussis-specific agglutinogen), treated with formaldehyde to inactivate the toxin into a toxoid. The 69-kDa protein is also called pertactin.

Antigen Type: Protein

> **Note:** Trivalent vaccines against diphtheria, tetanus and pertussis are the preferred immunizing agent for most children. Tetanus & diphtheria toxoids for adult use (Td) is the preferrred immunizing agent for adults and older children. Specific information about the individual components of this drug appear in the individual monographs on diphtheria toxoid, tetanus toxoid and pertussis vaccine.

Use Characteristics

Indications: Induction of active immunity against diphtheria, tetanus and pertussis in infants and children, from age 6 weeks up to the seventh birthday.

Refer to CDC's wound-management guidelines in the DTP Overview.

Unlabeled Uses: Acellular pertussis vaccines are being investigated for immunizing adults against pertussis (Edwards et al, 1993).

Contraindications:

Absolute: Do not give further doses of a vaccine containing pertussis antigens to children who have recovered from culture-confirmed pertussis. Do not vaccinate patients with a history of serious adverse reactions to a previous dose of a pertussis-containing vaccine. Do not vaccinate patients hypersensitive to any component of the vaccine, including thimerosal.

Data are not available on the use of DTaP in children for whom whole-cell pertussis vaccine is contraindicated. Until such data are available, consider contraindications to whole-cell pertussis vaccine administration adopted by ACIP and AAP to be contraindications to DTaP also. These contraindications include an immediate anaphylactic reaction or encephalopathy occurring within 7 days following DTP vaccination. Such encephalopathies may include major alterations in consciousness, unresponsiveness, generalized or focal seizures that persist more than a few hours and failure to recover within 24 hours, or other generalized or focal neurological signs.

If a contraindication to the pertussis-vaccine component occurs, substitute diphtheria and tetanus toxoids for pediatric use (DT) for each of the remaining doses.

Relative: Defer immunization during the course of any febrile illness or acute infection. A minor respiratory illness such as a mild upper respiratory infection is not usually reason to defer immunization. Give DTaP or DTwP with caution to children with thrombocytopenia or any coagulation disorder that would contraindicate IM injection.

Several events were previously listed as contraindications, but are now listed simply as precautions, warranting careful consideration: Temperature >40.5°C (105°F) within 48 hours after DTP administration not due to another identifiable cause, collapse or shock-like state (hypotonic-hyporesponsive episode) within 48 hours, persistent inconsolable crying lasting ≥3 hours within 48 hours, or convulsions with or without fever within 3 days. There may be circumstances, such as a high local incidence of pertussis, in which the potential benefits outweigh possible risks, particularly because these events are not associated with permanent sequelae.

The occurrence of any type of neurological symptoms or signs, including one or more convulsions, following DTaP administration is generally a contraindication to further use. The presence of any evolving or changing disorder affecting the CNS contraindicates administration of pertussis vaccine regardless of whether the suspected neurological disorder is associated with occurrence of seizure activity of any type.

ACIP and AAP recognize certain circumstances in which children with stable CNS disorders, including well controlled seizures or satisfactorily explained single seizures, may receive pertussis vaccine. ACIP and AAP do not consider a family history of seizures to be a contraindication to pertussis vaccine. Studies suggesting that infants and children with a history of convulsions in first-degree family members (ie, siblings and parents) have an increased risk for neurologic events, compared with those without such histories (Noble et al, 1987; Livengood et al, 1989) may be flawed by selection bias or genetic confounding.

Elderly: DTwP and DTaP are generally contraindicated after the seventh birthday.

Adults: DTwP and DTaP are generally contraindicated after the seventh birthday. Tetanus and diphtheria toxoids for adult use (Td) is the preferred immunizing agent for adults and older children. The benefit of routine pertussis immunization of adults to reduce their role as community disease reservoirs is being investigated.

Pregnancy: *Category* C. DTwP and DTaP are generally contraindicated after the seventh birthday. It is not known if DTP antigens or corresponding antibodies cross the placenta. Generally, most IgG passage across the placenta occurs during the third trimester.

Lactation: It is not known if DTP antigens or corresponding antibodies cross into human breast milk. Problems in humans have not been documented.

Children: For use from infancy until a child's seventh birthday. Do not reduce or divide the DTwP or DTaP dose for preterm infants or any other children. DTwP and DTaP are contraindicated in children <6 weeks, because the product may not be immunogenic. DTwP and DTaP are also contrindicated in children >7 years of age, because of their decreased risk of pertussis and increased likelihood of adverse effects. Trivalent DTwP or DTaP is the preferred immunizing agent for most children up to their seventh birthday. Tetanus & diphtheria toxoids for adult use (Td) is the preferred immunizing agent for adults and older children.

Children who have recovered from culture-confirmed pertussis do not need further doses of a pertussis-containing vaccine. Tetanus and diphtheria toxoids for adult use (Td) is the preferred immunizing agent for adults and older children.

Adverse Reactions:
Some adverse reactions following DTaP occur less frequently than in recipients of DTwP, especially less pain and tenderness, erythema, induration,

swelling and warmth at the injection site. Less drowsiness, fretfulness or irritability, and fever also followed DTaP use, compared with DTwP. *Tripedia* cites less frequent fever, irritability, drowsiness, injection site reactions, vomiting, anorexia and high-pitched unusual cry. *Acel-Imune* cites less frequent antipyretic drug use, compared to DTwP. The relative frequency of rare events can only be determined in large post-marketing surveillance studies currently underway.

Among children ≥1 year of age, fever of ≥38°C (100.4°F) or higher occurred in 7% to 19% of recipients within 72 hours of DTaP administration. Fever >39°C (102.2°F) occurred in 1.5% of recipients. Other occasional reactions that occurred included upper respiratory infection or rhinitis (6%), diarrhea or loose stools (3.5%), vomiting (2%) or rash (1.2%). As with other aluminum-containing vaccines, a nodule may occasionally be palpable at the injection site for several weeks. Sterile abscess formation or SC atrophy at the injection site may also occur.

Among infants 2 to 6 months old, *Tripedia* was associated with erythema (9% to 17%), swelling (4.5% to 6.5%), tenderness (6% to 12%).

Reactions not noted with DTaP in clinical trials, but noted with broader use of other drugs containing diphtheria, tetanus or pertussis antigens included urticaria, erythema multiforme, other rashes, arthralgias, or more rarely a severe anaphylactic reaction (eg, urticaria with swelling of the mouth, difficulty breathing, hypotension, shock). Other possible reactions: Neurological complications such as convulsions, encephalopathy, various mono- or polyneuropathies, including Guillain-Barré syndrome. Permanent neurological disability and death occurred rarely in temporal association to immunization with a pertussis antigen.

An expert panel assembled by the Institute of Medicine has concluded that no causal association exists between pertussis vaccination and autism, infantile spasms, hypsarrhythmia, Reye's syndrome, SIDS, aseptic meningitis, chronic neurologic damage, erythema multiforme or other rash, Guillain-Barré syndrome, hemolytic anemia, juvenile diabetes, learning disabilities, attention deficit disorder, peripheral mononeuropathy or thrombocytopenia.

The panel found evidence consistent with a causal association between DTwP and acute encephalopathy, shock and "unusual shock-like state," anaphylaxis and protracted, inconsolable crying.

When a child returns for the next dose in a series of either pertussis or DTwP or DTaP vaccine injections, question the adult accompanying the child about possible side effects following the prior dose. If any of the effects that contraindicate additional pertussis vaccine doses occur, continue childhood immunization with bivalent diphtheria and tetanus toxoids for pediatric use (DT).

Pharmacologic & Dosing Characteristics

Dosage: Shake vial well to obtain a uniform suspension before withdrawing each dose.

Primary Immunizing Series: Typically, 4 doses are given at 2, 4, 6 and 15 to 20 months of age. Give 0.5 ml at 6 to 8 weeks of age, then a second 0.5 ml dose 4 to 8 weeks later, then a third 0.5 ml dose 4 to 8 weeks later, then a fourth reinforcing 0.5 ml dose 1 year after the third dose. Study of the need for a fifth 0.5 ml dose at 4 to 6 years of age, preferably prior to entrance into kindergarten or elementary school, is ongoing. But, if the fourth primary dose (ie, the reinforcing dose) is given after a child's fourth birthday, a booster prior to school entry is not necessary.

DTaP may be used for doses in series begun with DTwP. In such cases, give a total of five DTP doses.

Do not use partial or fractional doses of DTwP or DTaP since the immunogenicity and clinical efficacy of such practices have not been adequately studied. Give preterm infants a full 0.5 ml dose at the normal chronologic age after birth. Do not dilute.

Refer to CDC's wound-management guidelines in the DTP overview.

Route & Site: IM; use no other route. The anterolateral aspect of the thigh or the deltoid muscle of the upper arm is preferred. Do not inject DTaP in the gluteal area or other areas where there may be a major nerve trunk.

Documentation Requirements: Federal law requires that (1) the manufacturer and lot number of this vaccine, (2) the date of its administration, and (3) the name, address and title of the person administering the vaccine be documented in the recipient's permanent medical record or in a permanent office log. Certain adverse events must be reported to the VAERS system, 1-800-822-7967.

Efficacy: Acellular pertussis vaccines have been used in Japan since 1981, mostly in 2-year-old children. The decline in pertussis with routine use of acellular vaccines in this setting provides evidence of the efficacy of these vaccines as a group. The vaccines were rated 88% effective among household contacts in protecting against clinical pertussis (95% CI: 79% to 93%).

In Swedish and German studies of the Connaught formulation among children 5 to 11 months old, the estimate of vaccine efficacy was 69% (95% CI: 47% to 82%) for all cases of culture-confirmed pertussis and 80% (95% CI: 84% to 96%) for culture-confirmed cases with cough persisting longer than 30 days. The anti-PT and anti-FHA antibody responses to *Tripedia* in US trials of 15- to 20-month-old children who had previously received three doses of DTwP were similar to responses in children in the Swedish trial. The role of specific serum antibodies in clinical protection is not known at present. Antibody responses to PT and FHA were significantly higher after *Tripedia* than after Connaught's brand to DTwP.

In a study of the Wyeth-Lederle formulation among 2-year-old children in Japan, efficacy was 79% (95% CI: 60% to 89%), or 97% using stricter disease criteria (95% CI: 82% to 99%). These estimates of efficacy are comparable to that for whole-cell pertussis vaccine studied in the US. Immunogenicity comparisons between DTaP and whole-cell DTP (*Tri-Immunol*) in about 1000 American children demonstrated similar antibody response for LPF, 69-kd and agglutinins. Antibody response to FHA was higher after *Acel-Imune* than after *Tri-Immunol*.

Onset: After multiple doses

Duration: Adequate immunization

against diphtheria and tetanus generally persists for 10 years. Protection against pertussis persists about 4 to 6 years.

Drug Interactions: Like all inactivated vaccines, administration of DTP to persons receiving immunosuppressant drugs, including high-dose corticosteroids, or radiation therapy may result in an insufficient response to immunization. They may remain susceptible despite immunization. Several routine pediatric vaccines may safely and effectively be administered simultaneously at separate injection sites (eg, DTP, MMR, OPV or e-IPV, Hib, hepatitis B). National authorities recommend simultaneous immunization at separate sites as indicated by age or health risk, if return of a vaccine recipient for a subsequent visit is doubtful. Delay diphtheria toxoid administration until 3 to 4 weeks after diphtheria antitoxin use, to avoid the hypothetical possibility of antitoxin-toxoid interference.

Several routine pediatric vaccines may safely and effectively be administered simultaneously at separate injection sites (eg, DTP, MMR, OPV or e-IPV, Hib, hepatitis B, varicella).

A Canadian DTwP vaccine evoked a higher pertussis antibody response given with e-IPV or OPV than did a tetravalent, parenteral DTwP-IPV vaccine from the same manufacturer or DTwP and IPV given as separate injections (Baker et al, 1992).

Concurrent administration of tetanus toxoid and tetanus immune globulin may delay development of active immunity by several days through partial antigen-antibody antagonism. But this interaction is not clinically significant and does not preclude concurrent administration of both drugs if both are needed.

Systemic chloramphenicol therapy may impair anamnestic response to tetanus toxoid. Avoid concurrent use of these two drugs.

As with other drugs administered by IM injection, give DTaP with caution to persons on anticoagulant therapy.

Pharmaceutical Characteristics

Concentration:

Connaught: 6.7 Lf units of diphtheria toxoid, 5 Lf units of tetanus toxoid and 46.8 mcg of pertussis antigens (23.4 mcg each of pertussis toxin and filamentous hemagglutinin) per 0.5 ml

Wyeth-Lederle: 7.5 Lf units of diphtheria toxoid, 5 Lf units of tetanus toxoid and 300 hemagglutinating (HA) units of acellular pertussis vaccine per 0.5 ml

Packaging:
Connaught: 15 doses per 7.5 ml multidose vial; five single-dose vials

Wyeth-Lederle: 10 doses per 5 ml multidose vial

Dose Form: Suspension

Solvent: Phosphate-buffered saline

Storage/Stability: Store at 2° to 8°C (35° to 46°F). Discard frozen vaccine. Contact manufacturers regarding exposures to prolonged room temperature or elevated temperatures. Temperature extremes may adversely affect resuspendability of this vaccine. Shipped in insulated containers with coolant packs.

Diphtheria & Tetanus Toxoids Adsorbed, for Pediatric Use (DT)

BACTERIAL VACCINES AND TOXOIDS

NAME:
Generic

MANUFACTURERS:
Generic, Connaught Laboratories; *Purogenated,* Wyeth-Lederle Vaccines & Pediatrics; Massachusetts Public Health Biologic Laboratories; Michigan Department of Public Health; Medeva Pharmaceuticals, Inc. (distributed by IMS); ⚜ Connaught; ⚜ Wyeth-Ayerst

Synonym: DT

Comparison: Generically equivalent

Viability: Inactivated
Antigenic Form: Toxoid mixture

Antigenic Type: Protein

Note: Trivalent DTP is the preferred immunizing agent for most children. Tetanus and diphtheria toxoids for adult use (Td) is the preferred immunizing agent for most adults and older children.
Specific information about the individual components of this drug appear in the individual monographs on diphtheria toxoid and tetanus toxoid.

Use Characteristics

Indications: Selective induction of active immunity against both tetanus and diphtheria in infants and children from age 2 months up to the seventh birthday. All persons should maintain tetanus immunity by means of booster doses throughout life since tetanus spores are ubiquitous. Trivalent DTP is the preferred immunizing agent for most children up to their seventh birthday. Use diphtheria and tetanus toxoids for pediatric use (DT) only for children for whom pertussis vaccination alone is contraindicated.

Refer to CDC's wound-management guidelines in the DTP Overview.

Contraindications:
Absolute: Patients >7 years of age; persons with a history of serious adverse reaction to constituents of this drug.

Relative: An acute infection is reason for deferring administration of routine primary immunizing or recall booster doses, but not emergency recall booster doses.

Elderly: Use of DT is contraindicated after the seventh birthday. Tetanus and diphtheria toxoids for adult use (Td) is the preferred immunizing agent for most adults and older children.

Adults: Use of DT is contraindicated after the seventh birthday. Tetanus and diphtheria toxoids for adult use (Td) is the preferred immunizing agent for most adults and older children.

Pregnancy: Use of DT is contraindicated after the seventh birthday.

Lactation: It is not known if DT antigens or corresponding antibodies are excreted in breast milk. Problems in humans have not been documented.

Children: DT is indicated for children >6 weeks and <7 years of age in whom pertussis vaccination is contraindicated. Trivalent DTwP or DTaP is the preferred immunizing agent for most children up to their seventh birthday. Td is the preferred immunizing agent for most adults and children from 7 years of age.

Adverse Reactions:
A small amount of erythema, induration, pain, tenderness, heat, and edema surrounding the injection site, persisting for a few days, is not unusual. Temperatures >38°C (100°F) following DT administration are unusual. A nodule may be palpable at the injection site for a few weeks. Allow such nodules to recede spontaneously and do not incise. Sterile abscesses (incidence, 6 to 10 cases per million doses) and SC atrophy may also occur. Adverse reactions often associated with multiple prior booster doses may be manifested by erythema, boggy edema, pruritus, lymphadenopathy, and induration surrounding the point of injection, 2 to >12 hours after administration. Pain and tenderness, if present, are usually not the primary complaints.

Systemic Manifestations: Transient low-grade fever, chills, malaise, generalized aches and pains, headaches, flushing, generalized urticaria or pruritus, tachycardia, anaphylaxis, hypotension, neurological complications. Although the cause is unknown, hypersensitivity to the toxin or bacillary protein of the tetanus organism itself is assumed to be possible. In other persons, interaction between the injected antigen and high levels of preexisting tetanus antibody from prior booster doses seems to be the most likely cause of the Arthus-like response. Do not give these persons even emergency doses of tetanus toxoid more frequently than every 10 years.

Pharmacologic & Dosing Characteristics

 Dosage: Shake well before withdrawing each dose.

Primary Immunizing Series: For children, beginning at 6 to 8 weeks of age, two 0.5 ml doses, at an interval of 4 to 8 weeks, followed by a third reinforcing 0.5 ml dose 6 to 12 months later. The third dose is an integral part of the primary series. Do not consider basic immunization complete until the third dose has been given.

When immunization with DT begins in the first year of life (rather than immunization with DTwP), the primary series consists of three 0.5 ml doses, 4 to 8 weeks apart, followed by a fourth reinforcing 0.5 ml dose 6 to 12 months after the third dose.

Immunization of infants normally

starts at 6 weeks to 2 months of age; always start immunization at once if diphtheria is present in the community. Give unimmunized children 1 year of age or older in whom pertussis immunization is contraindicated two 0.5 ml DT doses 4 to 8 weeks apart, followed by a third 0.5 ml dose 6 to 12 months after the second dose, to complete the primary series.

Refer to CDC's wound-management guidelines in the DTP Overview.

Route & Site: IM. Give injections in the deltoid area of the upper arm or the midlateral muscle of the thigh (the vastus lateralis). Take care to avoid major peripheral nerve trunks. Do not inject the same muscle site more than once during the course of primary immunization. To avoid deposition of this product along the needle track, expel the antigen slowly and terminate the dose with a small bubble of air (0.1 to 0.2 ml) before withdrawing the needle. Do not inject ID or into superficial SC tissues.

Documentation Requirements: Federal law requires that (1) the manufacturer and lot number of this vaccine, (2) the date of its administration, and (3) the name, address and title of the person administering the vaccine be documented in the recipient's permanent medical record or in a permanent office log. Certain adverse events must be reported to the VAERS system, 1-800-822-7967.

Efficacy: Extremely high, >99%

Onset: After third dose

Duration: Approximately 10 years, if a complete primary immunizing series was given.

 Drug Interactions: Like all inactivated vaccines, administration of DT to persons receiving immunosuppressant drugs, including high-dose corticosteroids, or radiation therapy may result in an insufficient response to immunization. They may remain susceptible despite immunization.

Several routine pediatric vaccines may safely and effectively be administered simultaneously at separate injection sites (eg, DTP or DT, MMR, OPV or e-IPV, Hib, hepatitis B). National authorities recommend simultaneous immunization at separate sites as indicated by age or health-risk, if return of a vaccine recipient for a subsequent visit is doubtful. Delay diphtheria toxoid administration until 3 to 4 weeks after diphtheria antitoxin use, to avoid the hypothetical possibility of antitoxin-toxoid interference.

Concurrent administration of tetanus toxoid and tetanus immune globulin may delay development of active immunity by several days through partial antigen-antibody antagonism. But this interaction is not clinically significant and does not preclude concurrent administration of both drugs if both are needed.

Systemic chloramphenicol therapy may impair anamnestic response to tetanus toxoid. Avoid concurrent use of these two drugs.

As with other drugs administered by IM injection, give DT with caution to persons receiving anticoagulant therapy.

Pharmaceutical Characteristics

Concentration:

Connaught-US: 6.6 Lf units diphtheria toxoid and 5 Lf units tetanus toxoid per 0.5 ml

Connaught-Canada: 25 Lf units diphtheria toxoid and 5 Lf units tetanus toxoid per 0.5 ml

Wyeth-Lederle: 5 Lf units tetanus toxoid and 12.5 Lf units diphtheria toxoid per 0.5 ml

Wyeth-Ayerst-Canada: 25 Lf units diphtheria toxoid and 5 Lf units tetanus toxoid per 0.5 ml

Massachusetts: 7.5 Lf units diphtheria toxoid and 7.5 Lf units tetanus toxoid per 0.5 ml

Michigan: Data not provided

Medeva: 10 Lf units diphtheria toxoid and 5 Lf units tetanus toxoid per 0.5 ml

Packaging:

Connaught: 10 doses per 5 ml multidose vial

Wyeth-Lederle: 10 doses per 5 ml multidose vial

Massachusetts: Unspecified multidose vial

Michigan: Unspecified multidose vial

Medeva: 10 doses per 5 ml multidose vial, ten 0.5 ml *Tubex* single-dose cartridge-needle units with 25 gauge, $^5/_8$ inch needle

Dose Form: Suspension

Solvent: Variously formulated with sodium chloride, with or without phosphate buffers.

Storage/Stability: Store at 2° to 8°C (35° to 46°F). Discard frozen toxoids. Contact manufacturers regarding prolonged exposure to room temperature or elevated temperatures. Shipped in insulated containers with coolant packs.

Connaught: Product can tolerate 4 days at not more than 37°C (100°F).

Tetanus and Diphtheria Toxoids Adsorbed, for Adult Use (Td)

BACTERIAL VACCINES AND TOXOIDS

NAME:
Generic

MANUFACTURERS:
Connaught Laboratories; Massachusetts Public Health Biologic Laboratories; Wyeth-Lederle Vaccines & Pediatrics; Medeva Pharmaceuticals, Inc. (distributed by IMS); ✚ Connaught; ✚ IAF Biovac;

Synonym: Td

Comparison: Generically equivalent

Viability: Inactivated

Antigenic Type: Protein

Antigenic Form: Toxoid mixture

> **Note:** Trivalent DTP is the preferred immunizing agent for most children. Tetanus and diphtheria toxoids for adult use (Td) is the preferred immunizing agent for most adults and older children. Specific information about the individual components of this drug appear in the individual monographs on diphtheria toxoid and tetanus toxoid.

Use Characteristics

◎ **Indications:** Induction of active immunity against tetanus and diphtheria. Tetanus and diphtheria toxoids for adult use (Td) is the preferred immunizing agent for most adults and children after their seventh birthday. All persons should maintain tetanus immunity by means of booster doses throughout life since tetanus spores are ubiquitous. Tetanus immunity is especially important for military personnel, farm and utility workers, those working with horses, firemen and all individuals whose occupation or vocation renders them susceptible to even minor lacerations and abrasions. Advise travelers to developing nations to maintain active tetanus immunity to obviate any need for therapy with equine tetanus antitoxin and thus avoid associated complications.

Refer to CDC's wound-management guidelines in the DTP Overview.

Outmoded Practices: Do not conduct a Schick or diphtheria-toxoid-sensitivity test for susceptibility prior to administration.

🛑 **Contraindications:**

Absolute: Persons with a history of serious adverse reaction to constituents of this drug.

Relative: An acute infection is reason for deferring administration of routine primary immunizing or routine recall doses, but not emergency recall doses.

Elderly: The elderly develop lower to normal antitoxin levels following tetanus immunization than younger persons. No specific information is available about geriatric use of diphtheria toxoid.

Adults: Tetanus and diphtheria toxoids for adult use (Td) is the preferred immunizing agent for most adults and older children.

Pregnancy: *Category C.* Use only if clearly needed. Based on extensive human experience, there is no evidence that tetanus toxoid is teratogenic. Give a previously unimmunized pregnant woman who may deliver her child under nonhygienic conditions two properly spaced doses of a product containing tetanus toxoid (eg, Td), preferably during the last two trimesters. Incompletely immunized pregnant women should complete the 3 dose series. Give those immunized >10 years previously a booster dose. Generally, most IgG passage across the placenta occurs during the third trimester.

Lactation: It is not known if Td antigens or corresponding antibodies are excreted in breast milk. Problems in humans have not been documented.

Children: Trivalent DTwP or DTaP is the preferred immunizing agent for most children up to their seventh birthday. If pertussis vaccination is contraindicated, use diphtheria and tetanus toxoids for pediatric use (DT) until the child's seventh birthday. From 7 years of age through adulthood, tetanus and diphtheria toxoids for adult use (Td) is the preferred immunizing agent.

 Adverse Reactions:
A small amount of erythema, induration, pain, tenderness, heat, and edema surrounding the injection site, persisting for a few days, is not unusual. Temperatures >38°C (100°F) following Td administration are unusual. A nodule may be palpable at the injection site for a few weeks. Allow such nodules to recede spontaneously and do not incise. Sterile abscesses (incidence, 6 to 10 cases per million doses) and SC atrophy may also occur. Adverse reactions often associated with multiple prior booster doses may be manifested 2 to >12 hours after administration by erythema, boggy edema, pruritus, lymphadenopathy, and induration surrounding the point of injection. Pain and tenderness, if present, are usually not the primary complaints.

Systemic Manifestations: Transient low-grade fever, chills, malaise, generalized aches and pains, headaches, flushing, generalized urticaria or pruritus, tachycardia, anaphylaxis, hypotension, neurological complications. Although the cause is unknown, hypersensitivity to the toxin or bacillary protein of the tetanus organism itself is assumed to be possible. In other persons, interaction between the injected antigen and high levels of preexisting tetanus antibody from prior booster doses seems to be the most likely cause of the Arthus-like response. Do not give these persons even emergency doses of tetanus toxoid more frequently than every 10 years.

Pharmacologic & Dosing Characteristics

 Dosage: Shake vial well before withdrawing each dose.

Primary Immunizing Series: For adults and children after their seventh birthday, two 0.5 ml doses, at an interval of 4 to 8 weeks, followed by a third reinforcing 0.5 ml dose 6 to 12 months later. The third dose is an integral part of the primary series. Do not consider immunization complete until the third dose has been given. Start immunization at once if diphtheria is present in the community.

Refer to CDC's wound-management guidelines in the DTP Overview.

Route & Site: IM or jet injection. Give IM injections in the deltoid area of the upper arm or the midlateral muscle of the thigh (the vastus lateralis). Take care to avoid major peripheral nerve trunks. Do not inject the same muscle site more than once during the course of primary immunization. To avoid deposition of this product along the needle track, expel the antigen slowly and terminate the dose with a small bubble of air (0.1 to 0.2 ml) before withdrawing the needle. Do not inject ID or into superficial SC tissues.

Documentation Requirements: Federal law requires that (1) the manufacturer and lot number of this vaccine, (2) the date of its administration, and (3) the name, address and title of the person administering the vaccine be documented in the recipient's permanent medical record or in a permanent office log. Certain adverse events must be reported to the VAERS system, 1-800-822-7967.

Efficacy: Extremely high

Onset: After third dose

Duration: Approximately 10 years

Drug Interactions: Like all inactivated vaccines, administration of Td to persons receiving immuno-suppressant drugs, including high-dose corticosteroids, or radiation therapy may result in an insufficient response to immunization. They may remain susceptible despite immunization.

Several routine vaccines may safely and effectively be administered simultaneously at separate injection sites (eg, Td, MMR, OPV or e-IPV, Hib, hepatitis B). National authorities recommend simultaneous immunization at separate sites as indicated by age or health-risk, if return of a vaccine recipient for a subsequent visit is doubtful. Delay diphtheria toxoid administration until 3 to 4 weeks after diphtheria antitoxin use, to avoid the hypothetical possibility of antitoxin-toxoid interference.

Concurrent administration of tetanus toxoid and tetanus immune globulin may delay development of active immunity by several days through partial antigen-antibody antagonism. But this interaction is not clinically significant and does not preclude concurrent administration of both drugs if both are needed.

Systemic chloramphenicol therapy may impair anamnestic response to tetanus toxoid. Avoid concurrent use of these two drugs.

As with other drugs administered by IM injection, give Td with caution to persons receiving anticoagulant therapy.

Pharmaceutical Characteristics

Concentration:

Connaught-US & -Canada: 5 Lf units tetanus toxoid and 2 Lf units diphtheria toxoid per 0.5 ml

Wyeth-Lederle: 5 Lf units tetanus toxoid and 2 Lf units diphtheria toxoid per 0.5 ml

Massachusetts: 2 Lf units tetanus toxoid and 2 Lf units diphtheria toxoid per 0.5 ml

Medeva: 5 Lf units tetanus toxoid and 2 Lf units diphtheria toxoid per 0.5 ml

IAF Biovac: 5 Lf units tt and 2 Lf units dt per 0.5 ml

Wyeth-Ayerst-Canada: 5 Lf units tt and 2 Lf units dt per 0.5 ml

Packaging:

Connaught: 10 doses per 5 ml multidose vial, 30 ml multidose vial for jet injection

Wyeth-Lederle: ten 0.5 ml *Lederject* disposable single-dose syringes with 25 gauge, $\frac{5}{8}$ inch needle; 10 doses per 5 ml multidose vial

Massachusetts: Unspecified multidose vial. Distributed free of charge, but only within the State of Massachusetts.

Medeva: 10 doses per 5 ml multidose vial, ten 0.5 ml *Tubex* single-dose cartridge-needle units with 25 gauge, $\frac{5}{8}$ inch needle

Dose Form: Suspension

Solvent: Variously formulated with sodium chloride, with or without phosphate buffers

Storage/Stability: Store at 2° to 8°C (35° to 46°F). Discard frozen toxoids. Contact manufacturer regarding prolonged exposure to room temperature or elevated temperatures. Shipped in insulated containers with coolant packs.

Connaught: Product can tolerate 4 days at not more than 37°C (100°F).

Medeva: Product can tolerate 10 days at room temperature.

Handling: Maintain jet injectors properly. Discard jet-injector vials at the end of each day.

NAME:
Te Anatoxal Berna,
Generic

MANUFACTURER:
Berna Products (*Te Anatoxal Berna*
only); Connaught Laboratories;
Massachusetts Public Health Bio-
logic Laboratories; Michigan
Department of Public Health;
Wyeth-Lederle Vaccine & Pedi-
atrics; Medeva Pharmaceuticals,
Inc. (distributed by IMS);
🍁 Connaught; 🍁 IAF Biovac;
🍁 Wyeth-Ayerst

Synonyms: T, TT, tetanus vaccine. The
disease is also known as lockjaw.

Comparison: Generically equivalent.
While the rate of seroconversion and
promptness of antibody response are
essentially equivalent for both the
fluid and adsorbed forms of tetanus
toxoid, adsorbed toxoids induce higher antitoxin titers and, hence, more
persistent antitoxin levels. Therefore,
adsorbed tetanus toxoid is strongly

recommended for both primary and
booster immunizations. Use fluid
tetanus toxoid to immunize the rare
patient who is hypersensitive to the
aluminum adjuvant. The only other
rational use remaining for fluid
tetanus toxoid is in compounding dilutions of a reagent for delayed-hypersensitivity skin-testing (refer to
product information).

Viability: Inactivated
Antigenic Form: Toxoid

Antigenic Type: Protein

Note: Trivalent DTP is the preferred immunizing agent for most children.
Tetanus & diphtheria toxoids for adult use (Td) is the preferred immunizing agent for most adults and older children.

Use Characteristics

(◎) Indications: Selective induction
of active immunity against
tetanus in selected patients. Tetanus &
diphtheria toxoids for adult use (Td) is
the preferred immunizing agent for
most adults and children after their
seventh birthday. All persons should

maintain tetanus immunity by means
of booster doses throughout life since
tetanus spores are ubiquitous. Tetanus
immunity is especially important for
military personnel, farm and utility
workers, those working with horses,
firemen, and all individuals whose
occupation or vocation renders them
liable to even minor lacerations and

abrasions. Advise travelers to developing nations to maintain active tetanus immunity to obviate any need for therapy with equine tetanus antitoxin and thus avoid associated complications.

While the rate of seroconversion and promptness of antibody response are essentially equivalent for both the fluid and adsorbed forms of tetanus toxoid, adsorbed toxoids induce higher antitoxin titers and, hence, more persistent antitoxin levels. Therefore, selection of tetanus toxoid adsorbed is strongly recommended for both primary and booster immunizations. Use fluid tetanus toxoid to immunize the rare patient who is hypersensitive to the aluminum adjuvant.

Contraindications:

Absolute: Patients with a history of any type of neurological symptoms or signs following administration of this product. Use fluid tetanus toxoid to immunize the rare patient who is hypersensitive to the aluminum adjuvant.

Relative: An acute infection is reason for deferring administration of routine primary immunizing or routine recall doses, but not emergency recall doses.

The FDA recommends that elective tetanus immunization be deferred during any outbreak of poliomyelitis (Sutter et al, 1992) since injections are an important cause of provocative poliomyelitis. This recommendation presupposes that the patient has not sustained an injury that increases the risk of tetanus. The caution has largely been superseded, as poliomyelitis has been controlled in the U.S. by universal vaccination, but the warning persists in some drug labeling.

Elderly: Tetanus and diphtheria toxoids for adult use (Td) is the preferred immunizing agent for most adults and older children. The elderly develop lower to normal antitoxin levels following tetanus immunization than younger persons.

Adults: Tetanus and diphtheria toxoids for adult use (Td) is the preferred immunizing agent for most adults and older children.

Pregnancy: *Category* C. Use only if clearly needed, although Td is preferred. Based on extensive human experience, there is no evidence that tetanus toxoid is teratogenic. Give a previously unimmunized pregnant woman who may deliver her child under nonhygienic conditions 2 properly spaced doses of a product containing tetanus toxoid adsorbed (eg, Td), preferably during the last 2 trimesters. Incompletely immunized pregnant women should complete their 3 dose primary series. Give those immunized >10 years previously a booster dose. It is not known if tetanus toxoid or corresponding antibodies cross the placenta. Generally, most IgG passage across the placenta occurs during the third trimester.

Lactation: It is not known if tetanus toxoid or corresponding antibodies are excreted in human breast milk. Problems in humans have not been documented.

Children: Safety and efficacy of tetanus toxoid are known for children as young as 2 months. Nonetheless, trivalent DTwP or DTaP is the preferred immunizing agent for most children until their seventh birthday.

Tetanus and diphtheria toxoids for adult use (Td) is the preferred immunizing agent for most adults and older children.

Adverse Reactions:

A small amount of erythema and induration surrounding the injection site, persisting for a few days, is not unusual. A nodule may be palpable at the injection site for a few weeks. Allow such nodules to recede spontaneously and do not incise. Sterile abscesses (incidence, < 6 to 10 cases per million doses) and SC atrophy may also occur. Adverse reactions often associated with multiple prior booster doses may be manifested 2 to >12 hours after administration by erythema, boggy edema, pruritis, lymphadenopathy, and induration surrounding the site of injection. Pain and tenderness, if present, are usually not the primary complaints.

Systemic Manifestations: Low-grade fever, chills, malaise, generalized aches and pains, headaches, flushing, generalized urticaria or pruritus, tachycardia, anaphylaxis, hypotension, neurological complications.

Although the cause is unknown, hypersensitivity to the exotoxin or bacillary protein of the tetanus organism itself is assumed to be possible. In other persons, interaction between the injected antigen and high levels of preexisting tetanus antibody from prior booster doses seems to be the most likely cause of these Arthus-like responses. Do not give these persons even emergency doses of tetanus toxoid more frequently than every 10 years.

Pharmacologic & Dosing Characteristics

Dosage:

Primary Immunizing Series: For adults and children, beginning at 6 to 8 weeks of age, two 0.5 ml doses, at an interval of 4 to 8 weeks, followed by a third reinforcing 0.5 ml dose 6 to 12 months after the second dose. The third dose is an integral part of the primary series. Do not consider basic immunization complete until the third dose has been given. The dosage is the same for children and adults. Shake the vial vigorously before withdrawing each dose.

However, when immunization with tetanus toxoid adsorbed begins in the first year of life (rather than immunization with DTwP), the primary series consists of three 0.5 ml doses, 4 to 8 weeks apart, followed by a fourth reinforcing 0.5 ml dose 6 to 12 months after the third dose.

If doubt exists about the patient's tolerance of tetanus toxoid and if an emergency booster dose is indicated, give a small dose (eg, 0.05 to 0.1 ml) SC as a test dose. If no reaction occurs, give the balance of the full 0.5 ml dose 12 hours later (Edsall, 1959). If a marked reaction does occur, further toxoid injections at that time may safely be omitted, since reducing the dose of tetanus toxoid does not proportionately reduce the magnitude of the response obtained.

Route & Site: IM or jet injection. Give IM injections in the deltoid area of the upper arm or the midlateral muscle of the thigh (the vastus lateralis). Take care to avoid major peripheral nerve trunks. Do not inject the same muscle site more than once during the course of primary immunization. Expel the antigen slowly and terminate the dose with a small bubble of air (0.1 to 0.2 ml) to reduce the risk of nodules. Do not inject ID or into superficial SC tissues.

Documentation Requirements: Federal law requires that (1) the manufacturer and lot number of this vaccine, (2) the date of its administration, and (3) the name, address and title of the person administering the vaccine be documented in the recipient's permanent medical record or in a permanent office log. Certain adverse events must be reported to the VAERS system, 1-800-822-7967.

Efficacy: Nearly perfect

Onset: After multiple doses

Duration: Approximately 10 years

Drug Interactions: Like all inactivated vaccines, administration of tetanus toxoid adsorbed to persons receiving immunosuppressant drugs, including high-dose corticosteroids, or radiation therapy may result in an insufficient response to immunization. They may remain susceptible despite immunization.

Several routine vaccines may safely and effectively be administered simultaneously at separate injection sites (eg, DTP or Td, MMR, e-IPV, Hib, hepatitis B). National authorities recommend simultaneous immunization at separate sites as indicated by age or health risk, if return of a vaccine recipient for a subsequent visit is doubtful.

Concurrent administration of tetanus toxoid adsorbed and tetanus immune globulin may delay development of active immunity by several days through partial antigen-antibody antagonism. But this interaction is not clinically significant and does not preclude concurrent administration of both drugs if both are needed.

Systemic chloramphenicol therapy may impair anamnestic response to tetanus toxoid. Avoid concurrent use of these two drugs.

As with other drugs administered by IM injection, give tetanus toxoid with caution to persons on anticoagulant therapy.

Pharmaceutical Characteristics

Concentration:

Berna: 10 Lf units per 0.5 ml

Connaught-US &-Canada: 5 Lf units per 0.5 ml

Wyeth-Lederle: 5 Lf units per 0.5 ml

Massachusetts: 5 Lf units per 0.5 ml

Michigan: 5 to 10 Lf units per 0.5 ml

Medeva: 5 Lf units per 0.5 ml

IAF Biovac: 5 Lf units per 0.5 ml

Wyeth-Ayerst-Canada: 5 Lf units per 0.5 ml

Packaging:

Berna: 10 doses per 5 ml multidose vial, ten 0.5 ml disposable single-dose syringes with needles of unspecified length and gauge.

Connaught: 10 doses per 5 ml multidose vial

Wyeth-Lederle: 10 doses per 5 ml multidose vial, ten 0.5 ml *Lederject* disposable single-dose syringes with 25 gauge, $\frac{5}{8}$ inch needle

Massachusetts: 10 doses per 5 ml multidose vial. Distributed free of charge, but only within the State of Massachusetts.

Michigan: unspecified multidose vial

Medeva: ten 0.5 ml *Tubex* single-dose cartridge-needle units with 25 gauge, $\frac{5}{8}$ inch needle, 10 doses per 5 ml multidose vial

Dose Form: Suspension

Solvent: Variously formulated with sodium chloride, with or without phosphate buffers.

Storage/Stability: Store at 2° to 8°C (35° to 46°F). Discard frozen toxoid. Contact manufacturers regarding prolonged exposure to room temperature or elevated temperatures. Shipped in insulated containers with coolant packs.

Connaught: Product can tolerate 4 days at not more than 37°C (100°F).

Medeva: Product can tolerate 10 days at room temperature.

Handling: Maintain jet injectors properly. Discard jet-injector vials at the end of each day.

Pertussis Vaccine Adsorbed
BACTERIAL VACCINES & TOXOIDS

NAME:
Generic

Synonyms: P, whooping-cough vaccine. The disease is also known as whooping cough.

Viability: Inactivated
Antigenic Form: Whole bacterium

MANUFACTURER:
Michigan Department of Public Health (MDPH)

Antigenic Type: Protein

> Note: Trivalent DTP is the preferred immunizing agent for most children. Tetanus and diphtheria toxoids for adult use (Td) is the preferred immunizing agent for most adults and older children.

Use Characteristics

Indications: Selective induction of active immunity against pertussis.

Trivalent DTP is the preferred immunizing agent for most children. Tetanus and diphtheria toxoids for adult use (Td) is the preferred immunizing agent for most adults and older children.

Contraindications:

Absolute: Do not give further doses of a vaccine containing pertussis antigens to children who have recovered from culture-confirmed pertussis. Do not vaccinate patients with a history of serious adverse reactions to a previous dose of a pertussis-containing vaccine. Do not vaccinate patients hypersensitive to any component of the vaccine, including thimerosal.

Data on the use of DTaP in children for whom whole-cell pertussis vaccine is contraindicated are not available. Until such data are available, consider contraindications to whole-cell pertussis

vaccine administration adopted by ACIP and AAP to be contraindications to DTaP also. These contraindications include an immediate anaphylactic reaction or encephalopathy occurring within 7 days following DTP vaccination. Such encephalopathies may include major alterations in consciousness, unresponsiveness, generalized or focal seizures that persist more than a few hours and failure to recover within 24 hours or other generalized or focal neurological signs.

Relative: Until safety, immunogenicity and efficacy data are evaluated, administration of DTaP to children <15 months of age is not recommended. Defer immunization during the course of any febrile illness or acute infection. A minor respiratory illness such as a mild upper respiratory infection is not usually reason to defer immunization. Give DTaP with caution to children with thrombocytopenia or any coagulation disorder that would contraindicate IM injection.

If a contraindication to the pertussis-vaccine component occurs, substitute diphtheria and tetanus toxoids for pediatric use (DT) for each of the remaining doses.

Several events were previously listed as contraindications, but are now listed simply as precautions, warranting careful consideration: Temperature >40.5°C (105°F) within 48 hours after DTP administration not due to another identifiable cause, collapse or shock-like state (hypotonic-hyporesponsive episode) within 48 hours, persistent inconsolable crying lasting ≥3 hours occurring within 48 hours, or convulsions with or without fever within 3 days. There may be circumstances, such as a high local incidence of pertussis, in which the potential benefits outweigh possible risks, particularly because these events are not associated with permanent sequelae.

The occurrence of any type of neurological symptoms or signs, including one or more convulsions, following DTaP administration is generally a contraindication to further use. The presence of any evolving or changing disorder affecting the CNS contraindicates administration of pertussis vaccine regardless of whether the suspected neurological disorder is associated with occurrence of seizure activity of any type.

ACIP and AAP recognize certain circumstances in which children with stable CNS disorders, including well controlled seizures or satisfactorily explained single seizures, may receive pertussis vaccine. ACIP and AAP do not consider a family history of seizures to be a contraindication to pertussis vaccine. Studies suggesting that infants and children with a history of convulsions in first-degree family members (ie, siblings and parents) have an increased risk for neurologic events, compared with those without such histories (Noble et al, 1987; Livengood et al, 1989) may be flawed by selection bias or genetic confounding.

Relative: Until safety, immunogenicity and efficacy data are evaluated, administration of DTaP to children <15 months of age is not recommended. Defer immunization during the course of any febrile illness or acute infection. A minor respiratory illness such as a mild upper respiratory infection is not usually reason to defer immunization. Give DTaP with caution to children with thrombocytopenia or any coagulation disorder that would contraindicate IM injection.

If a contraindication to the pertussis-vaccine component occurs, substitute diphtheria and tetanus toxoids for pediatric use (DT) for each of the remaining doses.

Elderly: Pertussis vaccination with any product is generally contraindicated after the seventh birthday.

Adults: Since the incidence of and mortality due to pertussis decreases with advancing age, while some local and systemic reactions to DTwP or DTaP may increase, routine immunization of persons ≥7 years of age is not generally recommended. Tetanus and diphtheria toxoids for adult use (Td) is the preferred immunizing agent for most adults and older children.

Pregnancy: *Category C*. Pertussis vaccination with any product is generally contraindicated after the seventh birthday.

Lactation: Pertussis vaccination with any product is generally contraindicated after the seventh birthday.

Children: Contraindicated in children

<6 weeks of age since the product may not be immunogenic. Contraindicated in children ≥7 years of age because of decreased risk of disease and increased likelihood of adverse effects. Trivalent DTwP or DTaP is the preferred immunizing agent for most children until their seventh birthday. Tetanus and diphtheria toxoids for adult use (Td) is the preferred immunizing agent for most adults and older children.

Adverse Reactions:

Not all adverse events following administration of pertussis vaccine, DTwP or DTaP are causally related to the drug. Mild local and constitutional reactions (40% to 60%): Pain, induration and redness at the injection site, usually beginning within 72 hours after vaccination. Occasionally a nodule develops at the injection site that can persist for several weeks. These reactions are self-limiting and usually require no treatment. Rarely, an abscess develops at the injection site, with an incidence of 6 to 10 cases per million doses. Mild consitutional reactions consist chiefly of febrile reactions (38.2° to 40.4°C; 101° to 104.7°F). Constitutional reactions usually begin within 12 hours after vaccination, persist for 1 to 7 days, and may be accompanied by irritability, malaise, sleepiness and vomiting.

Several types of severe reactions have followed administration of both pertussis and DTwP vaccines. These illnesses are usually considered reactions to the vaccine because of the temporal association between administration of the drug and the onset of symptoms. Most of the reactions are usually attributed to the pertussis component. Reactions that constitute absolute contraindications to further

vaccination with the pertussis component include convulsions, encephalopathy, focal neurological disease, collapse, shock and altered consciousness. Reactions such as thrombocytopenic purpura and demonstrable hypersensitivity reactions such as anaphylaxis, generalized urticarial eruptions, or Arthus-type reactions after administration of either pertussis, DTwP or DTaP vaccines also constitute absolute contraindications to additional doses of these drugs. Other reported reactions: Excessive somnolence, excessive screaming (persistent crying or screaming for ≥3 hours) and temperature above 40.5°C (105°F). Peripheral neuropathy has followed DTwP vaccination, possibly due in some cases to injection of vaccine too close to a peripheral nerve.

An expert panel assembled by the Institute of Medicine has concluded that no causal association exists between pertussis vaccination and autism, infantile spasms, hypsarrhythmia, Reye's syndrome, SIDS, aseptic meningitis, chronic neurologic damage, erythema multiforme or other rash, Guillain-Barré syndrome, hemolytic anemia, juvenile diabetes, learning disabilities, attention deficit disorder, peripheral mononeuropathy or thrombocytopenia. The panel found evidence consistent with a causal association between DTwP and acute encephalopathy, shock and "unusual shock-like state," anaphylaxis, and protracted, inconsolable crying.

When a child returns for the next dose in a series of either pertussis, DTwP or DTaP vaccine injections, question the adult accompanying the child about possible side effects following previous doses. If any of the effects that contraindicate additional pertussis vaccine doses occurs, continue childhood immunization with bivalent diphtheria and tetanus toxoids for pediatric use (DT).

Pharmacologic & Dosing Characteristics

Dosage:

Primary Immunizing Series: 0.5 ml at age 8 weeks, then 0.5 ml 4 to 8 weeks later, then another 0.5 ml dose 4 to 8 weeks later, then a fourth (reinforcing) 0.5 ml dose 1 year after the third dose. If the fourth primary dose (ie, the reinforcing dose) is given after the fourth birthday, omit the fifth (booster) dose. Shake well before withdrawing each dose. Do not use if resuspension is not possible with vigorous shaking. Do not dilute.

Do not use partial or fractional doses of pertussis, DTwP or DTaP vaccines since the efficacy of such practices have not been adequately studied.

Route & Site: IM, preferably into the midlateral muscles of the thigh or the deltoid muscle of the upper arm. Preferably, do not inject the same muscle group for successive injections.

Documentation Requirements:: Federal law requires that (1) the manufacturer and lot number of this vaccine, (2) the date of its administration, and (3) the name, address and title of the person administering the vaccine be documented in the recipient's permanent medical record or in a permanent office log. Certain adverse events must be reported to the VAERS system, 1-800-822-7967.

Efficacy: Three doses of pertussis vaccine produce a 50% to 95% reduction in disease incidence. Pertussis vaccine is generally more effective at preventing disease than at preventing infection.

Onset: After multiple doses

Duration: Greater than 4 to 6 years

Drug Interactions: Like all inactivated vaccines, administration of pertussis vaccine to persons receiving immunosuppressant drugs, including high-dose corticosteroids, or radiation therapy may result in an insufficient response to immunization. They may remain susceptible despite immunization.

Several routine pediatric vaccines may safely and effectively be administered simultaneously at separate injection sites (eg, DTP, MMR, OPV or e-IPV, Hib, hepatitis B). National authorities recommend simultaneous immunization at separate sites as indicated by age or health risk, if return of a vaccine recipient for a subsequent visit is doubtful.

As with other drugs administered by IM injection, give pertussis vaccine with caution to persons receiving anticoagulant therapy.

Pharmaceutical Characteristics

Concentration: Each dose contains at least 4 but not >16 opacity units per 0.5 ml.

Packaging: 10 doses per 5 ml multidose vial

Dose Form: Suspension

Solvent: 0.85% sodium chloride

Storage/Stability: Store at $2°$ to $8°$C ($35°$ to $46°$F). Do not freeze. Contact manufacturer regarding prolonged exposure to room temperature or elevated or freezing temperatures. Shipping data not provided.

NAME:

Diphtheria Toxoid Conjugate, *Pro-HIBit*, PRP-D, Diphtheria CRM197 Protein Conjugate, *HibTITER*, PRP-HbOC, HbOC (oligosaccharide conjugate), Meningococcal Protein Conjugate, *PedvaxHIB*, PRP-OMP (outer membrane protein), PRP-OMPC (outer membrane protein conjugate), Tetanus Toxoid Conjugate, *OmniHIB*, PRP-T, 🍁 *Act-HIB*

MANUFACTURERS:

Diphtheria Toxoid Conjugate, *Pro-HIBit*, PRP-D, Connaught Laboratories; Diphtheria CRM197 Protein Conjugate, *HibTITER*, PRP-HbOC, HbOC (oligosaccharide conjugate), Wyeth-Lederle Vaccines & Pediatrics; Meningococcal Protein Conjugate, *PedvaxHIB*, PRP-OMP (outer membrane protein), PRP-OMPC (outer membrane protein conjugate), Merck Vaccine Division; Tetanus Toxoid Conjugate, *OmniHIB*, PRP-T, Manufactured by Pasteur-Mérieux and distributed by SmithKline Beecham; 🍁 *Act-HIB*, Connaught; 🍁 *ProHIBit*, Connaught; 🍁 *HibTITER*, Wyeth-Ayerst; 🍁 *PedvaxHIB*, Merck Frosst

Synonyms: Hib vaccine, HBcV. The bacterium was previously known as the influenza bacillus.

Comparison: Not generically equivalent, based on immunogenicity and dosage schedule. Each Hib vaccine is immunogenically unique. PRP-OMP induces higher antibody titers after the first dose than do the other Hib vaccines, but the extent of clinical protection is comparable for all licensed products.

OmniHIB and *ActHIB* are the same vaccine. *ActHIB* is marketed by Connaught Laboratories in combination with DTP vaccine, *ActHIB*/DTP.

Viability: Inactivated

Antigenic Form: Capsular polysaccharide fragments, conjugated to various protein carriers.

Antigenic Type: Polysaccharide conjugated to protein. The polysaccharide is a polymer of ribose, ribitol and phosphate (polyribosyl-ribitol-phosphate, PRP).

Use Characteristics

⊙ **Indications:** Induction of active immunity against invasive diseases caused by encapsulated *Haemophilus influenzae* type b. Routine immunization of all infants beginning at 2 months of age is recommended in the US, using either *HibTITER*, *Pedvax-HIB*, *ActHIB*, or *OmniHIB*. Risk groups with increased susceptibility to disease include children attending day-care facilities, persons of low socioeconomic status, blacks [especially those lacking the Km(1) Ig allotype], Caucasians lacking the G2m(n or 23) Ig allotype, Native Americans, household contacts of Hib disease cases, and individuals with asplenia, sickle-cell disease and antibody-deficiency syndromes.

Children who have invasive Hib disease when <24 months of age may not develop adequate anticapsular antibody concentrations and remain at risk of a second episode of disease. Vaccinate these children according to current age, ignoring previous Hib doses. Do not immunize children whose disease occurred at >24 months of age, since they are likely to develop a protective immune response.

 Contraindications:

Absolute: None.

Relative: Patients with a history of a hypersensitivity reaction to any component. Any febrile illness or acute infection is reason for delaying immunization with this vaccine. A mild afebrile illness such as a mild upper respiratory infection is not usually reason to defer immunization.

Elderly: No specific information is available about geriatric use of Hib vaccine.

Adults: The American College of Physicians (1990) suggests vaccination of older children and adults who have underlying conditions associated with increased susceptibility to infection with encapsulated bacteria. These conditions include splenectomy, sickle-cell disease, Hodgkin's disease and other hematologic neoplasms, and immunosuppression. Do not use Hib vaccine to prevent recurrent sinusitis or bronchitis in adults, since *Haemophilus* organisms associated with these conditions are almost always nontypable, nonencapsulated strains unaffected by anti-Hib antibody. Hib vaccination is not necessary for healthcare personnel or daycare workers who frequently come in contact with children with invasive disease.

Pregnancy: *Category C.* Use is not generally recommended, but is not contraindicated. It is not known if Hib vaccine or corresponding antibodies cross the placenta. Generally, most IgG passage across the placenta occurs during the third trimester.

Lactation: It is not known if Hib vaccine or corresponding antibodies are excreted in breast milk. Problems in humans have not been documented.

Children: Routine immunization of all infants beginning at 2 months of age is recommended in the US. Routinely vaccinate children as old as 5 years of age.

Adverse Reactions:
A fever >38.3°C (101°F) occurred at least once in 2% of recipients during clinical trials. Other possible reactions include erythema, swelling or tenderness, which are generally infrequent, mild, transient, with no serious sequelae. A cause-effect relationship between Hib vaccine and observed postvaccinal irritability, restless sleep, diarrhea, vomiting, loss of appetite, rash, hives, thrombocytopenia, convulsions, renal failure or Guillain-Barré syndrome has not been established.

Pharmacologic & Dosing Characteristics

Dosage: Each Hib conjugate vaccine is immunogenically unique. Pediatric dosage schedules vary for each of the products. Do not complete an immunizing series begun with one product with some other product, until specific studies have been published. The adult dose of any brand is a single dose of 0.5 ml.

Connaught: Effective for routine immunization of children 18 months to 5 years of age with a single 0.5 ml dose. *ProHIBiT* may be given to children as young as 12 months of age when it is expected that the child will not return at 18 months of age for Hib immunization. The proportion of children 15 to 17 months of age who develop protective antibody titers (53%) is not as high as in children 18 to 21 months of age (75%). Do not immunize infants with *ProHIBiT*, since adequate immunity may not develop.

Wyeth-Lederle: In infants 2 to 6 months of age, give three separate 0.5 ml doses at 2 month intervals. Give unvaccinated 7 to 11 month-old infants 2 separate 0.5 ml doses approximately 2 months apart. Give unvaccinated 12 to 14 month-old children one 0.5 ml dose. Give all vaccinated children a single booster dose at 15 months of age or older, but not sooner than 2 months after the previous dose. Give previously unvaccinated children 15 to 60 months of age a single dose in the thigh or deltoid muscle.

Merck: Give infants 2 to 14 months of age a 0.5 ml dose, optimally at 2 months of age, followed by 0.5 ml dose 2 months later, or as soon as possible thereafter. When the primary 2 dose regimen is completed before 12 months of age, a 0.5 ml booster dose is needed at 12 months of age, but not earlier than 2 months after the second dose. Give a single 0.5 ml dose to children ≥15 months of age who were previously unvaccinated against Hib disease.

Pasteur/SKB: In infants 2 to 6 months of age, give 3 separate 0.5 ml doses at 2-month intervals. Give all vaccinated children a single booster dose at 15 to 18 months of age.

Only limited data regarding interchange of brands of Hib vaccines to complete a dosage schedule are available. For booster doses, using the product used for the first dose is generally preferred. Nonetheless, the sequences PRP-OMP/PRP-T/PRP-T, PRP-OMP/HbOC/HbOC, or HbOC/-PRP-T/PRP-T, at 2 month intervals, are known to be immunogenic after the primary series is completed; other sequences may be effective as well. It is not necessary to give >3 doses to any child to complete the primary series.

Route & Site: IM, preferably in the outer aspect of the vastus lateralis, mid-thigh or the outer aspect of the upper arm. Do not administer IV or intradermally, nor into the gluteal area or areas where there may be a nerve trunk.

Pasteur/SKB: In patients with coagulation disorders, PRP-T may be given SC in the mid-lateral aspect of the thigh.

Efficacy: The initial unconjugated polysaccharide Hib vaccines produced roughly 45% to 88% reduction in disease incidence among children 18 to 24 months of age or older, although some reports that failed to demonstrate efficacy were also published.

Connaught: 88% disease reduction in

children ≥18 months of age. In infants, the vaccine has demonstrated mixed results: 87% fewer cases of disease in a Finnish study, but only 35% efficacy in a study of Alaskan Native infants.

Wyeth-Lederle: 2 months after the second dose of vaccine, 95% of infants' sera had bactericidal activity and 99.5% of infants vaccinated at 7 to 11 months of age responded with anti-*Haemophilus* polysaccharide antibody levels of at least 1 mcg/ml. One month after the third dose, 98% had bactericidal activity.

Merck: In a study of 3,486 Navajo infants, vaccination provided a 93% reduction in disease incidence. After the first dose, 88% and 52% of infants, respectively, developed antibody responses >0.15 mcg/ml or >1mcg/ml. After the second dose, those proportions rose to 91% and 60%.

Pasteur/SKB: Of infants receiving PRP-T doses at 2, 4 and 6 months of age, 90% develop a GMT of anti-Hib antibody >1 mcg/ml. More than 98% of infants exceeded this level after a booster dose.

Onset:

Connaught: Several days to 1 week after the last recommended dose.

Wyeth-Lederle: Several days to 1 week after the last recommended dose.

Merck: >1 week after the dose at 2 months of age.

Pasteur/SKB: As much as 2 weeks after the last recommended dose.

Duration: Antibody titers exceeding 1 mcg/ml correlate with prolonged protection from disease, generally implying several years of protection.

 Drug Interactions: Like all inactivated vaccines, administration of Hib vaccine to persons receiving immunosuppressant drugs, including high-dose corticosteroids, or radiation therapy may result in an insufficient response to immunization. They may remain susceptible despite immunization. Hib vaccine does not impair immunogenicity of DTP, OPV, e-IPV, hepatitis B, influenza or MMR vaccines. Rates of adverse reactions when Hib vaccine was administered concurrently with DTP and either OPV or e-IPV were comparable to rates when DTP was given alone. Hib, meningococcal and pneumococcal vaccines may safely and effectively be administered simultaneously at separate injection sites.

Concurrent administration of PRP-T and a DTP vaccine formulation that is not licensed in the US resulted in decreased antibody response to the pertussis component in a trial in Chile. The implications for PRP-T use in the US have yet to be determined.

As with other drugs administered by IM injection, give Hib vaccine with caution to persons receiving anticoagulant therapy.

Laboratory Interference: Antigenuria has been detected following receipt of Hib vaccines; therefore, antigen detection (eg, with latex agglutination kits) may have no diagnostic value in suspected Hib disease within a short period after immunization (Wyeth-Lederle: 2 weeks; Merck: 7 days; Pasteur/SKB: 3 days; Connaught: Data not provided). False-positive latex agglutination tests of cerebrospinal fluid have also been reported 1 to 21 days following Hib vaccination (Perkins, 1993).

Pharmaceutical Characteristics

Concentration:

Connaught: 25 mcg polysaccharide per 0.5 ml

Wyeth-Lederle: 10 mcg oligosaccharide per 0.5 ml

Merck: 15 mcg polysaccharide per 0.5 ml

Pasteur/SKB: 10 mg polysaccharide per 0.5 ml

Packaging:

Connaught: Package of five 0.5 ml single-dose vials, one 2.5 ml five-dose vial, one 5 ml ten-dose vial; package of six 0.5 ml single-dose disposable syringes with 25 gauge, $\frac{5}{8}$ inch needle.

Wyeth-Lederle: Package of four 0.5 ml single-dose vials, one 2.5 ml five-dose vial, one 5 ml 10 dose vial

Merck: Package of 1 single-dose package of powder and 0.7 ml aluminum-hydroxide diluent, box of 5 single-dose packages

Pasteur/SKB: Box of 5 single-dose packages containing a vial of powder and a 0.6 ml syringe of diluent with a 23-gauge, $\frac{5}{8}$ inch needle. Use a new syringe for injection.

Dose Form:

Connaught: Solution

Wyeth-Lederle: Solution

Merck: Powder for suspension

Pasteur/SKB: Powder for suspension

Solvent: *Connaught*: Sodium phosphate-buffered 0.9% sodium chloride

Wyeth-Lederle: 0.9% sodium chloride

Diluent for reconstitution:

Merck: Add entire contents (about 0.7 ml) of diluent vial to powder. Shake well to a uniform suspension before withdrawing each dose. Withdraw entire contents (about 0.5 ml) of reconstituted vaccine. Use only 0.9% sodium chloride with aluminum hydroxide. Use of plain saline diluents may increase the incidence of adverse reactions (eg, fever, persistent crying, erythema, pain, swelling). Shake well to a uniform suspension before withdrawing each dose.

Pasteur/SKB: 0.6 ml of 0.4% sodium chloride. Alternately, Connaught's DTwP vaccine may be used as the diluent.

Storage/Stability: Store at 2° to 8°C (35° to 46°F). Discard frozen vaccine. Contact manufacturer regarding exposures to prolonged room temperature or elevated temperatures.

Connaught: Shipped in insulated containers.

Wyeth-Lederle: Discard if frozen. Shipped at ambient temperature.

Merck: After reconstitution, refrigerate and discard within 24 hours. Discard diluent or reconstituted vaccine if frozen. Shipped at a temperature between 2° to 8°C (35° to 46°F).

Pasteur/SKB: Shipped from the manufacturer in insulated containers with temperature monitors. Use or discard within 30 minutes after reconstitution.

Comparison of *Haemophilus* b Conjugate Vaccines

	ProHIBiT	*HibTITER*	*PedvaxHIB*	*ActHIB, OmiHIB*
Manufacturer	Connaught	Wyeth-Lederle	Merck	Connaught; Pasteur/SKB
Synonyms	PRP-D	PRP-HbOC, HbOC	PRP-OMP	PRP-T
Polysaccharide concentration	25 mcg/0.5 ml	10 mcg/0.5 ml	15 mcg/0.5 ml	10 mcg/0.5 ml
Conjugate	Diphtheria toxoid	Diphtheria CRM_{197}protein	Meningococcal outer membrane protein	Tetanus toxoid
Conjugate concentration	18 mcg/0.5 ml	25 mcg/0.5 ml	250 mcg/0.5 ml	24 mcg/0.5 ml
Dose form	Solution	Solution	Powder for suspension	Powder for solution
Packaging	0.5, 2.5 ml vials 0.5 ml syringe	0.5, 2.5, 5 ml vials	Single-dose vial plus 0.7 ml diluent vial	0.6 ml syringe of diluent; or 10 Hib vials with 7.5 ml DTwP diluent
Diluent	none	none	0.9% NaCl with 225 mcg A1OH adjuvant per 0.5 ml	0.4% NaCl or Connaught's DTwP
Standard schedule	1 dose; age 12 months to 5 yrs	4 doses: age 2, 4, 6, 15 months	3 doses: age 2, 4, 12 months	4 doses: age 2, 4, 6 and 15 to 18 mos.
Route	IM	IM	IM	IM

Recommended Administration Schedules for Conjugated *Haemophilus* Vaccines

Vaccine formulation	Age at first dose (months)	Primary series	Age sequence	Age for booster dose[1]
HbOC[2] (*HibTITER*, **Wyeth-Lederle**)	2-6	3 doses, 2 months apart	2, 4, 6 months	12 to 15 months[3]
	7-11	2 doses, 2 months apart		12 to 15 months[3]
	12-14	1 dose		15 months[3]
	15-59	1 dose		
PRP-OMP (*PedvaxHIB*, **Merck**)	2-6	2 doses, 2 m apart	2, 4 months	12 to 15 months[3]
	7-11	2 doses, 2 m apart		12 to 15 months[3]
	12-14	1 dose		15 months[3]
	15-59	1 dose		
PRP-D (*ProHIBiT*, **Connaught**)	12-59	1 dose	12-59 months	none
PRP-T[2] (*ActHIB* or *OmniHIB*, **Connaught** or **Pasteur/SKB**)	2-6	3 doses, 2 m apart	2, 4, 6 months	12 to 18 months[3]
	7-11	2 doses, 2 m apart		12 to 15 months[3]
	12-14	1 dose		15 months[3]
	15-59	1 dose		

[1]Use any of the licensed vaccines for the booster dose. For booster doses, using the product used for the first dose is generally preferred. Nonetheless, it is not necessary to give >3 doses to any child to complete the primary series.

[2]PRP-T and HbOC are also available in combination with DTwP vaccine (*ActHIB*/DTP, Connaught; *Tetramune, Wyeth*-Lederle). See the DTwP-HIB monograph for details. For Hib immunity, the same schedule described here applies; additional DTP, DT or Td doses may be needed for immunity to diphtheria, tetanus and pertussis.

[3]At least 2 months after previous dose.

Meningococcal Polysaccharide Vaccine, Groups A, C, Y, and W-135

NAME:
Menomune-A/C/Y/W-135,
🍁 *Mencevax*

MANUFACTURER:
Menomune-A/C/Y/W-135, Connaught Laboratories, 🍁 Connaught, 🍁 Pasteur Mérieux; 🍁 *Mencevax,* SmithKline Beecham

Viability: Inactivated

Antigenic Form: Capsular polysaccharide fragments

Antigenic Type: Polysaccharide mixture. The group A polysaccharide consists of a polymer of N-acetyl-O-acetyl mannosamine phosphate; the group C polysaccharide is primarily N-acetyl-O-acetylneuraminic acid. Immunogenicity is correlated with molecular weight; the group C antigen weighs >100 kilodaltons.

Use Characteristics

Indications: Induction of active immunity against select serogroups of *Neisseria meningitidis.* Populations warranting immunization include military recruits during basic training; persons with anatomic or functional asplenia (because of their increased risk of developing meningococcal disease of high severity); and travelers to countries with epidemic meningococcal disease, particularly travelers who will have prolonged contact with the local populace (eg, travelers to sub-Saharan Africa, pilgrims to the Hajj in Saudi Arabia). In addition, consider this vaccine for household or institutional contacts of persons with meningococcal disease as an adjunct to antibiotic chemotherapy, medical and laboratory personnel at risk of exposure to meningococcal disease, and immunosuppressed persons, including those with terminal-complement defects or deficiency of properdin.

Contraindications:
Absolute: None

Relative: Defer immunization during the course of any acute illness.

Elderly: No specific information is available about geriatric use of meningococcal vaccine.

Pregnancy: *Category C.* Use only if clearly needed. The manufacturer recommends that this vaccine should not be used in pregnant women, especially in the first trimester, on theoretical grounds. The use of this vaccine in a large number of pregnant women during an epidemic in Brazil apparently resulted in no adverse effects. Vaccinate pregnant women only if a substantial risk of infection exists. It is not known if meningococcal vaccine or corresponding antibodies cross the placenta. Generally, most IgG passage across the placenta occurs during the third trimester.

Lactation: It is not known if meningococcal vaccine or corresponding antibodies are excreted in breast milk. Problems in humans have not been documented.

Children: Not recommended for children >2 years of age because they are unlikely to develop an adequate antibody response. Serogroup A polysaccharide induces antibody in some children as young as 3 months of age, although a response comparable to that seen in adults is not achieved until 4 or 5 years of age.

Adverse Reactions:

Reactions to vaccination are generally mild and infrequent, consisting of localized erythema lasting 1 to 2 days. Up to 2% of young children develop a transient fever after vaccination.

Pharmacologic & Dosing Characteristics

Dosage: 0.5 ml as a single dose.

Route: SC or jet injection. Do not inject intradermally, IM or IV.

Efficacy: Groups A and C vaccines reduce disease incidence by 85% to 95%. Clinical protection from the Y and W-135 strains have not been determined directly, but immunogenicity has been demonstrated in adults and children >2 years of age.

Onset: 10 to 14 days

Duration: Antibodies against group A and C polysaccharides decline markedly over the first 3 years after vaccination. This decline is more rapid in infants and young children than in adults; in a group of children >4 years of age, efficacy declined from >90% to 67% three years after vaccination.

Drug Interactions: Like all inactivated vaccines, administration of meningococcal vaccine to persons receiving immunosuppressant drugs, including high-dose corticosteroids, or radiation therapy may result in an insufficient response to immunization. They may remain susceptible despite immunization.

Meningococcal vaccine efficacy was slightly suppressed following live measles vaccination in one study. If possible, separate these vaccines by 1 month or more for optimal responses. Hib, meningococcal and pneumococcal vaccines may safely and effectively be administered simultaneously at separate injection sites.

Pharmaceutical Characteristics

Concentration: 50 mcg of each serogroup polysaccharide per 0.5 ml

Packaging: Package of single-dose vial with 0.78 ml diluent, package of 10 dose vial with 6 ml diluent, package of 50 dose vial with 27.5 ml diluent

Dose Form: Powder for solution

Diluent for reconstitution: Sterile water for injection with thimerosal

Storage/Stability: Store at 2° to 8°C (35° to 46°F); discard if frozen. Powder can tolerate 12 weeks at 37°C (98.6°F) and for 6 to 8 weeks at 45°C (113°F). Shipping data not provided. Reconstitute gently. Use single-dose vial within 24 hours after reconstitution. Refrigerate the multidose vial after reconstitution and discard within 5 days.

Handling: Maintain jet injectors properly. Discard jet-injector vials at the end of each day.

Pneumococcal Vaccine, 23-Valent
BACTERIAL VACCINES & TOXOIDS

NAME:
Pnu-Imune-23, Pneumovax 23

MANUFACTURER:
Pnu-Imune-23, Wyeth-Lederle Vaccine & Pediatrics; *Pneumovax 23*, Merck Vaccine Division, ♦ Merck Frosst

Comparison: Generically equivalent

Viability: Inactivated

Antigenic Form: Capsular polysaccharide fragments

Antigenic Type: Polysaccharide mixture

Use Characteristics

Indications: Induction of active immunity against pneumococcal disease caused by those pneumococcal types included in the vaccine. Vaccination offers protection against pneumococcal pneumonia, pneumococcal bacteremia and other pneumococcal infections.

Adults: Vaccinate all adults ≥65 years of age, emphasizing immunization of the older adult while still in good health. Vaccinate all immunocompetent adults who are at increased risk of pneumococcal disease or its complications because of chronic illnesses (eg, cardiovascular or pulmonary disease, impaired hepatic or renal systems, diabetes mellitus, alcoholism, cirrhosis, chronic cerebrospinal fluid leaks). Consider vaccinating persons ≥50 years of age. Refer to the tables of pertinent diagnoses and related indicator medications. Vaccinate immunocompromised adults at increased risk of pneumococcal disease or its complications (eg, splenic dysfunction or anatomic asplenia, sickle-cell anemia and other severe hemoglobinopathies, Hodgkin's disease, lymphoma, multiple myeloma, chronic renal failure, nephrotic syndrome, conditions such as organ transplantation associated with immunosuppression).

Children: Vaccinate children ≥2 years of age with chronic illness specifically associated with increased risk of pneumococcal disease or its complications (eg, splenic dysfunction or anatomic asplenia, sickle-cell disease, nephrotic syndrome, cerebrospinal fluid leaks). Pneumococcal immunization is specifically recommended for children ≥2 years of age with renal failure, diabetes or severe immunosuppression.

Members of Closed Groups: Pneumococcal vaccination is also indicated for adults or children living in closed groups (eg, residential schools, nursing homes, other institutions), to decrease the likelihood of acute outbreaks of pneumococcal disease where there is increased risk that the disease may be severe.

Contraindications:
Absolute: Patients with a history of any type of neurological symptom or sign following administration of this product.

Relative: Consider during a febrile respiratory illness or active infection. Do

57

not vaccinate patients <2 years of age, since they are unlikely to respond to the vaccine.

Elderly: Immune response in the elderly is generally good, although immunosuppressed elderly may exhibit an impaired response. The elderly may exhibit a lower IgM antibody response. Published data support giving pneumococcal vaccine to the "young elderly," before advancing age impairs immune response to vaccines such as this one.

Pregnancy: *Category C.* Use not recommended unless substantial risk exists. It is not known if pneumococcal vaccine or corresponding antibodies cross the placenta. Generally, most IgG passage across the placenta occurs during the third trimester.

Lactation: It is not known if pneumococcal vaccine or corresponding antibodies are excreted in breast milk. Problems in humans have not been documented.

Children: Children <2 years of age respond poorly to most capsular types. Children <5years of age may not respond to some antigens. Nonetheless, children >2 years of age with anatomical or functional asplenia and otherwise intact lymphoid function generally respond to pneumococcal vaccines with a serological conversion comparable to that observed in healthy individuals of the same age.

Adverse Reactions:
Local erythema and soreness at the injection site, usually shorter than 48 hours in duration, occur commonly. Local induration occurs less commonly. Rash, arthralgia, adenitis, fever >39°C (102°F), malaise, myalgia and asthenia occur rarely. Low-grade fever (<38.3°C; 100.9°F) occurs occasionally and usually subsides within 24 hours.

Patients with otherwise stabilized immune thrombocytopenic purpura have, on rare occasions, experienced a relapse in their thrombocytopenia, occurring 2 to 14 days after vaccination and lasting up to 2 weeks.

Systemic reactions of greater severity, duration or extent are unusual, although anaphylactoid reactions have been reported. Neurological disorders such as paresthesias and acute radiculoneuropathy, including Guillain-Barré syndrome, have occurred rarely in temporal association with administration of pneumococcal vaccine, but no cause-and-effect relationship has been established.

Patients who have had episodes of pneumococcal pneumonia or other pneumococcal infection may have high levels of preexisting pneumococcal antibodies to certain types that may result in increased reactions to pneumococcal vaccine, usually localized to the injection site, but occasionally systemic.

Pharmacologic & Dosing Characteristics

Dosage: 0.5 ml. When elective splenectomy is considered or when cancer chemotherapy or other immunosuppression is planned, give pneumococcal vaccine at least 2 weeks before surgery or immunosuppression, if possible. Following unplanned splenectomy, vaccinate after the immediate postoperative period.

Route & Site: SC or IM injection, preferably in the deltoid muscle or lateral mid-thigh. Severe reactions may follow intradermal (ID) or IV administration; do not use these routes.

Efficacy: Vaccination will reduce disease incidence by 60% to 80%. Strains represented in the 23-valent vaccine account for 90% of pneumococcal blood isolates and 85% of isolates from other normally sterile sites.

Seroconversion: More than 90% of healthy adults, including the elderly, demonstrate at least a 2-fold rise in type-specific geometric mean antibody titers within 2 to 3 weeks after immunization. Similar antibody responses occurred in patients with alcoholic cirrhosis and diabetes mellitus. In elderly individuals with chronic pulmonary disease and immunocompromised patients, the response to immunization may be lower.

Clinical Protection: In Austria's 1976 report of a 13-valent pneumococcal vaccine, pneumonias caused by the capsular types present in the vaccine were reduced by 79%. Reduction in type-specific pneumococcal bacteremia was 82%. Case-control studies usually show the vaccine to be efficacious, with point-estimates of efficacy (reduction in disease incidence) of 60% to 70% prospective. A prospective French study found pneumococcal vaccine 77% effective in reducing the incidence of pneumonia among nursing-home residents (Gaillat et al, 1985).

Onset: 14 days to 3 weeks

Duration: Protective antibody persists for ≥5 years in most recipients.

Drug Interactions: In patients anticipating immunosuppression, response to pneumococcal vaccine is best if administered 10 to 14 days prior to immunosuppressive chemo-therapy or radiation. Like all inactivated vaccines, administration of pneumo-coccal vac-

cine to persons receiving immunosuppressant drugs, including high-dose corticosteroids, or radiation therapy may result in an insufficient response to immunization. They may remain susceptible despite immunization.

Pneumococcal and influenza vaccines may safely and effectively be administered simultaneously at separate injection sites. While influenza vaccine is given annually, pneumococcal vaccine is given only once to all but those at highest risk of fatal pneumococcal disease. Hib, meningococcal and pneumococcal vaccines may safely and effectively be administered simultaneously at separate injection sites.

In a study of six patients, pneumococcal vaccine had no effect on the pharmacokinetics of theophylline (Cupit et al, 1988).

As with other drugs administered by IM injection, give pneumococcal vaccine with caution to persons receiving anticoagulant therapy.

Pharmaceutical Characteristics

Concentration: 25 mcg each of 23 polysaccharides per 0.5 ml

Packaging:

Wyeth-Lederle: Five 0.5 ml *Lederject* disposable single-dose syringes with 25 gauge, $\frac{5}{8}$ inch needle, 2.5 ml 5 dose vial

Merck: 2.5 ml 5 dose vial, box of five 0.5 ml single-dose vials, package of 1000 0.5 ml vials, package of 100 0.5 ml vials

Dose Form: Solution

Solvent: 0.9% sodium chloride

Storage/Stability: Store at 2° to 8°C (35° to 46°F). Do not freeze.

Wyeth-Lederle: Product can tolerate several days at room temperature. Discard frozen vaccine. Contact manufacturer regarding prolonged exposure to elevated temperatures. Shipped in insulated containers with coolant packs.

Merck: Product can tolerate 1 month at room temperature. Shipped in insulated containers with coolant packs.

Typhoid Vaccine (Parenteral)
BACTERIAL VACCINES & TOXOIDS

NAME:
Generic, *Typhim Vi*

Manufacturer:
Generic Typhoid Vaccine (Heat- & Phenol-Inactivated), Wyeth-Ayerst Laboratories; Generic Typhoid Vaccine (Acetone-Inactivated, Dried), Wyeth-Ayerst Laboratories; *Typhim Vi*, Typhoid Vi Capsular Polysaccharide Vaccine, Connaught Laboratories, ❧ Connaught.

Synonyms: The acetone-inactivated vaccine is known as the acetone-killed and dried (AKD) formulation. The heat- and phenol-inactivated form is abbreviated in this monograph as H-P. Typhoid Vi capsular polysaccharide vaccine may be abbreviated ViCPs. Typhoid fever is also known as enteric fever and typhus abdominalis.

Comparison: AKD and H-P vaccines are commonly considered generically equivalent, although the H-P vaccine may contain little of the important Vi antigen, which may reduce protective efficacy of the H-P vaccine. Efficacy of the AKD vaccine varies from 75% to 94%; efficacy of the H-P vaccine varies from 61% to 77% over 2.5 to 3 years.

Viability: Inactivated

Antigenic Form: Whole bacterium

Antigenic Type: *AKD & H-P*: Protein and polysaccharide Q. H-P vaccines contain the O and, to a lesser extent, Vi antigens. AKD vaccines contain the O and Vi antigens and, to a lesser extent, the H antigen.

Vi: Vi polysaccharide only.

AKD & H-P parenteral vaccines are inequivalent to the Vi polysaccharide vaccine and live, attenuated typhoid vaccine for oral administration. The Vi polysaccharide vaccine reduces disease incidence by 49% to 87%, whereas the capsules reduce disease by 60% to 77%.

Although each typhoid vaccine induces comparable immunity, the vaccines vary considerably in the side effects they induce. The AKD vaccine causes the most cases of pain at the injection site, while the oral vaccine causes the fewest adverse effects. Direct comparisons of various typhoid vaccines have not yet been performed.

Use Characteristics

◎ Indications: For induction of active immunity against typhoid fever. The vaccine regimen should be completed 2 weeks before potential exposure to typhoid bacteria. Persons at greatest risk include:

—travelers to endemic areas (especially Africa, Asia and South and Central America), especially if prolonged exposure to potentially contaminated food and water is likely

—people with intimate exposure (eg, prolonged household contact) to a known typhoid carrier

—laboratory personnel who work frequently with *Salmonella typhi*

For specific locations, consult specialty references or call one of the CDC's travel hotlines.

Contraindications:

STOP *Absolute*: A previous severe systemic or allergic reaction is a contraindication to future use. Do not vaccinate a person with typhoid fever or a chronic typhoid carrier.

Relative: Defer administration in the presence of acute respiratory or other active infection, or intensive physical activity (particularly when environmental temperatures are high).

Elderly: No specific information is available about geriatric use of typhoid vaccine.

Pregnancy: *Category C*. Specific information about use of typhoid vaccine during pregnancy is not available. Parenteral vaccination is not specifically contraindicated. Nonetheless, use typhoid vaccine only if clearly needed: If disease risk exceeds vaccination risks. It is not known if typhoid vaccine or corresponding antibodies cross the placenta. Generally, most IgG passage across the placenta occurs during the third trimester.

Lactation: It is not known if typhoid vaccine or corresponding antibodies cross into human breast milk. Problems in humans have not been documented.

Children: *AKD & H-P*: Reduce dosage volume to 0.25 ml for children <10 years of age. These vaccines are known to be effective in children as young as 6 months of age.

Vi: Vi vaccine is not recommended for children <2 years of age, because no safety or efficacy data are available for that age group.

Adverse Reactions: *AKD & H-P*: Local and systemic reactions may follow typhoid vaccination, usually beginning within 6 to 24 hours of administration and persisting 1 or 2 days. Local reactions, occurring in 50% to 80% of recipients, include erythema, induration and tenderness (6% to 40%). Expect these reactions when the vaccine is injected ID. Systemic manifestations may include malaise, headache (9% to 30%), myalgia and elevated temperature (14% to 29%). Hypotension has been reported rarely. Reactogenicity does not differ significantly for typhoid vaccines prepared using the AKD or H-P methods. Local reaction rates increase if vaccine is administered by jet injector.

Vi: Most adverse reactions to Vi polysaccharide are minor and transient local reactions. Local reactions may include erythema (4% to 11%) or induration (5% to 18%) at the injection site. Many recipients experience pain (26% to 56%) or tenderness (>93%) at the site. These almost always resolve within 48 hours. Systemic effects may include fever $\geq 37.8^{\circ}C$ ($\geq 100^{\circ}F$; 0% to 2%), malaise (4% to 37%), myalgia (2% to 7%), nausea (2% to 8%) or headache (11% to 27%). Rarely, lymphadenopathy, cervical pain, vomiting, diarrhea, abdominal pain, tremor, hypotension, loss of consciousness, allergic reactions including urticaria and other events have been reported. Since Vi vaccine contains negligible amounts of bacterial lipopolysaccharide, it produces reactions less than half as frequently as H-P or AKD vaccines. No statistically significant difference in reaction rates were seen between first and subsequent doses of Vi polysaccharide.

Pharmacologic & Dosing Characteristics

Dosage:
AKD & H-P: For adults and children >10 years of age: Two 0.5 ml doses SC ≥4 weeks apart.

For children <10 years of age: Two 0.25 ml doses SC ≥4 weeks apart. Shake vial vigorously before withdrawing each dose. In urgent situations, 3 doses of the appropriate volume have been given at weekly intervals although efficacy may be reduced.

Vi: A single 25-mcg dose in 0.5 ml.

Route & Site: *AKD & H-P:* Administer either AKD or H-P vaccine SC. Only H-P vaccine may be given ID and only for booster doses. Do not administer AKD vaccine ID because of a high frequency of local reactions. The AKD vaccine can be given by jet injection. Vials of HP vaccine are not compatible with jet injectors.

Vi: IM. Inject adults in the deltoid muscle. Inject children in either the deltoid or vastus lateralis. Do not inject in the gluteal area or where there may be a nerve trunk. There are no published data on safety and efficacy with administration by jet injection.

Efficacy: *AKD & H-P:* Complete immunization with the H-P vaccine reduces disease incidence by about 70%, depending on degree of exposure. The AKD vaccine is 70% to 90% effective in preventing typhoid fever, depending on degree of exposure. Food and water discipline are the most important measures to avoid disease, even for vaccine recipients. Efficacy of the AKD vaccine varies from 75% to 94%; efficacy of the H-P vaccine varies from 61% to 77% over 2 1/2 to 3 years.

Vi: A 25 mcg dose produced a fourfold rise in antibody titers in 88% to 96% of healthy American adults. The Vi polysaccharide vaccine reduced disease incidence by 49% to 87% in a trial among adults and children in Nepal. In a pediatric study in South Africa, blood culture-confirmed cases of typhoid fever were reduced 61%, 52% and 50% in the first, second and third years, respectively, after a single dose of Vi polysaccharide vaccine.

Onset: *AKD & H-P:* Protective antibody titers presumably develop within 1 to 2 weeks after the second dose.

Vi: Protective antibody titers develop within 2 weeks after a single dose.

Duration: *AKD & H-P:* >2 years

Vi: ≈2 years

Drug Interactions: Like all inactivated vaccines, administration of typhoid vaccine to persons receiving immunosuppressant drugs, including high-dose corticosteroids, or radiation therapy may result in an insufficient response to immunization. They may remain susceptible despite immunization.

Avoid concurrent administration with other reactogenic parenteral vaccines (eg, cholera, plague) if possible, to avoid the theoretical risk of additive adverse effects.

Concomitant therapy with phenytoin may decrease antibody response to SC typhoid vaccination. Anticipate the possibility of suboptimal antibody response and consider risk/benefit ratios for each drug. Counsel these persons especially to observe good food and water discipline.

Vi: As with other drugs administered by IM injection, give Vi polysaccharide vaccine with caution to persons receiving anticoagulant therapy.

Patient information: Advise vaccine recipients to take standard food and water precautions to avoid typhoid fever. Vaccine protection can be overwhelmed by swallowing a large dose of typhoid bacteria.

Pharmaceutical Characteristics

Concentration:

AKD & H-P: 8 units per ml; not >1 billion organisms per ml. *H-P*: Not >35 mcg nitrogen per ml. *AKD*: Not >23 mcg nitrogen per ml. *Vi*: 25 mcg of purified Vi polysaccharide per 0.5 ml.

Packaging: H-P and Vi vaccines are sold to civilian and military customers. AKD vaccine is available to military forces only.

H-P: 5 ml multidose vial, 10 ml multidose vial, 20 ml multidose vial

AKD: 50-dose multidose vial with 20 ml diluent

Vi: 0.5 ml single-use syringe with needle length of $5/8$ inch and gauge of 25. Vials are available on a special contract basis: 20 dose per 10 ml vial, 50 dose per 25 ml vial.

Dose Form:

H-P: Suspension

AKD: Powder for suspension

Vi: Solution

Solvent: *H-P*: Sodium phosphate-buffer 0.02 molar in 0.9% sodium chloride

Vi: Isotonic phosphate-buffered saline

Diluent for reconstitution: *AKD* Sodium-phosphate buffer 0.02 molar in 0.9% sodium chloride

Storage/Stability: *AKD & H-P*: Store at $2°$ to $8°$C ($35°$ to $46°$F). Do not freeze. Both AKD and H-P vaccine can tolerate 14 days at room temperature or 10 days at $46°$C ($114°$F). Contact the manufacturer regarding exposure to freezing temperatures. Shipped at ambient temperatures. Discard AKD vaccine 30 days after reconstitution.

Vi: Store at $2°$ to $8°$C ($35°$ to $46°$F). Discard frozen vaccine. Contact the manufacturer regarding exposure to freezing (extreme) temperatures. Shipped in insulated containers with coolant packs.

Typhoid Vaccine (Oral)
BACTERIAL VACCINES & TOXOIDS

NAME:

Typhoid Vaccine, Live, Oral, Ty2la Capsules, *Vivotif Berna*

Synonyms: Ty2la. Typhoid fever is also known as enteric fever and typhus abdominalis.

Comparison: AKD & H-P parenteral vaccines are inequivalent to the Vi polysaccharide vaccine and live, attenuated typhoid vaccine for oral administration. The Vi polysaccharide vaccine reduces disease incidence by 49% to 87%, while the capsules reduce disease by 60% to 77%.

Viability: Live, attenuated bacteria, plus nonviable cells

Antigenic Form: Whole bacterium

MANUFACTURER:

Manufactured by Swiss Serum and Vaccine Institute, distributed in US by Berna Products

Although each typhoid vaccine induces comparable immunity, the vaccines vary considerably in the side effects they induce. The AKD vaccine causes the most cases of pain at the injection site, while the oral vaccine causes the fewest adverse effects. Direct comparisons of various typhoid vaccines have not yet been performed.

Antigenic Type: Protein and polysaccharide

Use Characteristics

 Indications: Induction of active immunity against typhoid fever. Persons at greatest risk include:

—Travelers to endemic areas (especially Latin America, Asia and Africa);

—People with intimate exposure (eg, household contact) to a known typhoid carrier;

—Laboratory personnel who work frequently with *Salmonella typhi*.

For specific location, consult specialty references, the Disease Epidemiology section in the Typhoid Fever monograph, or call one of CDC's travel hotlines.

Contraindications:

Absolute: Patients with a history

of hypersensitivity to any component of the vaccine or the capsule. Do not vaccinate a person with typhoid fever or a chronic typhoid carrier.

Relative: Do not give typhoid vaccine capsules during an acute febrile illness or during an acute GI illness (eg, persistent diarrhea, vomiting).

Elderly: No specific information is available about geriatric use of typhoid vaccine capsules.

Pregnancy: *Category* C. Use only if clearly needed. It is not known if attenuated typhoid vaccine or corresponding antibodies cross the placenta. Generally, most IgG passage across the placenta occurs during the third trimester. Consider using parenteral inactivated typhoid vaccine in pregnant women at risk of typhoid fever.

Lactation: It is not known if attenuated typhoid vaccine or corresponding antibodies cross into breast milk. Problems in humans have not been documented.

Children: Typhoid vaccine capsules are not recommended for children <6 years of age, since no safety or efficacy data are available for that age group.

 Adverse Reactions: Nausea, abdominal cramps, diarrhea, vomiting, skin rash or urticaria on trunk or extremities may occur, although they are generally self-resolving. At five times the recommended dose, no significant reactions were noted. Bacteria are not shed in feces at the normal dose, but overdosages increase the possibility of shedding.

Pharmacologic & Dosing Characteristics

Dosage: 1 capsule orally every other day on days 1, 3, 5 and 7. Swallow each capsule whole, 1 hour before meals, with cold or luke-warm water (not to exceed body temperature). Do not chew capsules. Swallow as soon as possible after placing in mouth. Encourage compliance with complete regimen.

Route: Oral

Efficacy: Vaccination reduces disease incidence by 60% to 70%. Counsel vaccinated travelers to take all necessary precautions to avoid contact or ingestion of potentially contaminated food or water. Ty2la trials were conducted in Alexandria, Egypt; Santiago, Chile; and Plaju, Indonesia.

Onset: Finish the fourth capsule at least 1 week before travel.

Duration: Approximately 5 years

Drug Interactions: Like all live bacterial vaccines, administration to patients receiving immunosuppressant drugs, including steroids, or radiation may predispose patients to disseminated infections or insufficient response to immunization. They may remain susceptible despite immunization. Sulfonamides and other antibiotics (eg, amoxicillin, chloramphenicol, ciprofloxacin) may be active against the Ty2la oral vaccine strain and reduce vaccine efficacy. Therefore, give the vaccine capsules at least 24 hours before or after the antibiotic.

If indicated, give mefloquine (*Lariam*) tablets at least 24 hours before or after the vaccine. Chloroquine can be taken simultaneously with the vaccine. Immune globulin (eg, IGIM) and other live vaccines (eg, yellow fever) can be taken simultaneously with this vaccine without loss of antibody response.

Concomitant therapy with phenytoin may decrease antibody response to parenteral typhoid vaccination, although no effect on oral vaccination has been reported. Anticipate suboptimal antibody response and consider risk/benefit ratios for each drug. Counsel these persons to especially observe good food and water discipline.

No evidence of interaction between simultaneous administration of live virus vaccines (eg, MMR, OPV, yellow fever vaccines) and oral live typhoid (Ty2la) vaccine has been documented. If both drugs are needed (eg, prior to international travel), both vaccines may be administered simultaneously or at any interval between each other.

Pharmaceutical Characteristics

Patient Information: Advise vaccine recipients to take standard food and water precautions to avoid typhoid fever.

Concentration: 2 to 6 x 10^9 CFU of viable *Salmonella typhi* organisms per capsule, plus 5 to 50 x 10^9 nonviable bacterial cells

Packaging: Unit-dose blister package of 4 capsules

Dose Form: Enteric-coated oral capsules

Storage/Stability: Store at 2° to 8°C (35° to 46°F) prior to use and between doses. If frozen, thaw the capsules before administration. Product can tolerate 48 hours at 25°C (77°F). Shipped at 2° to 8°C (36° to 46°F).

Comparison of Typhoid Vaccines

	H-P Vaccine	AKD Vaccine	ViCPs Vaccine	Oral Vaccine
Proprietary name	generic	generic	*Typhim Vi*	*Vivotif Berna*
Manufacturer	Wyeth-Lederle	Wyeth-Lederle	Connaught Laboratories	Berna Products
Strain	Ty-2	Ty-2	Ty-2	Ty21a
Process	heat- and phenol-inactivated bacteria	acetone-inactivated bacteria	precipitation with hexadecyltrimeth-ylammonium	bacteria attenuated
Concentration	8 units/ml, ≤1 billion organisms/ml	8 units/ml, ≤1 billion organisms/ml	25 mcg/0.5 ml	2 to 6 billion CFU/capsule
Packaging	5, 10, 20 ml vials	50 dose vial for 20 ml	0.5 ml syringe, 20- and 50-dose vials	blister package of 4 capsules
Dose Form	suspension	powder for suspension	solution	oral capsule
Standard Schedule	2 doses at least 4 weeks apart: 0.5 ml each for people ≥10 years of age; 0.25 ml if <10 years of age	2 doses at least 4 weeks apart: 0.5 ml each for people ≥10 years of age; 0.25 ml if <10 years of age	one 0.5 ml dose	one capsule every other day for 4 doses
Boosters	one dose every 3 years	one dose every 3 years	one dose every 2 years	4 capsules every 5 years
Route of adminstration	SC, intradermal (booster doses only)	SC, jet	IM	oral
Side effect rates	Local reactions: 50% to 80%	Local reactions: 50% to 80%	Local reactions: 4% to 18%	GI symptoms rarely

Viral Vaccines

Hepatitis A Vaccine (HAV)

Hepatitis B Vaccine (HBV)

Influenza Virus Vaccine, Trivalent,
  Types A & B

Measles, Mumps & Rubella Virus
  Vaccine Live

Measles & Rubella Virus Vaccine Live

Mumps & Rubella Virus Vaccine Live

Measles Virus Vaccine Live

Mumps Virus Vaccine Live

Rubella Virus Vaccine Live

Poliovirus Vaccine Inactivated

Poliovirus Vaccine Live Oral Trivalent

Rabies Vaccine

Vaccinia (Smallpox) Vaccine, Dried,
  Calf-lymph Type

Varicella Virus Vaccine Live

Yellow Fever Vaccine

Hepatitis A Vaccine (HAV)
VIRAL VACCINES

NAME:
Havrix, Vaqta

MANUFACTURER:
Havrix, Manufactured by Smith-Kline Beecham Biologicals, Rixensart, Belgium, distributed by SmithKline Beecham Pharmaceuticals; Vaqta, Merck Vaccine Division

Synonyms: HAV. The disease is also known as infectious hepatitis, epidemic jaundice and catarrhal jaundice.

Comparison: Hepatitis A vaccine is considered more effective than IGIM in reducing the frequency and severity of hepatitis A infection. Hepatitis A vaccine provides more persistent protection, although induction of protective antibody levels may be delayed

several days after that which can be obtained with IGIM.

Havrix and *Vaqta* are comparably safe and effective. They can be considered prophylactically equivalent, although their potencies are measured in differing systems, using units with different bases. No data about using one brand to boost initial immunity from the other brand is available.

Viability: Inactivated

Antigenic Form: Lysed whole viruses

Antigenic Type: Protein

Use Characteristics

Indications: For induction of active immunity against infection caused by hepatitis A virus. The quality of antibodies induced by hepatitis A vaccine is indistinguishable from that found in human immune globulin products by in vitro assays. The quantity of antibodies induced by immunization is considerably higher than that induced after a standard dose of IGIM or clinical infection. Persons who are or will be at increased risk of infection or transmission of hepatitis A virus include:

Travelers: Persons traveling to areas of higher endemicity for hepatitis A, such as Africa, Asia (except Japan), the Mediterranean basin, eastern Europe, the Middle East, Central and South

America, Mexico and parts of the Caribbean. Consult specialty references for exact locations, or call one of CDC's travel hotlines. Hepatitis A prophylaxis is not needed by travelers to Australia, Canada, Japan, New Zealand and countries in Western Europe and Scandinavia.

Military personnel.

People living in, or relocating to, areas of high endemicity (eg, missionaries, diplomats, engineers).

Certain ethnic or geographical populations that experience cyclic hepatitis A epidemics: Native peoples of Alaska, the Americas and the Pacific Islands.

Other persons: Persons engaging in high-risk sexual activity (such as homosexually active males); users of illicit injectable drugs; residents of a community experiencing an outbreak of hepatitis A; persons with chronic liver disease.

Although the epidemiology of hepatitis A does not permit the identification of other specific populations at high risk of disease, outbreaks of hepatitis A or exposure to hepatitis A virus have been described in a variety of populations in which hepatitis A vaccine may be useful: Certain institutional workers (eg, caretakers for the developmentally challenged), employees of child day-care centers, laboratory workers who handle live hepatitis A virus or handlers of primate animals that may be harboring hepatitis A virus.

People exposed to hepatitis A through household and sexual contacts with persons having hepatitis A infection. For those desiring both immediate and long-term protection, hepatitis A vaccine may be administered concomitantly with IGIM.

Unlabeled Uses: The value of vaccination for people described below is less clear:

Other people for whom hepatitis A is an occupational hazard: Individuals in frequent contact with human fecal matter as a result of their occupationally related activities (eg, sewage workers, certain hospital workers such as neonatal ICU workers).

Other people who, if infected, could transmit the disease to others: Food handlers, children in day-care settings.

Other people at risk of hepatitis A: Carriers of hepatitis B virus (in whom the morbidity of hepatitis A would be increased). Patients with hemophilia A or B receiving plasma-derived clotting factors (the solvent-detergent production method does not reliably inactivate hepatitis A virus, a non-enveloped virus).

Contraindications:
Absolute: Persons with known hypersensitivity to any component of the vaccine. Persons who experience hypersensitivity reactions to hepatitis A vaccine should not receive further injections.

Relative: Defer administration of hepatitis A vaccine, if possible, in people with any febrile illness or active infection. Administer with caution to people with thrombocytopenia or a bleeding disorder, as bleeding may occur following an IM injection.

Elderly: No specific information is available about geriatric use of hepatitis A vaccine. Persons born prior to 1945 are more likely to already be immune to disease, but those who are infected later in life will have greater morbidity and mortality.

Adults: *SKB:* In three clinical studies of >400 adults given a single 1440 ELu dose of hepatitis A vaccine, specific anti-HAV antibodies developed in >96% of subjects when measured 1 month after vaccination. By day 15, 80% to 98% of vaccinees had already seroconverted (defined as anti-HAV ≥20 mIU/ml). GMTs among seroconverters varied from 264 to 339 mIU/ml at day 15 and increased to 335 to 637 mIU/ml by 1 month after immunization.

Merck: In clinical trials, 98% of adults seroconverted at 24 weeks after an ≈50 u dose, with a GMT of 134 mIU/ml. They were then given an ≈50 u booster dose. Four weeks later, 100% of adults had seroconverted, with a GMT of 6010 mIU/ml.

Pregnancy: *Category C.* Use only if clearly needed. It is not known if hepatitis A vaccine or corresponding antibodies cross the placenta. Generally, most IgG passage across the placenta occurs during the third trimester. Problems in pregnant women have not been documented and are unlikely.

Lactation: It is not known if hepatitis A vaccine or corresponding antibodies cross into human breast milk. Problems in humans have not been documented and are unlikely.

Children: Safety and efficacy in children <2 years of age have not been established. Hepatitis A antibodies in infants that were contributed from the mother's circulation may interfere with the immune response to hepatitis A immunization. These children appear to be immunologically primed for future viral exposures, but the antibody titers they achieve are lower than those of children without circulating maternal antibodies.

SKB: In six clinical trials around the world, involving 762 children ranging from 1 to 18 years of age, the GMT following two 360 ELu doses of hepatitis A vaccine given 1 month apart ranged from 197 to 660 mIU/ml. Seroconversion occurred in 99% of subjects after the second dose. When the second dose was administered 6 months after the first, all subjects were seropositive at month 7, with GMTs ranging from 3388 mIU/ml to 4643 mIU/ml. In one study in which children were followed for 6 more months, all subjects remained seropositive.

Merck: In clinical trials, 97% of children and adolescents seroconverted at 24 weeks after an ≈25 u dose, with a GMT of 109 mIU/ml. They were then given an ≈25 u booster dose. Four weeks later, 100% of them had seroconverted, with a GMT of 10,609 mIU/ml. Another group showed 91% seroconversion, with a GMT of 48 mIU/ml, when they received a booster dose 52 weeks after initial vaccination. Four weeks later, 100% had seroconverted, with a GMT of 12,308 mIU/ml. A third group showed 90% seroconversion, with a GMT of 50 mIU/ml, when they received a booster dose 78 weeks after initial vaccination. Four weeks later, 100% had seroconverted, with a GMT of 9591 mIU/ml.

Adverse Reactions:

SKB: Generally well tolerated during clinical trials involving >26,000 subjects receiving doses from 360 to 1440 ELu. The frequency of solicited adverse events tends to decrease with successive doses of vaccine. Most events reported were rated by subjects as mild and did not last >24 hours. The most frequent reaction reported was injection-site soreness (56% of adults and 15% of children; <0.5% of soreness was reported as severe). Headache was reported by 14% of adults and <5% of children.

Incidence 1% to 10% of Injections: Induration, redness or swelling of the injection site; fatigue, fever (>37.5°C) or malaise, anorexia or nausea.

Incidence <1% of Injections: Hematoma at injection site; pruritus, rash or urticaria; pharyngitis or other upper respiratory tract symptoms; abdominal pain, diarrhea, dysgeusia or vomiting; arthralgia, elevated creatinine phosphokinase or myalgia; lymphadenopathy; hypertonic episode, insomnia, photophobia or vertigo.

While no causal relationship has been established, spontaneous voluntary reports of adverse events include localized edema, anaphylaxis or anaphylactoid reactions, somnolence, syncope, jaundice, hepatitis, erythema multiforme, Guillain-Barré syndrome, hyperhydrosis, angioedema, dyspnea, convulsions, transient encephalopathy, dizziness, neuropathy, myelitis, paresthesia, multiple sclerosis, and a report of a child born with a deformed ear to a mother vaccinated during pregnancy.

Merck: In combined clinical trials, 16,252 doses were given to 9181 healthy children, adolescents and adults. No serious vaccine-related adverse experiences were observed during clinical trials. In the Monroe Efficacy Study, subjects were observed for 5 days for fever and local complaints and for 14 days for systemic complaints. Injection-site complaints, generally mild and transient, were the most frequently reported complaints. There were no significant differences in the rates of any complaints between vaccine and placebo recipients.

Among children and adolscents in all studies, these are the events reported (≥1%), without regard to causality: Pain (18.7%), tenderness (16.8%), warmth (8.6%), erythema (7.5%), swelling (7.3%), fever (≥102°F, oral) (3.1%), headache (2.3%), abdominal pain (1.6%), pharyngitis (1.5%), ecchymosis (1.3%), upper respiratory infection (1.1%), cough (1%), diarrhea (1%) and vomiting (1%). Very few laboratory abnormalties were reported and included isolated reports of elevated liver function tests, eosinophilia and increased urine protein.

Among adults in all studies, these are the events preported (1%), without regard to causality: Tenderness (52.6%,

generally mild and transient), pain (51.1%), warmth (17.3%), headache (16.1%), swelling (13.6%), erythema (12.9%), asthenia/fatigue (3.9%), upper respiratory infection (2.8%), pharyngitis (2.7%), fever (101°F, oral) (2.6%), diarrhea (2.4%), nausea (2.3%), myalgia (2%), ecchymosis (1.5%), abdominal pain (1.3%), arm pain (1.3%), pain/soreness (1.2%), back pain (1.1%), nasal congestion (1.1%), menstruation disorder (1.1%) and stiffness (1%).

Local or systemic allergic reactions that occured in <1% of children, adolescents or adults in clinical trials, regardless of causality included injection site pruritus or rash, bronchial constriction, asthma, wheezing, edema/swelling, rash, generalized erythema, urticaria, pruritus, eye irritation/itching and dermatitis.

Pharmacologic & Dosing Characteristics

 Dosage: Shake product well before withdrawing a dose.

SKB Adult: 1440 ELu on day 0. In Europe, other schedules have been used, including 720 ELu on days 0 and 30. Most countries have now adopted the single 1440 ELu dose. A single 1440 ELu/1 ml booster dose is recommended 6 to 12 months later, if persistent antibody titers are desired. A 1 inch to 1$^{1}/_{2}$ inch needle is recommended.

Pediatric: For children 2 to 18 years of age, give one dose of 720 ELu. The initial recommendation was to give 360 ELu on days 0 and 30. A single booster dose of 720 ELu is recommended 6 to 12 months later, if persistent antibody titers are desired. Children started on the 360 ELu dose should complete a 3-dose series at that dose.

Merck: Adult: 50 u on day 0. A single 50 u/1 ml booster dose is rocmmended 6 months later, if persistent antibody titers are desired.

Pediatric: 25 u on day 0. A single 25 u/0.5 ml booster dose is recommended 6 to 18 months later, if persistent antibody titers are desired. A $^7/_8$ inch to 1 inch needle is recommended.

Route & Site: IM. In adults, inject the deltoid region. Do not inject into the gluteal region, to avoid a suboptimal immune response. Do not inject IV, ID or SC. Jet injection induces higher antibody responses for the first 8 months after immunization; immune responses are similar to IM adminis-tration thereafter (Hoke et al, 1992). Sore arms occasionally occur from jet injection.

Efficacy: *SKB:* In an efficacy trial of 40,119 children at high risk of hepatitis A infection, 41 cases of clinical hepati-tis A occurred in the control group, compared with two markedly attenu-ated cases in the vaccinated group. The calculated rate of disease prevention was 94% (95% CI: 81% to 98%). A 96% efficacy rate for protection against inapparent or subclinical infection was observed. In outbreak investiga-tions during the study, protection against hepatitis A infection, both symptomatic and asymptomatic cases, was 97%.

Merck: In combined clinical studies, 97% of 1214 healthy children and ado-lescents 2 to 17 years of age serocon-verted with a GMT of 43 mIU/ml within 4 weeks after a single ≈25 u/0.5 ml IM dose. Similarly, 95% of 1428 aldults ≥18 years of age seroconverted with a GMT of 37 mIU/ml within 4 weeks after a single ≈50 u/1 ml IM dose. Two weeks after a single dose, 69%

(n=744) of adults seroconverted with a GMT of 16 mIU/ml. Immune memory was demonstrated by an anamnestic antibody response in people who received a booster dose.

A very high degree of protection was shown after a single dose in children and adolescents. In a randomized, double-blind, placebo controlled study invoving 1037 susceptible healthy children and adolescents 2 to 16 years of age in a US community with recur-rent outbreaks of hepatitis A (the Monroe Efficacy Study), each child received an IM dose (≈ 25 u) or place-bo. The protective efficacy of a single dose of vaccine was 100%, with 21 cases of hepatitis A in the placebo group and none in the vaccine group (p <0.001). No cases of confirmed hepatitis A occured in the vaccine group after day 16.

Onset: Protective antibody titers develop within 15 to 30 days after immunization. By day 15, 80% to 98% of vaccinees seroconverted (anti-HAV ≥20 mIU/ml, the lower limit of the antibody assay).

Duration: *SKB:* In 89 vaccinees, a single 1440 ELu dose of hepatitis A vaccine elicited anti-HAV neutralizing anti-bodies in >94% of vaccinees when measured 1 month after vaccination. These antibodies persisted through at least 6 months. After a second dose given at month 6, 100% of vaccinees had neutralizing antibodies when measured at month 7.

In two clinical trials in which a boost-er dose of 1440 ELu was given 6 months after the initial dose, 100% of vaccinees (n =269) were seropositive 1 month after the booster dose, with GMTs ranging from 3318 to 5925 mIU/ml. The titers obtained from the second dose approximate those observed several years after natural infection.

Merck: Seropositivity persisted up to 18 months after a single ≈25 u dose in a cohort of 35 out of 39 children and adolescents who participated in the Monroe Efficacy Study; 95% of this cohort responded anamnestically following a booster at 18 months. To date, no cases of hepatitis A disease 250 days after vaccination have occured in those vaccinees from the Monroe Efficacy Study monitored for up to 4 years.

Pharmacokinetic models of anti-hepatitis A antibodies suggest that clinical protection may persist 10 to 20 years or longer. More data is needed to make definitive recommendations about booster doses for lifelong immunity.

Drug Interactions: Like all inactivated vaccines, administration of hepatitis A vaccine to persons receiving immunosuppressant drugs (including high-dose corticosteroids)or radiation therapy may result in an inadequate response to immunization. They may remain susceptible despite immunization.

For persons desiring both immediate and long-term protection, hepatitis A vaccine may be administered concomitantly with IGIM, with separate syringes and at different injection sites. Simultaneous administration of hepatitis A vaccine and parenteral immune globulin products may reduce the ultimate antibody titer obtained from vaccination compared with vaccine alone. In a study using 2.5 to 5 times the standard IGIM dose, the anti-hepatitis A GMT was 146 mIU/ml 5 days after IGIM administration, 77 mIU/ml after 1 month and 63 mIU/ml 2 months after IGIM. Lower antibody titers might result in protection of less duration than that without IGIM administration.

Havrix brand of hepatitis A vaccine has been administered simultaneously with *Engerix-B* brand of hepatitis B vaccine without impairing immune response to either. Concomitant administration with other inactivated vaccines (eg, tetanus-diphtheria, rabies, poliovirus, typhoid) also has not interfered with immune responses to either vaccine.

In preliminary studies, recipients of yellow-fever vaccine were slightly less likely to seroconvert if they also received hepatitis A vaccine. Yellow-Fever vaccine does not interfere with the antibody response to hepatitis A vaccine. Hepatitis A vaccine did not affect the immunogenicity of, nor was it affected by, oral poliovirus vaccine or oral typhoid vaccine.

Concomitant administration of mefloquine (*Lariam*) did not impair antibody response to hepatitis A vaccine.

As with other drugs administered by IM injection, give hepatitis A vaccine with caution to persons receiving anticoagulant therapy.

Patient Information: No vaccine is perfect. Advise vaccine recipients that food and water precautions are essential to avoid infection. Refer to the section on Recommendations for International Travel.

Pharmaceutical Characteristics

Concentration:

SKB: Adult: 1440 ELu/ml

Pediatric: 720 ELu/0.5ml

Merck: Adult: 50 u per 1 ml

Pediatric: 25 u per 0.5 ml

Packaging:

SKB: Adult: 1440 ELu per 1 ml single-dose vial. Disposable, prefilled single-dose 1 ml syringe of 1440 ELu with 23-gauge, 1 inch needle.

Pediatric: 720 ELu per 0.5 ml single-dose vial. Disposable, prefilled single-dose 0.5 ml syringe of 720 ELu with 25-gauge, ⅝ inch needle.

Merck: Adult: 50 u per 1 ml single-dose vial. Disposable, prefilled singe-dose 1 ml syringe of 50 u with 23-gauge, 1 inch needle, five single-dose vials, five pre-filled syringes.

Pediatric/Adolescent: 25 u per 0./5 ml single-dose vial. Disposable, prefilled single-dose 0.5 ml syringe of 25 u with 25-gauge, ⅝ inch needle, five single-dose vials, five prefilled syringes.

Dose Form: Suspension

Solvent: *SKB:* Phosphate-buffered saline solution

Merck: Solution of sodium borate 70 mcg/ml and sodium chloride 0.9%

Storage/Stability: Store at 2° to 8°C (35° to 46°F). Discard frozen vaccine.

SKB: In one study, immunogenicity was not affected by storage for 7 days at 37°C (98.6°F; Wiedermann, et al. 1993). Shipped in insulated containers with coolant packs and temperature monitoring strips.

Merck: Contact manufacturer regarding prolonged exposures to room temperature or elevated temperatures. Shipping procedure information not provided by manufacturer.

Comparison of Hepatitis A Vaccines

	Vaqta	Havrix
Manufacturer	Merck	SKB
Strain	Attenuated CR326F' strain	HM-175 strain
Concentration	50 u/ml	1440 ELu/ml
Packaging	Single-dose vial or syringe	Single-dose vial or syringe
Dose Form	Suspension	Suspension
Cell culture	MRC-5	MRC-5
Standard schedule Children (2-18 years) Adults	Single dose 25 units 50 units	Single dose 720 ELu 1440 ELu
Booster dose	6-18 months later	6-12 months later
Route	IM	IM

Hepatitis B Vaccine (HBV)
VIRAL VACCINES

NAME:
Recombivax HB, Engerix-B

MANUFACTURER:

Recombivax HB, Merck Vaccine Division, under license from Biogen and Chiron, ✳ Merck Frosst; *Energix-B,* Manufactured by SmithKline Beecham Biologicals, Rixensart, Belgium, distributed by SmithKline Beecham Pharmaceuticals, under license from Biogen, ✳ SmithKline Beecham

Synonyms: Hepatitis B surface antigen (HBsAg) is also called the Dane particle and the Australia antigen. Hepatitis B was initially called "serum hepatitis," to differentiate it from "infectious hepatitis" (IH, hepatitis A). The acronym HBV may refer either to hepatitis B virus or hepatitis B vaccine.

Comparison: Either hepatitis B vaccine is prophylactically interchangeable with any other (including the original plasma-derived vaccine, *Heptavax-B*, Merck) for completion of a basic immunizing series or for booster

Viability: Inactivated

Antigenic Form: Purified antigen, a 226 amino acid polypeptide, 22 nm particles possessing antigenic epitopes of the hepatitis B virus surface-coat (S) protein.

doses, but the quantity of antigen or the dosage volume will vary between comparably potent *Recombivax HB* and *Engerix-B*. Immunogenic potency of the two current products varies because of antigenic differences in their three-dimensional epitopes, effects of the purification process on the hepatitis B surface antigen particles, and other factors. Although the two vaccines contain the same aluminum concentration, *Recombivax HB* has a higher ratio of hepatitis B surface antigen to aluminum.

Antigenic Type: Lipoprotein complex containing the S protein

Use Characteristics

◎ **Indications:** Induction of active immunity against hepatitis B virus among persons of all ages who are currently or who will be at increased risk of infection with this virus.

Because hepatitis D virus (delta hepatitis, the delta agent) can only infect and cause illness in persons infected with hepatitis B, and since hepatitis D virus requires a coat of hepatitis B surface antigen to become infectious, immunity to hepatitis B also protects against hepatitis D. Hepatitis D virus is a circular RNA-containing virus.

CDC, ACIP, AAP, Canada's National Advisory Committee on Immunization (NACI), and the Canadian Paediatric Society recommend routine vaccination of all infants against hepatitis B, with 3 doses either:

(1) at birth (prior to discharge from a hospital), at 1 to 2 months of age, and at 6 to 18 months of age; or

(2) at 1 to 2 months of age, at 4 months of age, and at 6 to 18 months of age.

Special efforts should be made to vaccinate all children <11 years of age who are Alaskan natives, Pacific Islanders, or who reside in households of first-generation immigrants from countries where hepatitis B virus is of high or intermediate endemicity.

Vaccinate all children 11 to 12 years of age, if they were not previously vaccinated earlier in childhood. Vaccination of adolescents is most important in high-risk settings, including communities where use of illicit injectable drugs, teenage pregnancy or sexually transmitted diseases are common. These steps are important to more quickly control the rate of hepatitis B infection among young adults.

Vaccination is indicated for several major groups of persons:

(1) Healthcare workers exposed to blood or blood products: Dentists and oral surgeons, physicians and surgeons, nurses, podiatrists, paramedical personnel, dental hygienists and nurses, laboratory personnel, students in these occupations, and cleaning staff who handle potentially infectious waste.

(2) Selected patients and patient contacts: Patients and staff of hemodialysis and hematology/oncology units; persons with hemophilia, thalassemia or similar conditions requiring large-volume transfusions of blood or blood products; residents and staff in institutions for the mentally handicapped; classroom contacts of deinstitutionalized mentally handicapped persons with persistent hepatitis B antigenemia who demonstrate aggressive behavior; and household and other intimate contacts of persons with persistent hepatitis B antigenemia.

(3) Social groups with a known high incidence of disease, such as Alaskan Eskimos, Indochinese refugees and Haitian refugees.

(4) Persons at increased risk because of their sexual practices: Persons who have heterosexual activity with multiple partners (eg, >1 partner in a 6 month period), persons who repeatedly contract sexually transmitted diseases, homosexually active males and female prostitutes.

(5) Other persons at increased risk, including certain military personnel, morticians and embalmers, blood-bank and plasma-fractionation workers, prisoners, adopted children from countries of high hepatitis-B endemicity, and users of contaminated injectable drugs (eg, through needle sharing).

OSHA requires that hepatitis B vaccine be offered for occupational protection to anyone at risk from blood-borne pathogens. Vaccine must be made available within 10 working days of initial assignment to all employees who have the potential for occupational exposure to blood, at no cost to the employee, at a reasonable time and place, under the supervision of a healthcare professional, and according to the latest recommendations of the US PHS; antibody screening may not be required as a condition of receiving the vaccine (29 CFR 1910.1030).

Unlabeled Uses: Hepatitis B vaccination is appropriate for persons expected to receive human alpha 1-proteinase inhibitor (*Prolastin*, Miles). If insufficient time is available for adequate antibody responses to active vaccination to develop, give a single dose of HBIG with the initial dose of vaccine. Prolastin is produced from heat-treated, pooled human plasma that may contain the causative agents of hepatitis and other viral diseases. Manufacturing procedures at plasma collection centers, plasma testing laboratories, and fractionation facilities are designed to reduce the risk of transmitting viral infection, but that risk cannot be totally eliminated. Hepatitis B vaccination will further reduce the risk of this disease, but not of other hepatic viral diseases that might be transmitted by *Prolastin*.

Contraindications:

Absolute: Do not give further injections to persons who develop symptoms of hypersensitivity after an injection of hepatitis B vaccine.

Relative: Patients with a history of hypersensitivity to yeast or other components. Defer vaccination until after resolution of any serious active infection.

Elderly: Immunogenicity of hepatitis B vaccines is somewhat reduced in persons >40 years of age.

Pregnancy: *Category* C. Use if clearly needed. It is not known if hepatitis B vaccine or corresponding antibodies cross the placenta. Generally, most IgG passage across the placenta occurs during the third trimester.

Lactation: It is not known if hepatitis B vaccine or corresponding antibodies are excreted in breast milk. Problems in humans have not been documented.

Children: Hepatitis B vaccine is well tolerated and highly immunogenic in newborns, infants and children. Maternal antibodies do not interfere with pediatric immunogenicity.

Adverse Reactions:

Adverse effects are comparable for the two hepatitis B vaccines. Injection site (17% to 22%) and systemic complaints (14% to 15%) may involve pain, tenderness, pruritus, induration, erythema, ecchymosis, swelling, warmth or nodule formation.

Systemic reactions: Fatigue, weakness, headache, fever >37.5°C (100°F), malaise, nausea, diarrhea, dizziness, pharyngitis, upper respiratory infection, abnormal liver functions, thrombocytopenia, eczema, purpura, tachycardia or palpitations, erythema multiforme (eg, Stevens-Johnson syndrome) by temporal association. Reactions following <1% of injections: Sweating, achiness, chills, tingling, hypertension, anorexia, abdominal pain or cramps, constipation, flushing, vomiting, paresthesia, rash, alopecia, angioedema, urticaria, arthralgia, arthritis, myalgia, back pain, lymphadenopathy, hypotension, anaphylaxis, bronchospasm, Guillain-Barré syndrome. Some of these events may simply have been temporally associated with immunization.

No published reports of delayed hypersensitivities have been noted yet, as were seen with the serum-based vaccine, despite the yeast source of the vaccine antigen.

Pharmacologic & Dosing Characteristics

Dosage: Shake product well before withdrawing each dose. Dosage (both quantity of antigen and fluid volume) varies between the licensed products. The harmonized pediatric schedule is to give the first dose from birth to 2 months of age, the second dose from 1 to 4 months of age, and the third dose from 6 to 18 months of age. Either brand may be used on this schedule. At least 4 weeks between doses is needed for proper immune response.

Pre-Exposure Prophylaxis

Merck: Give patients 3 doses, with the second dose 1 month after the first and the third dose 6 months after the first (ie, at 0, 1 and 6 months). At each dose, give recipients an amount of vaccine corresponding to their age, see table.

Give dialysis patients and other immunocompromised persons 40 mcg at each dose.

Although not described in the product labeling, *Recombivax HB* may be administered on an alternate schedule with doses at 0, 1 and 2 months to provide rapid induction of immunity. On this alternate schedule, give an additional dose 12 months after the first dose if prolonged protection is needed (*Jilg et al, 1989*).

Hepatitis B Vaccine Dose Based on Age

	Recombivax HB	Engerix-B
Dialysis and immunocompromised patients	40 mcg/1 ml (0, 1, 6 mos)	40 mcg/2 ml (0, 1, 2, 6 mos)
Adults (>19 years of age)	10 mcg/1 ml	20 mcg/1 ml
Adolescents (11-19 years of age)	5 mcg	10 mcg
Infants & children (birth to 10 years of age)	2.5 mcg[1]	10 mcg[2]

[1]Unless the infant is born of an HBsAg-positive mother. Give these infants 0.5 ml HBIG at birth and 5 mcg *Recombivax HB* within 7 days of birth, with an additional 5 mcg vaccine dose 1 month and 6 months later.

[2]If the infant is born of an HBsAg-positive mother, give 0.5 ml HBIG at birth and 10 mcg *Engerix-B* within 7 days of birth, with an additional 10 mcg vaccine dose 1 month and 6 months later. Or the vaccine can be given on a schedule of 0, 1, 2 and 12 months.

SKB: Give patients 3 doses, with the second dose 1 month after the first and the third dose 6 months after the first (ie, at 0, 1 and 6 months). At each dose, give recipients an amount of vaccine corresponding to their age, according to the table.

An alternate schedule of doses at 0, 1 and 2 months will provide rapid induction of immunity (eg, in neonates born of hepatitis B infected mothers, others who may have been exposed to the virus, and travelers to high-risk areas wanting prompt attention). On this alternate schedule, give an additional dose 12 months after the first dose to infants born of infected mothers and to others for whom prolonged protection is desired. Also give these infants 0.5 ml of HBIG at birth and 10mcg/0.5 ml of vaccine within 7 days of birth, with additional 10 mcg/0.5 ml vaccine doses either 1 and 6 months later or 1, 2 and 12 months later.

Give dialysis patients and other immunocompromised persons 40 mcg/2 ml, with additional doses 1, 2 and 6 months after the first dose. Although not described in either manufacturers' labeling, the most persistently elevated antibody titers may result from a 3 dose series in months 0, 1 and 12 (Bryan et al, 1991). Such a schedule may be appropriate for health students whose current risk is small, but who will need prolonged immunity.

Post-Exposure Prophylaxis: See also the HBIG monograph.

In response to known or presumed exposure to hepatitis B surface antigen (eg, needle-stick, ocular or mucous-membrane exposure; human bites that penetrate the skin; sexual contact; infants born of HBsAg-positive mothers), give previously unvaccinated persons post-exposure prophylaxis. This consists of 0.06 ml/kg HBIG as soon as possible or within 24 hours after exposure, if possible (within 14 days in the case of sexual contact). Give the appropriate volume of either hepatitis B vaccine based on age within 7 days of exposure, with additional vaccine doses either 1 and 6 months after the first dose or 1, 2 and 12 months later.

Route & Site: IM in deltoid muscle or, for infants and young children, in the anterolateral thigh. Avoid gluteal injection into the buttock, which may result in less than optimal immune response, due to vaccine deposition in fatty tissue rather than muscle. Never inject IV. SC injection may be used in patients who risk hemorrhage following IM injection (eg, persons with hemophilia or thalassemia), but the SC route may produce a less than optimal response and may lead to an increased incidence of local reactions, including nodules.

Both Merck and SKB recommend not administering a reduced (usually one-tenth) dose of hepatitis B vaccine via the ID route. CDC has reported several programs where suboptimal immune response followed ID injection, probably due to improper technique. Nonetheless, some practitioners have successfully used the ID route to immunize large groups of people, when appropriate attention was paid to proper technique. Inadvertent SC injection into fat will impair the immune response. Proper ID technique may not achieve antibody titers as high (or perhaps as persistent) as from IM injection of either plasma-derived or recombinant vaccines. Additionally, seroconversion may be less when using recombinant vaccines ID. Delayed-hypersensitivity reactions at the injection site may follow ID administration.

Efficacy:

Merck: 94% to 98% immunogenicity among adults 20 to 39 years of age, 1 to 2 months after the third dose; 89% immunogenicity in adults ≥40 years of age; 96% to 99% immunogenicity among infants, children and adolescents.

SKB: Among healthy adults and adolescents who received three doses at months 0, 1 and 6, seroprotection (defined as titers ≥10mIU/ml) of 79% was seen at month 6 and 96% at month 7; the geometric mean antibody titer for seroconverters at month 7 was 2204 mIU/ml.

On the alternate month 0, 1 and 2 schedule, 99% of recipients were seroprotected at month 3 and remained protected through month 12. An additional dose after 12 months produced a GMT for seroconverters at month 13 of 9163 mIU/ml.

Neonates immunized with 10 mcg at 0, 1 and 2 months of age produced a sero-protection rate of 93% in infants by month 4, with a GMT among seroconverters of 210 mIU/ml; an additional dose at month 12 produced a GMT among seroconverters of 2941 mIU/mL at month 13. Immunization at 0, 1 and 6 months of age resulted in 100% sero-conversion of infants by month 7 with a GMT of 713 mIU/ml and a seropro-tection rate of 97%. In a study of clin-ical protection, only 3.4% of 58 infants became chronic carriers in the 12 month follow-up period, compared to an expected rate of 70%, a protective efficacy rate of 95%.

Among children 6 months to 10 years of age who received three 10 mcg doses at months 0, 1 and 6, 98% seroprotec-tion occurred 1 to 2 months after the third dose; the GMT among seroconverters was 4023 mIU/ml.

Among older subjects given 20 mcg at months 0, 1 and 6, 88% seroprotection resulted 1 month after the third dose. In adults >40 years of age, the GMT among seroconverters 1 month after the third dose was 610 mIU/ml.

Hemodialysis patients respond to hepatitis B vaccine with lower titers that remain at protective levels for shorter durations than normal sub-jects. Among chronic hemodialysis patients who received 40 mcg of *Hep-tavax-B* at months 0, 1 and 6, only about 50% of patients were seroprotected.

Onset: 70% to 80% of recipients are protected after the second dose and >95% after the third dose.

Duration: Duration of protection is undetermined, but apparently lasts >5 to 7 years in most healthy recipients. Studies of Alaskan Eskimos suggest that clinical protection may persist even after circulating anti-HBs antibodies can no longer be detected.

Drug Interactions: Like all inac-tivated vaccines, administration of hepatitis B vaccine to persons receiving immunosuppressant drugs, including high-dose corticosteroids, or radiation therapy may result in an insufficient response to immuniza-tion. They may remain susceptible despite immunization.

Several routine vaccines may safely and effectively be administered simul-taneously at separate injection sites (eg, DTP, MMR, e-IPV, Hib, hepatitis B, influenza). National authorities rec-ommend simultaneous immunization at separate sites as indicated by age or health risk, if return of a vaccine recipient for a subsequent visit is doubtful.

There is no significant interaction between hepatitis B vaccines and HBIG, if administered at separate sites. Maternal antibodies do not interfere with immunogenicity in newborn infants. *Havrix* brand of hepatitis A vac-cine has been administered simultane-ously with *Engerix-B* brand of hepatitis B vaccine without impairing immune response to either.

Concurrent vaccination against hepati-tis B and yellow fever viruses in one study reduced the antibody titer oth-erwise expected from yellow fever vaccine. Separate these vaccines by 1 month, if possible.

As with other drugs administered by IM injection, give hepatitis B vaccine with caution to persons receiving anti-coagulant therapy.

Natural interleukin-2 may boost systemic immune response to HBsAg in immunodeficient nonresponders to hepatitis B vaccination (*Meuer et al, 1989*), but the recombinant interleukin-2 known as teceleukin did not augment response to hepatitis B vaccine in healthy adults in another study (*Rose et al, 1992*).

IM hepatitis B immunization of 153 hemophiliacs with a 23-gauge needle, followed by steady pressure (without rubbing) to the injection site for 1 to 2 minutes, resulted in a 4% bruising rate, with no patients requiring factor supplementation.

Pharmaceutical Characteristics

Concentration:

Merck: 5, 10 and 40 mcg/ml, depending on package

SKB: 20mcg/ml

Packaging:

Merck: Adult Formulation (10mcg/ml, with green caps): 1 ml single-dose vial, 3 ml multi-dose vial

Pediatric Formulation: (2.5 mcg/0.5 ml, with brown caps): 0.5 ml single-dose vial, 3 ml multi-dose vial

Adolescent/High-Risk Infant Formulation: (5 mcg/0.5 ml, with yellow caps): 0.5 ml single-dose vial

Dialysis Formulation: (40 mcg/ml, with blue caps): 1 ml single-dose vial

SKB Adult Formulation: (20 mcg/ml, with orange caps): 1 ml single-dose vial; 10 ml multi-dose vial; package of five 1 ml disposable single-dose syringes with 23-gauge, 1 inch needles

Pediatric/High-Risk Infant/Adolescent Formulation: (10 mcg/0.5 ml, with blue caps): 0.5 ml single-dose vial; package of five 0.5 ml disposable single-dose syringes with 23-gauge, 1-inch needles; package of five 0.5 ml disposable single-dose syringes with 25-gauge, $\frac{5}{8}$ inch needles

Dose Form: Suspension

Solvents: Do not dilute prior to administration.

Merck: Sterile water

SKB: 0.9% sodium chloride and phosphate buffer

Storage/Stability: Store at $2°$ to $8°$C ($36°$ to $46°$F). Discard vaccine if frozen; freezing destroys potency.

Merck: Product can tolerate 7 days at room temperature when prefilled into syringes without significant loss of potency. Shipped by routine courier in insulated containers with coolant packs.

SKB: Product can tolerate $37°$C ($98.6°$F) for 7 days according to the Belgian package insert. Shipped by overnight courier in insulated containers with coolant packs and temperature monitor.

Comparison of Hepatitis B Vaccines

	Recombivax HB	*Engerix-B*
Manufacturer	Merck	SKB
Packaging	2.5 mcg/0.5 ml, 7.5 mcg/3 ml, 5 mcg/0.5 ml, 10 mcg/ml, 30 mcg/3 ml, 40 mcg/ml vials	10 mcg/0.5 ml vial or syringe, 20 mcg/ml vial or syringe, 200 mcg/10 ml vial
Source	Product of *Saccharomyces cerevisiae*	Product of *Saccharomyces cerevisiae*

Recommended Schedule for Prophylaxis of Perinatal Hepatitis B

Infant born to monther known to be HBsAg-positive

Age of infant	Vaccine dose	HBIG dose
Birth (within 12 hours)	First	First
1 month	Second	
6 months[1]	Third	

Infant born of mother not screened or known to be HBsAg-negative

Age of infant	Vaccine dose[2]	HBIG dose
Birth to 2 months of age	First	See footnote 3
1 to 4 months[4]	Second	
6 to 18 months[1]	Third	

[1]If the 4-dose schedule for *Engerix-B* is used, give the third dose at 2 months of age and the fourth dose at 12 to 18 months.

[2]If mother was not screened, use appropriate dose for an infant of a HBsAg-positive mother. If the mother is later found to be HBsAg-positive, continue that dose. If the mother is later found to be HBsAg-negative, decrease Merck vaccine dose to appropriate level.

[3]If mother is later found to be HBsAg-positive, administer HBIG to infants as soon as possible, not later than 1 week after birth.

[4]Vaccinate infants of women who are HBsAg-negative beginning at birth or at 2 months of age.

Dosage Recommendations of FDA, CDC, ACIP & AAP
(for both pre- and post-exposure prophylaxis)

	Recombivax HB	Energix-B
Infants of HBsAg-positive mothers	5 mcg/0.5 ml	10 mcg/0.5 ml
Other infants/children <11 years	2.5 mcg/0.25 ml or 0.5 ml	10 mcg/0.5 ml
11-19 years	5 mcg/0.5 ml	10 mcg/0.5 ml
Adults	10 mcg/ml	20 mcg/ml
Dialysis patients & other immunocompromised persons	40 mcg/ml	40 mcg/2 ml
Administration Schedules		
Labeled	0, 1, 6 months	0, 1, 6, months 0, 1, 2 (12) months
Unlabeled	0, 1, 2 (12) months 0, 1, 12 months	0, 1, 12 months
Measures of Immunogenicity		
Seroconversion[1] (titer ≥1 ml mIU/ml)	99% to 100%	98% to 100%
Seroprotection[1] (titer ≥10 mIU/ml)	94% to 98%	96% to 100%
Antibody Titers[1] (GMT, mIU/ml)	3154 to 3846	944 to 7488

[1]Among healthy adults, <40 years of age, using a 0, 1 and 6 month schedule.

Influenza Virus Vaccine, Trivalent, Types A & B
VIRAL VACCINES

NAME:
Fluzone subvirion or whole-virion vaccines, *Fluvirin* purified surface antigen, *Fluogen* subvirion vaccine/immunizing antigen, *Flu-Shield* purified subvirion antigen, ✿ *Fluviral*

MANUFACTURERS:
Fluzone subvirion or whole-virion vaccines manufacturered by Connaught Laboratories; *Fluvirin* purified surface antigen manufactured by Evans Medical Limited, distributed by Adams Laboratories; *Fluogen* subvirion vaccine/immunizing antigen manufacured by Parke-Davis, ✿ CSL Limited, ✿ Evens Medical; *Flu-Shield* purified subvirion antigen manufactured by Wyeth-Lederle Vaccines & Pediatrics; ✿ Fluviral, IAF Biovac, Merck Frosst

Synonyms: Flu vaccine. Split-virion, split-virus, subvirion and purified surface antigen are comparable terms.

Comparison: Split-virion influenza vaccines are generically equivalent to each other, as whole-virion influenza vaccines are generically equivalent to each other. Split vaccines are slightly less reactogenic in children than whole vaccines, although they are comparable in immunogenicity in both adults and children. Use only split vaccines in children <13 years of age.

Viability: Inactivated. Influenza vaccine cannot cause influenza, despite this widely held belief. Occasional cases of respiratory disease following vaccination represent coincidental viral infection unrelated to vaccination or the lethargy associated with any vaccination.

Antigenic Form: Either split- or whole-virus

Antigenic Type: Protein

Use Characteristics

◎ **Indications:** Induction of active immunity against influenza viruses corresponding to the strains in the vaccine formula. Give influenza vaccine to any person >6 months of age who, because of age or underlying medical condition, is at increased risk for complications of influenza. Also vaccinate healthcare workers and others (including household members) in close contact with high-risk persons. In addition, give influenza vaccine to any person who wishes to reduce the chance of becoming infected with influenza.

Target Groups for Special Vaccination Programs:

Groups at increased risk of influenza-related complications:

(1) Otherwise healthy persons ≥65 years of age;

(2) residents of nursing homes and other chronic-care facilities housing patients of any age with chronic medical conditions;

(3) adults and children with chronic disorders of the pulmonary or cardiovascular systems requiring regular medical follow-up or hospitalization during the preceding year, including children with asthma. Refer to tables of pertinent diagnoses and related indicator medications (see Vaccine Indications by Risk Group in the Resources Section).

(4) adults and children who required medical follow-up or hospitalization during the preceding year because of chronic metabolic diseases (including diabetes mellitus), renal dysfunction, hemoglobinopathies or any form of immunosuppresion;

(5) children and teenagers (6 months to 18 years of age) who are receiving long-term aspirin therapy and, therefore, may be at risk of developing Reye's syndrome after influenza infection.

Groups potentially capable of nosocomial transmission of influenza to high-risk persons:

Individuals attending high-risk persons can transmit influenza infections to them while they are themselves incubating infection, undergoing subclinical infection or working despite the existence of symptoms. Some high-risk persons (eg, the elderly, transplant recipients, AIDS patients) can have relatively low antibody responses to influenza vaccine. Efforts to protect them against influenza may be improved by reducing the chances that their care providers may expose them to influenza. Therefore, vaccinate the following groups:

(1) Physicians, nurses and other personnel in both hospital and outpatient-care settings who have contact with high-risk persons in all age groups, including infants;

(2) providers of home care to high-risk persons (eg, visiting nurses, volunteer workers) as well as all household members of high-risk persons, including children, whether or not they provide care.

Vaccination of other groups:

(1) Persons who provide essential community services and students or other healthy individuals in institutional settings (ie, schools and colleges), to minimize disruption of routine activities during outbreaks;

(2) persons preparing for travel to the tropics at any time of year or to the Southern Hemisphere from April to September, especially if they have other risk factors. Use the most current vaccine. Risk of exposure to influenza during international travel varies, depending on season of travel, destination and other factors. Because of the short incubation period for influenza, exposure to the virus during travel will often result in clinical illness that begins during travel, an inconvenience or potential danger, especially for persons at increased risk for complications. Revaccinate high-risk travelers given the previous season's vaccine prior to departure with the current vaccine the following autumn.

If influenza vaccine is used in an immunization program sponsored by an organization where a traditional physician/patient relationship does not exist, advise each participant or guardian of the possible risks associated with influenza vaccination.

Contraindications:

STOP *Absolute*: Do not vaccinate persons with a history of anaphylactoid or other immediate reactions (eg, hives, swelling of the mouth or throat, difficulty breathing, hypotension, shock) following ingestion of eggs unless desensitization is appropriate. Skin test persons suspected of being hypersensitive to egg protein, using a dilution of the vaccine as the antigen (*Murphy & Strunk*, 1985). Refer to detailed instructions in the Introduction section. Do not vaccinate persons with adverse reactions to such testing unless benefits outweigh risks. Persons are apparently not at risk if they have egg allergies that are not anaphylactoid in nature; vaccinate such persons in the usual manner. There is no evidence that persons with allergies to chickens or feathers are at increased risk of reaction to the vaccine. If influenza vaccine contains residual neomycin, the amount would be less than used in a skin test to assess hypersensitivity. Neomycin allergy is usually a contact dermatitis, a manifestation of cell-mediated immunity rather that anaphylaxis and does not contraindicate administration.

Relative: Do not routinely vaccinate persons with acute febrile illness until their symptoms abate. Delay immunization in persons with an active neurological disorder characterized by changing neurological findings, but reconsider immunization when the disease process has stabilized. The occurence of any neurological symptoms or signs after vaccination with this product is a contraindication to further use. Conflicting advice is offered regarding vaccination of persons with a history of Guillain-Barré syndrome (GBS). The FDA and the manufacturer include this contraindication in the product labeling, but it is not included in ACIP recommendations.

Elderly: Elderly persons and persons with certain chronic diseases may develop lower postvaccination antibody titers than healthy young adults and thus remain susceptible to influenza upper-respiratory-tract infections. Nevertheless, even if such persons develop influenza illness, vaccination is effective in preventing lower-respiratory-tract involvement or other complications, thereby reducing the risk of hospitalization and death.

Pregnancy: *Category* C. Use only if clearly needed. Influenza-associated excess mortality among pregnant women has not been documented, except in the largest pandemics of 1918-19 and 1957-58. However, additional case reports and limited studies suggest that women in the third trimester of pregnancy and shortly after pregnancy, including women without underlying risk factors, may be at increased risk for serious complications from influenza. Vaccinate pregnant women who have medical conditions increasing their risk of complications from influenza, regardless of the stage of pregnancy, since the vaccine is considered safe for pregnant women. Consider vaccinating all women who would be in the third trimester of pregnancy or early puerperium during the influenza season. Influenza vaccine is considered safe at any stage of pregnancy. It is not known if influenza vaccine or corresponding antibodies cross the placenta. Generally, most IgG passage across the placenta occurs during the third trimester.

Lactation: It is not known if influenza vaccine or corresponding antibodies are excreted in breast milk. Problems in humans have not been documented.

Children: Give previously unvaccinated children <9 years of age 2 doses at least 1 month apart. Give the second dose before December, if possible. Use only split-virion vaccine in children <13 years of age.

Vaccinate children and teenagers (6 months to 18 years of age) who are receiving long-term aspirin therapy, and therefore at risk of developing Reye's syndrome after influenza infection.

Adverse Reactions:
Influenza vaccine contains only noninfectious, inactivated viruses. It cannot cause influenza. The most likely side effect of influenza vaccine is fever or tenderness at the injection site (20% to 30%).

Side effects of influenza vaccine are generally inconsequential in adults and occur at low frequency, but side effects may be more common in younger recipients. As many as two-thirds of recipients experience soreness around the vaccination site for 2 days. Fever, malaise, myalgia and other systemic symptoms occur infrequently and usually affect persons with no prior exposure to the antigens in the vaccine (eg, young children). The effects usually begin 6 to 12 hours after vaccination and persist 1 to 2 days. Immediate, probably allergic, reactions such as hives, angioedema, allergic asthma or systemic anaphylaxis occur extremely rarely after influenza vaccination. Do not vaccinate persons with severe egg allergy (eg, hives, swelling of lips or tongue, acute respiratory distress, collapse).

Increased risk of Guillain-Barré syndrome (GBS) was noted among recipients of the 1976-77 A/New Jersey/76 (swine flu) influenza vaccine. An active surveillance system for GBS was initiated in 1978 and data were collected for 3 years. A statistically significant excess risk of contracting GBS after receipt of the 1978-79, 1979-80 and 1980-81 influenza vaccine formulations could not be demonstrated. Unlike the 1976 swine influenza vaccine, subsequent influenza vaccines prepared from other virus strains have not been associated with an increased frequency of GBS.

Before modern purification techniques were adopted, split-virion vaccine induced fewer side effects than whole-virion vaccine, although possibly at the cost of reduced immunogenicity. Modern split- and whole-virion vaccines are comparably immunogenic and reactogenic in adults. Use split vaccine in children to reduce the likelihood of inducing fever.

Pharmacologic & Dosing Characteristics

Dosage: Shake product well before withdrawing each dose.

Vaccination: Give adults and children ≥9

years of age one 0.5 ml dose annually, so long as indications persist. Give children ≤12 years of age only the split-virion vaccine.

Give previously unvaccinated children ≤8 years of age 2 doses at least 1 month apart. Give the second dose before December 1, if possible. For children 6 to 35 months of age, give 0.25 ml at each injection. For children 3 to 8 years of age, give two 0.5 ml injections. Give children 9 to 12 years old one 0.5 ml injection. Give children ≤12 years of age only the split-virion vaccine. Use either the split-virion or whole-virion vaccine in persons ≥13 years of age or older.

Offer the new annual vaccine formula to high-risk individuals, such as those presenting for routine care or hospitalization, beginning each September. Organized vaccination campaigns where high-risk persons are routinely accessible (eg, nursing homes) are optimally undertaken between October 15 and November 15 each year. Continue to offer vaccine to both children and adults up to and even after influenza virus activity is documented in a community, as late as April in some years.

Route & Site: IM or jet injection. Use the deltoid muscle for adults and older children. For infants and young children, the anterolateral aspect of the thigh is preferred. Do not inject IV.

Efficacy: Vaccination will reduce disease incidence by approximately 70%. Influenza vaccine is more effective at preventing mortality than at preventing morbidity.

Onset: 2 to 4 weeks

Duration: Declines during the year following immunization.

Drug Interactions: Like all inactivated vaccines, administration of influenza vaccine to persons receiving immunosuppressant drugs, including high-dose corticosteroids, or radiation therapy may result in an insufficient response to immunization. They may remain susceptible despite immunization. Chemoprophylaxis may be indicated in such persons.

Pneumococcal and influenza vaccines may safely and effectively be administered simultaneously at separate injection sites. While influenza vaccine is given annually, pneumococcal vaccine is given only once to all but those at highest risk of fatal pneumococcal disease.

Although no studies are published, influenza vaccine is not expected to diminish immunogenicity or enhance adverse reactions with other routine pediatric vaccines (eg, OPV or e-IPV, Hib, MMR, hepatitis B).

Several vaccine-drug interactions have been attributed to influenza vaccine, although independent researchers have often been unable to corroborate the interactions. The vaccine-drug interaction may be clinically significant only in a few isolated individuals (Grabenstein, 1990). Influenza vaccine, like some other vaccines and other drugs, may be able to depress drug-metabolizing pathways by induction of endogenous interferon production. Influenza vaccine can decrease elimination and increase the biological half-life of aminopyrine, a probe chemical not used therapeutically, by inhibiting the P-450 metabolic pathway in the liver.

Theophylline elimination, which includes the P-450 pathway, has been noted by several clinicians to decline following influenza vaccination, but their work has been contradicted by others. This effect may be greatest in persons with higher pre-vaccination theophylline metabolism. Watch patients on chronic theophylline therapy for the symptoms of theophylline toxicity (eg, nausea, vomiting, palpitations).

A few patients treated with warfarin have shown prolonged prothrombin time after influenza vaccination (incidence, 10 of 208 patients reported). None of the studies published to date preclude the possibility of isolated cases of significant bleeding events, but there is insufficient evidence to substantiate a systemic interaction between warfarin and influenza vaccine. Watch patients on chronic warfarin therapy for the symptoms of toxicity. As with other drugs administered by IM injection, give influenza vaccine with caution to persons receiving anticoagulant therapy.

Anticonvulsants: Phenytoin steady-state plasma concentrations rose, fell or remained unchanged after influenza vaccination in several studies. Carbamazepine and phenobarbital levels rose after influenza vaccination in one study. Phenytoin and phenobarbital are metabolized by the P-450 pathway, but carbamazepine is not. Watch patients on chronic anticonvulsant therapy for the symptoms of drug toxicity.

Methacholine inhalation challenge may be falsely positive for a few days after influenza or other immunization. This effect appears to mimic the bronchospastic effect associated with acute respiratory infections. The effect has been observed in 44% to 90% of asthmatic patients, but apparently not among normal subjects.

Laboratory Interference: The 1991 influenza vaccine formulation was associated with a transient slight increase in the incidence of false-positive serologic tests for human immunodeficiency virus (HIV), human T-cell lymphotrophic virus type 1 (HTLV-1) and hepatitis C virus (*MacKenzie et al, 1992*). No infections occurred as a result of vaccination and there is no apparent need to defer vaccinees from blood donation. This effect has not been seen with more recent influenza vaccine formulations.

Pharmaceutical Characteristics

Concentration: 3 hemagglutinin antigens, each at a concentration of 15 mcg per 0.5ml dose

Packaging:

Connaught: 0.5 ml prefilled single-dose syringe with 25-gauge, $\frac{5}{8}$ inch needle, 10 doses per 5 ml multidose vial, 50 doses per 25 ml multidose vial for jet injection

Evans: 0.5 ml prefilled single-dose syringe with needle of unspecified gauge and length, 10 doses per 5 ml multidose vial

Parke-Davis: 0.5 ml prefilled single-dose syringe with 25-gauge, $\frac{3}{4}$ inch needle, 10 doses per 5 ml multidose vial

Wyeth-Lederle: Box of ten 0.5 ml prefilled *Tubex* single-dose cartridge-needle units with 25 gauge, $\frac{5}{8}$ inch needle, 10 doses per 5 ml multidose vial, 50 doses per 25 ml multidose vial for jet injection

Dose Form: Solution

Storage/Stability: Store at 2° to 8°C (35° to 46°F); discard frozen vaccine.

Connaught: Contact manufacturer regarding prolonged exposure to room temperature or elevated temperatures. Shipped by second-day courier in insulated containers with coolant packs.

Evans: Contact manufacturer regarding prolonged exposure to room temperature or elevated temperatures. Shipped in insulated containers with coolant packs.

Parke-Davis: Stability data suggest the product will tolerate 14 days at room temperature. Shipped at ambient temperature.

Wyeth-Lederle: Product can tolerate 10 days at room temperature or 7 days at 37°C (98.6°F). Shipped by overnight courier in insulated containers with coolant packs and temperature monitor.

Handling: Maintain jet injectors properly to prevent blood-borne diseases. Discard jet-injector vials at the end of each day.

Influenza Vaccine Comparison

	Split-virion vaccine	Whole-virion vaccine
Manufacturer	Connaught Evans Parke-Davis Wyeth-Lederle	Connaught
Concentration	3 antigens, 15 mcg/0.5 ml each	3 antigens, 15 mcg/0.5 ml each
Packaging	Vials and syringes	Vials and syringes
Age range	Any person >6 months old	Any person >12 years old
Immunogenicity	Comparable	Comparable
Reactogenicity	Fewer fevers in very young children	

Influenza Vaccine Dosage by Age

Age group	Product	Volume	# of doses[1]	Route
6 to 35 months	Split vaccine only	0.25 ml	1 or 2	IM
3 to 8 years	Split vaccine only	0.5 ml	1 or 2	IM
9 to 12 years	Split vaccine only	0.5 ml	1	IM
>12 years	Either whole or split vaccine	0.5 ml	1	IM

[1]Two doses administered at least 1 month apart are recommended for children <9 years old who receive influenza vaccine for the first time.

Measles, Mumps & Rubella Virus Vaccine Live

NAME:
M-M-R II

MANUFACTURER:
Merck Vaccine Division, ⬩ Merck Frosst

Viability: Live, attenuated

Antigenic Type: Protein

Antigenic Form: Whole viruses

> This vaccine is a simple combination of its component vaccines.
> For complete descriptions, refer to each individual monograph.

Use Characteristics

Indications: Simultaneous active immunization against mumps, rubella and especially measles. The national rubella immunization program is intended to reduce the occurrence of congenital rubella syndrome (CRS) among offspring of women who contract rubella during pregnancy. Trivalent measles-mumps-rubella (MMR) vaccine is the preferred immunizing agent for most children and many adults. Almost all children and some adults need >1 dose of MMR vaccine.

Prior to international travel, give individuals known to be susceptible to measles, mumps or rubella either a single-antigen vaccine or a combined-antigen vaccine, as appropriate. Trivalent MMR vaccine is preferred for persons likely to be susceptible to mumps and rubella. If single-antigen vaccines are not readily available, give travelers trivalent MMR regardless of their immune status to mumps or rubella.

Contraindications:

Absolute: Pregnant patients, patients with a personal history of a hypersensitivity reaction to this vaccine or any of its components (eg, eggs), patients receiving immunosuppressive therapy, patients with a blood dyscrasia, leukemia, lymphoma of any type, or other malignant neoplasms affecting the bone marrow or lymphatic systems, patients with primary or acquired immunodeficiency, any febrile illness or infection, active untreated tuberculosis, and persons with a family history of congenital or hereditary immunodeficiency, until the immune competence of the potential vaccine recipient is demonstrated. Refer to individual monographs for details.

Do not vaccinate persons who are immunosuppressed in association with AIDS or other clinical manifestations of infection with HIV, cellular immune deficiencies, and hypogammaglobulinemic and dysgammaglobulinemic states. Nonetheless, vaccinate asymptomatic children with HIV infection.

Do not vaccinate persons with a history of anaphylactoid or other immediate reactions (eg, hives, swelling of the mouth or throat, difficulty breathing, hypotension, shock) following egg ingestion. Give persons suspected of being hypersensitive to egg protein a skin test using a dilution of the vaccine as the antigen. Refer to Introduction section. Do not vaccinate persons with adverse reactions to such testing. Persons are apparently not at risk if they have egg allergies that are not anaphylactoid in nature; vaccinate such persons in the usual manner. There is no evidence to indicate that persons with allergies to chickens or feathers are at increased risk of reaction to the vaccine.

Relative: Defer immunization during the course of any acute illness.

Elderly: Most persons born in 1956 or earlier are likely to have been infected naturally and generally are considered not susceptible.

Adults: Vaccinate persons born more recently than 1956, unless they have a personal contraindication to vaccination, since they are considered susceptible. Vaccinate persons who may be immune but who lack adequate documentation of immunity as evidenced by physician diagnosis, laboratory evidence of immunity, or adequate immunization with live vaccine on or after the first birthday.

Pregnancy: *Category C.* Contraindicated. Measles—Contracting natural measles during pregnancy enhances fetal risk. There are no adequate studies of attenuated measles vaccine in pregnant females. Do not intentionally give measles vaccine to pregnant females, since the possible effects of the vaccine on fetal development are unknown at this time. If postpubertal females are vaccinated, counsel these women to avoid pregnancy for 3 months following vaccination. It is not known if attenuated measles virus or corresponding antibodies cross the placenta.

Mumps—Although mumps virus can infect the placenta and fetus, there is no good evidence that it causes congenital malformations in humans. Attenuated mumps vaccine virus can infect the placenta, but the virus has not been isolated from fetal tissues of susceptible women who were vaccinated and underwent elective abortions. Nonetheless, do not intentionally give attenuated mumps vaccine to pregnant females. If postpubertal females are vaccinated, counsel these women to avoid pregnancy for 3 months following vaccination.

Rubella—Natural rubella infection of the fetus may result in congenital rubella syndrome (CRS). There is evidence suggesting transmission of attenuated rubella virus to the fetus, although the vaccine is not known to cause fetal harm when administered to pregnant women. Nonetheless, do not intentionally give attenuated rubella vaccine to pregnant females. If postpubertal females are vaccinated, counsel these women to avoid pregnancy for 3 months following vaccination. It may be convenient to vaccinate rubella-susceptible women in the immediate postpartum period.

In counseling women who are inadvertently vaccinated when pregnant or who become pregnant within 3 months of vaccination, the following information may be useful. In a 10 year survey of >700 pregnant women who received rubella vaccine within 3 months before or after conception (of whom 189 received the Wistar RA 27/3 strain), none of the newborns had abnormalities compatible with congenital rubella syndrome.

Generally, most IgG passage across the placenta occurs during the third trimester.

Lactation: It is not known if attenuated measles virus or corresponding antibodies are excreted in breast milk. Problems in human mothers or children have not been documented.

It is not known if mumps virus or corresponding antibodies are excreted in breast milk. Problems in humans have not been documented.

Vaccine-strain rubella virus is secreted in milk and may be transmitted to infants in this manner. In the infants with serologic evidence of rubella infection, none exhibited severe disease. However, one exhibited mild clinical illness typical of acquired rubella.

Children: Trivalent MMR vaccine is safe and effective for children ≥12 months of age. Vaccination is not recommended for children <12 months of age since remaining maternal virus neutralizing antibody may interfere with the immune response. Trivalent MMR is the preferred agent for children and many adults.

Adverse Reactions:
MMR vaccine may cause burning or stinging of short duration at the injection site. One of the most common side effects is fever >39.4°C (103°F) 5 to 12 days after vaccination (5% to 15%). Symptoms of the same kind as seen following natural measles or rubella infection may occur after vaccination: Mild regional lymphadenopathy, urticaria, rash, malaise, sore throat, fever, headache, dizziness, nausea, vomiting, diarrhea, polyneuritis, arthralgia or arthritis (usually transient and rarely chronic). Local pain, induration and erythema may occur at the site of injection. Reactions are usually mild and transient. Moderate fever (38.3° to 39.4°C; 101° to 102.9°F) occurs occasionally; high fever (>39.4°C or 103°F) occurs less commonly.

Rarely, erythema multiforme has followed vaccination, as have allergic reactions at the injection site, urticaria, diarrhea, febrile and afebrile convulsions or seizures, thrombocytopenia and purpura and optic neuritis. Very rarely, encephalitis and encephalopathy have occurred within 30 days after measles vaccination, but no cause-and-effect relationship has been established. The risks of encephalitis and encephalopathy are far less after vaccination than after natural measles infection. A similar relationship has been seen between attenuated measles vaccine and risk of subacute sclerosing panencephalitis (SSPE).

Rarely, parotitis or orchitis may occur. In most of these cases, prior exposure to natural mumps was established.

Local reactions characterized by swelling, redness and vesiculation at the injection site and systemic reactions (including atypical measles), have occurred in persons who previously received killed measles vaccine. Rarely, more severe reactions requiring hospitalization, including prolonged high fevers, panniculitis and extensive local reactions, have occurred. There have been no published reports of transmission of attenuated measles virus from vaccinees to susceptible contacts.

Children under treatment for tuberculosis have not experienced exacerbation of that disease when immunized with attenuated measles vaccine. No studies have reported the effect of attenuated measles vaccine on untreated tuberculosis in children.

Isolated cases of polyneuropathy, including Guillain-Barré syndrome, have been reported after immunization with rubella-containing vaccines. Encephalitis and other nervous-system reactions have occurred very rarely in subjects given this vaccine, but a cause-and-effect relationship has not been established. In view of reported decreases in platelet counts, thrombocytopenic purpura is a theoretical hazard of rubella vaccination. Chronic arthritis is associated with natural rubella infection. Only rarely have vaccine recipients developed chronic joint symptoms, but an Institute of Medicine (IOM) report classified the association as consistent with a causal relation. Following vaccination in children, reactions in joints are uncommon (0% to 3%) and generally of brief duration. In adult women, incidence rates for arthritis and arthralgia are generally higher (12% to 20%) and the reactions tend to be more marked and of longer duration. Symptoms may persist for months or, on rare occasions, for years. In adolescent girls, the reactions appear to be intermediate in incidence between those seen in children and in adult women. Even in older women (35 to 45 years of age), these reactions are generally well tolerated and rarely interfere with normal activities. Myalgia and paresthesia have been reported rarely. Advise postpubertal females of the frequent occurrence of generally self-limited arthralgia or arthritis beginning 2 to 4 weeks after vaccination.

There have been no published reports of transmission of attenuated mumps virus from vaccinees to susceptible contacts.

Excretion of small amounts of attenuated rubella virus from the nose or throat has occurred in the majority of susceptible individuals 7 to 28 days after vaccination. There is no firm evidence that vaccine virus is transmitted to susceptible persons who are in contact with vaccinees. Transmission through close personal contact, while accepted as a theoretical possibility, is not considered a significant risk. However, transmission of attenuated rubella virus to infants through breast milk has been documented.

Pharmacologic & Dosing Characteristics

Dosage:

Vaccination: 0.5 ml, for both children and adults, preferably at 12 to 15 months of age. Trivalent MMR vaccine is the preferred product for most vaccinations. A booster dose is recommended under certain conditions.

In some other countries, measles vaccine is routinely administered at 9 months of age, even though seroconversion rates are lower than at ages 12 to 15 months. Revaccinate those children who were vaccinated against measles before their first birthday.

Minimum intervals between doses of the same vaccine: 4 weeks (except 6 weeks for OPV). Typically, 6 months should elapse before giving the final dose in a vaccine series. Do not count doses within the minimum interval, because too short an interval may interfere with antibody response and protection from disease. Increasing the interval beyond the recommended timing does not affect the ultimate efficacy of immunization, but waiting does delay achieving adequate protection from infection.

Route & Site: SC, preferably in the outer aspect of the upper arm, with a 25 gauge, $\frac{5}{8}$ inch needle. The 10 dose vial may be used with either syringe or jet injector.

Documentation Requirements: Federal law requires that (1) the manufacturer and lot number of this vaccine, (2) the date of its administration, and (3) the name, address and title of the person administering the vaccine be documented in the recipient's permanent medical record or in a permanent office log. Certain adverse events must be reported to the VAERS system, 1-800-822-7967.

Efficacy: Induces measles hemagglutination-inhibiting (HI) antibodies in 97%, mumps-neutralizing antibodies in 97%, and rubella HI antibodies in 97% of children. Seroconversion is somewhat less in adults. Disease incidence is typically reduced by 95% in family and classroom cohorts.

Onset: 2 to 6 weeks

Duration: Antibody levels persist ≥11 years in most recipients without substantial decline.

Drug Interactions: Reconstitute trivalent MMR vaccine with the diluent provided. Addition of a diluent with an antimicrobial preservative may inactivate the attenuated viruses.

Like all live viral vaccines, administration to patients receiving immunosuppressant drugs, including steroids, or radiation may predispose patients to disseminated infections or insufficient response to immunization. They may remain susceptible despite immunization.

To avoid inactivation of the attenuated virus, administer live virus vaccines at least 14 to 30 days before or 6 to 8 weeks after administration of any immune globulin or other blood product. Alternately, check antibody titers or repeat the vaccine dose 3 months after immune globulin administration. Base the interval on the dose of IgG administered: 3 months for 3 to 10 mg/kg, 4 months for 20 mg/kg, 5 months for 40 mg/kg, 6 months for 60 to 100 mg/kg, 7 months for 160 mg/kg, 8 months for 300 to 400 mg/kg, 10 months for 1 g/kg, 11 months for 2 g/kg (*CDC, 1994*).

To avoid the hypothetical concern over antigenic competition, administer measles vaccine after or not less than 1 month before administration of other virus vaccines, except those given simultaneously. Several routine vaccines may safely and effectively be administered simultaneously at separate injection sites (eg, DTP, MMR, OPV or e-IPV, Hib, hepatitis B, influenza). National authorities recommend simultaneous immunization at separate sites as indicated by age or health-risk, if return of a vaccine recipient for a subsequent visit is doubtful. Give two live vaccines simultaneously or wait at least 4 weeks between immunizations (does not apply to MMR-OPV or OPV-oral typhoid).

Live virus vaccines may cause delayed-hypersensitivity skin tests (eg, tuberculin, histoplasmin) to appear falsely negative. Evaluate such tests knowingly. The effect may persist for several weeks after vaccination. ACIP and AAP recommend that tuberculin tests be given prior to live-virus vaccination, simultaneously, or 6 or more weeks after vaccination.

Concurrent administration of a live-virus vaccine and an interferon product may inhibit antibody response to the vaccine, although this is poorly studied. Avoid concurrent use.

Concurrent immunization with measles vaccine and meningococcal polysaccharide vaccine resulted in a reduced seroconversion rate to meningococci in one study. If possible, separate these two vaccinations by 1 month or more for optimal response.

Anti-Rh₀ (D) immune globulin does not appear to impair rubella vaccine efficacy. Susceptible postpartum women who received blood products or anti-Rh₀ (D) immune globulin may receive attenuated rubella vaccine prior to discharge, provided that a repeat HI titer is drawn 6 to 8 weeks after vaccination to assure seroconversion.

Methacholine inhalation challenge may be falsely positive for a few days after influenza, measles or other immunization (but not after rubella vaccine). This effect appears to mimic the bronchospastic effect associated with acute respiratory infections. The effect has been observed in 44% to 90% of asthmatic patients, but apparently not among normal subjects.

Simultaneous administration of large doses of vitamin A impaired the response to Schwarz-strain measles vaccine in a group of Indonesian infants at 6 months of age (Semba et al, 1995).

Pharmaceutical Characteristics

Concentration: Not <1000 measles $TCID_{50}$, not <20,000 mumps $TCID_{50}$, and not <1000 rubella $TCID_{50}$ per 0.5 ml dose

Packaging: Single-dose package of separate vials of powder and diluent, box of 10 single-dose vial sets. Package for government agencies: 10 dose vial with 7 ml diluent

Dose Form: Powder for solution

Diluent for Reconstitution: Sterile water for injection without preservative

Storage/Stability: Store at 2° to 8°C (35° to 46°F). Freezing does not harm this vaccine, although diluent vials may crack. Store diluent at room temperature or in the refrigerator. Shipped at 10°C (50°F) or colder.

Protect vaccine from light. Contact manufacturer regarding prolonged exposure to room temperature or elevated temperatures. Reconstituted vaccine can tolerate 8 hours in the refrigerator.

Handling: Maintain jet injectors properly. Discard jet-injector vials at the end of each day.

Measles & Rubella Virus Vaccine Live

VIRAL VACCINES

NAME:

M-R-Vax II, ❦ *Moru-Viraten*

MANUFACTURER:

Merck Vaccine Division; ❦ Swiss Serum & Vaccine Institute

Synonym: MR vaccine. Do not use this abbreviation, to avoid confusion with mumps-rubella vaccine *(Biavax II)*.

This vaccine is a simple combination of its component vaccines. For complete descriptions, refer to each individual monograph.

Viability: Live, attenuated

Antigenic Form: Whole viruses

Antigenic Type: Protein

Note: Trivalent measles-mumps-rubella (MMR) vaccine is the preferred immunizing agent for most children and many adults.

Use Characteristics

Indications: Simultaneous active immunization against measles and rubella. The national rubella immunization program is intended to reduce the occurrence of congenital rubella syndrome (CRS) among offspring of women who contract rubella during pregnancy. Trivalent measles-mumps-rubella (MMR) vaccine is the preferred immunizing agent for most children and many adults. Almost all children and some adults need >1 dose of MMR vaccine.

Prior to international travel, give individuals known to be susceptible to measles, mumps or rubella either a single-antigen vaccine or a polyvalent vaccine, as appropriate. Trivalent MMR vaccine is preferred for persons likely to be susceptible to mumps and rubella. If single-antigen vaccines are not readily available, give travelers trivalent MMR regardless of their immune status to measles or rubella.

Contraindications:

Absolute: Pregnant patients, patients with a personal history of hypersensitivity reactions to this vaccine or any of its components (eg, eggs), patients receiving immunosuppressive therapy, patients with a blood dyscrasia, leukemia, lymphoma of any type, or other malignant neoplasms affecting the bone marrow or lymphatic systems, persons with primary or acquired immunodeficiency, any febrile illness or infection, active untreated tuberculosis, and persons with a family history of congenital or hereditary immunodeficiency, until the immune competence of the potential vaccine recipient is demonstrated. Refer to individual monographs for details.

Do not vaccinate persons who are immunosuppressed in association with AIDS or other clinical manifestations of infection with HIV, cellular immune deficiencies, and hypogammaglobulinemic and dysgammaglobulinemic states. Nonetheless, vaccinate asymptomatic children with HIV infection.

Do not vaccinate persons with a history of anaphylactoid or other immediate reactions (eg, hives, swelling of the mouth or throat, difficulty breathing, hypotension, shock) following egg ingestion. Skin test persons suspected of being hypersensitive to egg protein, using a dilution of the vaccine as the antigen. Refer to the Introduction section. Do not vaccinate persons with adverse reactions to such testing. Persons are apparently not at risk if they have egg allergies that are not anaphylactoid in nature. Vaccinate such persons in the usual manner. There is no evidence that persons with allergies to chickens or feathers are at increased risk of reaction to the vaccine.

Relative: Defer immunization during the course of any acute illness.

Elderly: Most persons born in 1956 or earlier are likely to have been infected naturally and generally are considered not susceptible.

Adults: Vaccinate persons born more recently than 1956, unless they have a personal contraindication to vaccination, since they are considered susceptible. Vaccinate persons who may be immune but who lack adequate documentation of immunity as evidenced by physician diagnosis, laboratory evidence of immunity, or adequate immunization with live vaccine on or after the first birthday.

Pregnancy: *Category C*. Contraindicated. Measles—Contracting natural measles during pregnancy enhances fetal risk. There are no adequate studies of attenuated measles vaccine in pregnant females. Do not intentionally give measles vaccine to pregnant females, since the possible effects of the vaccine on fetal development are unknown at this time. If postpubertal females are vaccinated, counsel these women to avoid pregnancy for 3 months following vaccination. It is not known if attenuated measles virus or corresponding antibodies cross the placenta.

Rubella—Natural rubella infection of the fetus may result in congenital rubella syndrome (CRS). There is evidence suggesting transmission of attenuated rubella virus to the fetus, although the vaccine is not known to cause fetal harm when administered to pregnant women. Nonetheless, do not intentionally give attenuated rubella vaccine to pregnant females. If postpubertal females are vaccinated, counsel these women to avoid pregnancy for 3 months following vaccination. It may be convenient to vaccinate rubella-susceptible women in the immediate postpartum period.

In counseling women who are inadvertently vaccinated when pregnant or who become pregnant within 3 months of vaccination, the following information may be useful. In a 10 year survey of >700 pregnant women who received rubella vaccine within 3 months before or after conception (of whom 189 received the current RA 27/3 strain), none of the newborns had abnormalities compatible with congenital rubella syndrome.

Generally, most IgG passage across the placenta occurs during the third trimester.

Lactation: It is not known if attenuated measles virus or corresponding antibodies are excreted in breast milk. Problems in human mothers or children have not been documented.

Vaccine-strain rubella virus is secreted in milk and may be transmitted to infants in this manner. In the infants with serologic evidence of rubella infection, none exhibited severe disease. However, one exhibited mild clinical illness typical of acquired rubella.

Children: Safe and effective for children ≥12 months of age. Vaccination is not recommended for children <12 months of age since remaining maternal virus-neutralizing antibody may interfere with the immune response. Trivalent MMR vaccine is the preferred agent for children and many adults.

Adverse Reactions:

Burning or stinging of short duration at the injection site have occurred. Symptoms of the same kind as seen following natural measles or rubella infection may occur after vaccination: Mild regional lymphadenopathy, urticaria, rash, malaise, sore throat, fever, headache, dizziness, nausea, vomiting, diarrhea, polyneuritis, and arthralgia or arthritis (usually transient and rarely chronic). Local pain, induration and erythema may occur at the site of injection. Reactions are usually mild and transient. Moderate fever (38.3° to 39.4°C; 101° to 102.9°F) occurs occasionally; high fever (>39.4°C or 103°F) occurs less commonly.

Rarely, erythema multiforme has followed vaccination, as have allergic reactions at the injection site, urticaria, diarrhea, febrile and afebrile convulsions or seizures, thrombocytopenia and purpura, optic neuritis. Very rarely, encephalitis and encephalopathy have occurred within 30 days after measles vaccination, but no cause-and-effect relationship has been established. The risks of encephalitis and encephalopathy are far less after vaccination than after natural measles infection. A similar relationship has been seen between attenuated measles vaccine and risk of subacute sclerosing panencephalitis (SSPE).

Local reactions characterized by swelling, redness and vesiculation at the injection site and systemic reactions (including atypical measles), have occurred in persons who previously received killed measles vaccine. Rarely, more severe reactions requiring hospitalization, including prolonged high fevers, panniculitis and extensive local reactions, have been reported. There have been no published reports of transmission of attenuated measles virus from vaccinees to susceptible contacts.

Children under treatment for tuberculosis have not experienced exacerbation of that disease when immunized with attenuated measles vaccine. No studies have reported the effect of attenuated measles vaccine on untreated tuberculosis in children.

Isolated cases of polyneuropathy, including Guillain-Barré syndrome, have been reported after immunization with rubella-containing vaccines.

Encephalitis and other nervous-system reactions have occurred very rarely in subjects given this vaccine, but a cause-and-effect relationship has not been established. In view of reported decreases in platelet counts, thrombocytopenic purpura is a theoretical hazard of rubella vaccination. Chronic arthritis has been associated with natural rubella infection. Only rarely have vaccine recipients developed chronic joint symptoms, but an Institute of Medicine (IOM) report classified the association as consistent with a causal relation. Following vaccination in children, reactions in joints are uncommon (0% to 3%) and generally of brief duration. In adult women, incidence rates for arthritis and arthralgia are generally higher (12% to 20%) and the reactions tend to be more marked and of longer duration. Symptoms may persist for months or, on rare occasions, for years.

In adolescent girls, the reactions appear to be intermediate in incidence between those seen in children and in adult women. Even in older women (35 to 45 years of age), these reactions are generally well tolerated and rarely interfere with normal activities. Myalgia and paresthesia have been reported rarely. Advise postpubertal females of the frequent occurrence of generally self-limited arthralgia or arthritis beginning to 4 weeks after vaccination.

Excretion of small amounts of attenuated rubella virus from the nose or throat has occurred in the majority of susceptible individuals 7 to 28 days after vaccination. There is no firm evidence that such virus is transmitted to susceptible persons in contact with vaccinees. Transmission through close personal contact, while accepted as a theoretical possibility, is not regarded as a significant risk. However, transmission of attenuated rubella virus to infants through breast milk has been documented.

Pharmacologic & Dosing Characteristics

Dosage:

Vaccination: 0.5 ml, for both children and adults, preferably at 12 to 15 months of age. Trivalent MMR vaccine is the preferred product for most vaccinations. A booster dose is recommended under certain conditions.

In some other countries, measles vaccine is routinely administered at 9 months of age, even though seroconversion rates are lower than at ages 12 to 15 months. Revaccinate those children who were vaccinated against measles before their first birthday.

Minimum intervals between doses of the same vaccine: 4 weeks (except 6 weeks for OPV). Typically, 6 months should elapse before giving the final dose in a vaccine series. Do not count doses within the minimum interval, because too short an interval may interfere with antibody response and protection from disease. Increasing the interval beyond the recommended timing does not affect the ultimate efficacy of immunization, but waiting does delay achieving adequate protection from infection.

Route & Site: SC, preferably in the outer aspect of the upper arm, with a 25 gauge, $\frac{5}{8}$ inch needle. The 10 dose vial may be used with either syringe or jet injector. Use the 50 dose vial by jet injection only.

To avoid inactivation of the attenuated virus, administer live virus vaccines ar least 14 to 30 days before or 6 to 8 weeks after administration of any immune globulin or other blood product. Alternately, check antibody titers or repeat the vaccine dose 3 months after IG administration. Base the interval on the dose of IgG administered: 3 months for 3 to 10 mg/kg, 4 months for 20 mg/kg, 5 months for 40 mg/kg, 6 months for 60 to 100 mg/kg, 7 months for 160 mg/kg, 8 months for 300 to 400 mg/kg, 10 months for 1 g/kg, 11 months for 2 mg/kg (*CDC, 1994*).

Several routine pediatric vaccines may safely and effectively be administered simultaneously at separate injection sites (eg, DTP, MMR, OPV or e-IPV, Hib, hepatitis B, influenza).

Simultaneous administration of large doses of vitamin A impaired the response to Schwarz-strain measles vaccine in a group of Indonesian infants at 6 months of age (Semba et al, 1995).

Documentation Requirements:: Federal law requires that (1) the manufacturer and lot number of this vaccine, (2) the date of its administration, and (3) the name, address and title of the person administering the vaccine be documented in the recipient's permanent medical record or in a permanent office log. Certain adverse events must be reported to the VAERS system, 1-800-822-7967.

Efficacy: Induces measles and rubella hemagglutination-inhibiting (HI) antibodies in 97% of children. Seroconversion is somewhat less in adults. Disease incidence is typically reduced by 95% in family and classroom cohorts.

Onset: 2 to 6 weeks

Duration: Antibody levels persist ≥11 years in most recipients without substantial decline.

Drug Interactions: Reconstitute MMR vaccine with the diluent provided. Addition of a diluent with an antimicrobial preservative may inactivate the attenuated viruses.

Like all live viral vaccines, administration of this vaccine to patients receiving immunosuppressant drugs, including steroids, or radiation may predispose patients to disseminated infections or insufficient response to immunization. They may remain susceptible despite immunization. To avoid inactivation of the attenuated virus, administer live virus vaccines at least 14 to 30 days before or 6 to 8 weeks after administration of any immune globulin or other blood product. Alternately, check antibody titers or repeat the vaccine dose 3 months after IG administration. *Siber et al (1993)* recommend basing the interval on the dose of IgG administered.

To avoid the hypothetical concern over antigenic competition, administer measles vaccine after or ≥1 month before administration of other virus vaccines, except those given simultaneously. Several routine vaccines may safely and effectively be administered simultaneously at separate injection sites (eg, DTP, MMR, OPV or e-IPV, Hib, hepatitis B). National authorities recommend simultaneous immunization at separate sites as indicated by age or health-risk, if return of a vaccine recipient for a subsequent visit is doubtful. Give two live vaccines simultaneously or wait at least 4 weeks between immunizations (does not apply to MMR-OPV or OPV-oral typhoid).

Live virus vaccines may cause delayed-hypersensitivity skin tests (eg, tuberculin, histoplasmin) to appear falsely negative. Evaluate such tests knowingly. The effect may persist several weeks after vaccination. ACIP and AAP recommend that tuberculin tests be given prior to live-virus vaccination, simultaneously with it, or 6 or more weeks after vaccination.

Concurrent administration a live-virus vaccine and an interferon product may inhibit antibody response to the vaccine, although this is poorly studied. Avoid concurrent use.

Concurrent immunization with measles vaccine and meningococcal polysaccharide vaccine resulted in a reduced seroconversion rate to meningococci in one study. If possible, separate these two vaccinations by ≥1 month.

Anti-Rh$_0$ (D) immune globulin does not appear to impair rubella vaccine efficacy. Susceptible postpartum women who received blood products or anti-Rh$_0$ (D) immune globulin may receive attenuated rubella vaccine prior to discharge, provided that a repeat HI titer is drawn 6 to 8 weeks after vaccination to assure seroconversion.

Methacholine inhalation challenge may be falsely positive for a few days after influenza, measles or other immunization (but not after rubella vaccine). This effect appears to mimic thebronchospastic effect associated with acute respiratory infections. The effect has been observed in 44% to 90% of asthmatic patients, but apparently not among normal subjects.

Pharmaceutical Characteristics

Concentration: Not less than 1000 measles TCID$_{50}$ and not less than 1000 rubella TCID$_{50}$ per 0.5 ml dose

Packaging: Single-dose package of separate vials of powder and diluent, box of 10 single-dose packages. Packages for government agencies: 10 dose vial with 7 ml diluent, 50 dose vial with 30 ml diluent for jet injection only.

Dose Form: Powder for solution

Diluent for Reconstitution: Sterile water for injection without preservative.

Storage/Stability: Store at 2° to 8°C (35° to 46°F). Freezing does not affect this vaccine, although diluent vials may crack. Store diluent at room temperature or in the refrigerator. Shipped at ≤10°C (50°F). Protect vaccine from light. Contact manufacturer regarding prolonged exposure to room temperature or elevated temperatures. Reconstituted vaccine can tolerate 8 hours if stored in a refrigerator.

Handling: Maintain jet injectors properly to prevent blood-borne diseases. Discard jet-injector vials at the end of each day.

Mumps & Rubella Virus Vaccine Live
VIRAL VACCINES

NAME:
Biavax II

MANUFACTURER:
Merck Vaccine Division

Synonym: MR usually, but not always, refers to measles-rubella vaccine (*M-R-Vax II*). Do not use this abbreviation, to avoid confusion with measles-rubella vaccine.

> This vaccine is a simple combination of its component vaccines. For complete descriptions, refer to each individual monograph.

Viability: Live, attenuated
Antigenic Form: Whole viruses

Antigenic Type: Protein

> NOTE: Trivalent measles-mumps-rubella (MMR) vaccine is the preferred immunizing agent for most children and many adults.

Use Characteristics

Indications: Simultaneous, selective active immunization against mumps and rubella. The national rubella immunization program is intended to reduce the occurrence of congenital rubella syndrome (CRS) among offspring of women who contract rubella during pregnancy. Trivalent measles-mumps-rubella (MMR) vaccine is the preferred immunizing agent for most children and many adults. Almost all children and some adults need >1 dose of MMR vaccine.

Prior to international travel, give individuals known to be susceptible to measles, mumps or rubella either a single-antigen vaccine or a polyvalent vaccine, as appropriate. Trivalent MMR vaccine is preferred for persons likely to be susceptible to mumps and rubella. If single-antigen vaccines are not readily available, give travelers triva-

lent MMR regardless of their immune status to mumps or rubella.

Contraindications:
Absolute: Pregnant patients, patients with a personal history of a hypersensitivity reaction to this vaccine or any of its components (eg, eggs), patients receiving immunosuppressive therapy, patients with a blood dyscrasias, leukemia, lymphoma of any type, or other malignant neoplasms affecting the bone marrow or lymphatic systems, patients with primary or acquired immunodeficiency, any febrile illness or infection, active untreated tuberculosis, and persons with a family history of congenital or hereditary immunodeficiency, until the immune competence of the potential vaccine recipient is demonstrated. Refer to individual monographs for details.

Do not vaccinate persons who are immunosuppressed in association with AIDS or other clinical manifestations of infection with HIV, cellular immune deficiencies, and hypogammaglobulinemic and dysgammaglobulinemic states.

Nonetheless, vaccinate asymptomatic children with HIV infection.

Do not vaccinate persons with a history of anaphylactoid or other immediate reactions (eg, hives, swelling of the mouth or throat, difficulty breathing, hypotension, shock) following egg ingestion. Skin test persons suspected of being hypersensitive to egg protein, using a dilution of the vaccine as the antigen. Refer to the Introduction section. Do not vaccinate persons with adverse reactions to such testing. Persons are apparently not at risk if they have egg allergies that are not anaphylactoid in nature; vaccinate such persons in the usual manner. There is no evidence that persons with allergies to chickens or feathers are at increased risk of reaction to the vaccine.

Relative: Defer immunization during the course of any acute illness.

Elderly: Most persons born in 1956 or earlier are likely to have been infected naturally and generally are considered not susceptible.

Adults: Vaccinate persons born more recently than 1956, unless they have a personal contraindication to vaccination, since they are considered susceptible. Vaccinate persons who may be immune but who lack adequate documentation of immunity as evidenced by physician diagnosis, laboratory evidence of immunity, or adequate immunization with live vaccine on or after the first birthday.

Pregnancy: *Category* C. Contraindicated. Mumps—Although mumps virus can infect the placenta and fetus, there is no good evidence that it causes congenital malformations in humans. Attenuated mumps vaccine virus can infect the placenta, but the virus has not been isolated from fetal tissues of susceptible women who were vaccinated and underwent elective abortions. Nonetheless, do not intentionally give attenuated mumps vaccine to pregnant females. If postpubertal females are vaccinated, counsel these women to avoid pregnancy for 3 months following vaccination.

Rubella—Natural rubella infection of the fetus may result in congenital rubella syndrome (CRS). There is evidence suggesting transmission of attenuated rubella virus to the fetus, although the vaccine is not known to cause fetal harm when administered to pregnant women. Nonetheless, do not intentionally give attenuated rubella vaccine to pregnant females. If postpubertal females are vaccinated, counsel these women to avoid pregnancy for 3 months following vaccination. It may be convenient to vaccinate rubella-susceptible women in the immediate postpartum period.

In counseling women who are inadvertently vaccinated when pregnant or who become pregnant within 3 months of vaccination, the following information may be useful. In a 10 year survey of >700 pregnant women who received rubella vaccine within 3 months before or after conception (of whom 189 received the current RA 27/3 strain), none of the newborns had abnormalities compatible with congenital rubella syndrome.

Generally, most IgG passage across the placenta occurs during the third trimester.

Lactation: It is not known if mumps virus or corresponding antibodies are excreted in breast milk. Problems in humans have not been documented.

Vaccine-strain rubella virus is secreted in milk and may be transmitted to infants in this manner. In the infants with serologic evidence of rubella infection, none exhibited severe disease. However, one exhibited mild clinical illness typical of acquired rubella.

Children: Safe and effective for children ≥12 months of age. Vaccination is not recommended for children <12 months of age since remaining maternal virus neutralizing antibody may interfere with the immune response. Trivalent MMR vaccine is the preferred agent for children and many adults.

Adverse Reactions:

Burning or stinging of short duration at the injection site has occurred. Symptoms of the same kind as seen following natural mumps or rubella infection may occur after vaccination: Mild regional lymphadenopathy, urticaria, rash, malaise, sore throat, fever, headache, dizziness, nausea, vomiting, diarrhea, polyneuritis, arthralgia or arthritis (usually transient and rarely chronic). Local pain, induration and erythema may occur at the site of injection. Reactions are usually mild and transient. Moderate fever (38.3° to 39.4°C; 101° to 102.9°F) occurs occasionally; high fever (>39.4°C or 103°F) occurs less commonly.

Erythema multiforme occurs rarely following both mumps and rubella vaccination, as does optic neuritis. Rarely, parotitis or orchitis may occur. In most of these cases, prior exposure to natural mumps was established.

Isolated cases of polyneuropathy, including Guillain-Barré syndrome, have been reported after immunization with rubella-containing vaccines.

Encephalitis and other nervous-system reactions have occurred very rarely in subjects given this vaccine, but a cause-effect relationship has not been established. In view of reported decreases in platelet counts, thrombocytopenic purpura is a theoretical hazard of rubella vaccination. Chronic arthritis has been associated with natural rubella infection. Only rarely have vaccine recipients developed chronic joint symptoms, but an Institute of Medicine (IOM) report classified the association as consistent with a causal relation. Following vaccination in children, reactions in joints are uncommon (0% to 3%) and generally of brief duration. In adult women, incidence rates for arthritis and arthralgia are generally higher (12% to 20%) and the reactions tend to be more marked and of longer duration. Symptoms may persist for months or, on rare occasions, for years.

In adolescent girls, the reactions appear to be intermediate in incidence between those seen in children and in adult women. Even in older women (35 to 45 years of age), these reactions are generally well tolerated and rarely interfere with normal activities. Myalgia and paresthesia have been reported rarely. Advise postpubertal females of the frequent occurrence of generally self-limited arthralgia or arthritis beginning 2 to 4 weeks after vaccination. There have been no published reports of transmission of attenuated mumps virus from vaccinees to susceptible contacts.

Excretion of small amounts of attenuated rubella virus from the nose or throat has occurred in the majority of susceptible individuals 7 to 28 days after vaccination. There is no firm evidence that such virus is transmitted to susceptible persons in contact with vaccinees. Transmission through close personal contact, while accepted as a theoretical possibility, is not regarded as a significant risk. However, transmission of attenuated rubella virus to infants through breast milk has been documented.

Pharmacologic & Dosing Characteristics

Dosage:

Vaccination: 0.5 ml for children and adults, preferably at 12 to 15 months of age. Trivalent MMR vaccine is the preferred product for most vaccinations.

Minimum intervals between doses of the same vaccine: 4 weeks (except 6 weeks for OPV). Typically, 6 months should elapse before giving the final dose in a vaccine series. Do not count doses within the minimum interval, because too short an interval may interfere with antibody response and protection from disease. Increasing the interval beyond the recommended timing does not affect the ultimate efficacy of immunization, but waiting does delay achieving adequate protection from infection.

Give a booster dose under certain conditions.

Route & Site: SC, preferably in the outer aspect of the upper arm, with a 25 gauge, $^5/_8$ inch needle.

Although not labeled for this route, this product can probably be given safely and effectively by jet injection. Each of its component vaccines can be so given, as can trivalent MMR vaccine.

Documentation Requirements: Federal law requires that (1) the manufacturer and lot number of this vaccine, (2) the date of its administration, and (3) the name, address and title of the person administering the vaccine be documented in the recipient's permanent medical record or in a permanent office log. Certain adverse events must be reported to the VAERS system, 1-800-822-7967.

Efficacy: Induces mumps-neutralizing antibodies and rubella hemagglutination-inhibiting antibodies in 97% of children. Seroconversion is somewhat less in adults. Disease incidence is typically reduced by 95% in family and classroom cohorts.

Onset: 2 to 6 weeks

Duration: Antibody levels induced with the original Biavax formula persisted 10 years or longer in most recipients. *Biavax II* is expected to perform similarly.

Drug Interactions: Reconstitute mumps-rubella vaccine with the diluent provided. Addition of a diluent with an antimicrobial preservative may inactivate the attenuated vaccine.

Like all live viral vaccines, administration to patients receiving immunosuppressant drugs, including steroids, or radiation may predispose patients to disseminated infections or insufficient response to immunization. They may remain susceptible despite immunization.

To avoid inactivation of the attenuated virus, administer live virus vaccines at least 14 to 30 days before or 6 to 8 weeks after administration of any immune globulin or other blood product. Alternately, check antibody titers or repeat the vaccine dose 3 months after IG administration. Base the interval on the dose of IgG administered: 3 months for 3 to 10 mg/kg, 4 months for 20 mg/kg, 5 months for 40 mg/kg, 6 months for 60 to 100 mg/kg, 7 months for 160 mg/kg, 8 months for 300 to 400 mg/kg, 10 months for 1 g/kg, 11 months for 2 g/kg (*CDC, 1994*).

Several routine vaccines may safely and effectively be administered simultaneously at separate injection sites (eg, DTP, MMR, OPV or e-IPV, Hib, hepatitis B, influenza). National authorities recommend simultaneous immunization at separate sites as indicated by age or health-risk, if return of a vaccine recipient for a subsequent visit is doubtful. Give two live vaccines simultaneously or wait at least 4 weeks between immunizations (does not apply to MMR-OPV or OPV-oral typhoid).

Live virus vaccines may cause delayed-hypersensitivity skin tests (eg, tuberculin, histoplasmin) to appear falsely negative. The effect may persist for several weeks after vaccination. ACIP and AAP recommend that tuberculin tests be given prior to live-virus vaccination, simultaneously with it, or 6 or more weeks after vaccination.

Concurrent administration of a live-virus vaccine and an interferon product may inhibit antibody response to the vaccine, although this is poorly studied. Avoid concurrent use.

Anti-Rh$_o$(D) immune globulin does not appear to impair rubella vaccine efficacy. Susceptible postpartum women who received blood products or anti-Rh$_o$(D) immune globulin may receive attenuated rubella vaccine prior to discharge, provided that a repeat HI titer is drawn 6 to 8 weeks after vaccination to assure seroconversion.

Pharmaceutical Characteristics

Concentration: Not less than 20,000 mumps TCID$_{50}$ and not less than 1000 rubella TCID$_{50}$ per 0.5 ml dose

Packaging: Single-dose package of separate vials of powder and diluent, box of 10 single-dose vial sets

Dose Form: Powder for solution

Diluent for Reconstitution: Sterile water for injection without preservative

Storage/Stability: Store at 2° to 8°C (35° to 46°F). Freezing does not harm this product, although diluent vials may crack. Store diluent at room temperature or in the refrigerator. Shipped at ≤10°C (50°F).

Protect vaccine from light. Contact manufacturer regarding prolonged exposure to room temperature or elevated temperatures.

Reconstituted vaccine can tolerate 8 hours in the refrigerator.

Measles Virus Vaccine Live
VIRAL VACCINES

NAME:
Attenuvax, Generic

MANUFACTURER:
Attenuvax, Merck Vaccine Division;
🍁 Generic, Connaught-Canada

Synonyms: Measles is also known as rubeola, hard measles, red measles and morbilli. Do not use the term rubeola, to avoid confusion with rubella (which is also called German measles, another source of confusion).

Viability: Live, attenuated
Antigenic Form: Whole virus

Antigenic Type: Protein

Note: Trivalent measles-mumps-rubella (MMR) vaccine is the preferred immunizing agent for most children and many adults.

Use Characteristics

Indications: Selective induction of active immunity against measles. Trivalent measles-mumps-rubella (MMR) vaccine is the preferred immunizing agent for most children and many adults. Almost all children and some adults need >1 dose of MMR.

Prior to international travel, give individuals known to be susceptible to measles, mumps or rubella either a single-antigen vaccine or a polyvalent vaccine, as appropriate. Trivalent MMR vaccine is preferred for persons likely to be susceptible to mumps and rubella. If single-antigen vaccines are not readily available, give travelers trivalent MMR regardless of their immune status to mumps or rubella.

Contraindications:

STOP

Absolute: Pregnant patients, patients with a personal history of a hypersensitivity reaction to this vaccine or any of its components (eg, eggs), patients receiving immunosuppressive therapy, patients with a blood dyscrasia, leukemia, lymphoma of any type, or other malignant neoplasms affecting the bone marrow or lymphatic systems, patients with primary or acquired immunodeficiency, active untreated tuberculosis, and persons with a family history of congenital or hereditary immunodeficiency, until the immune competence of the potential vaccine recipient is demonstrated.

Do not vaccinate persons who are immunosuppressed in association with AIDS or other clinical manifestations of infection with HIV, cellular immune deficiencies, and hypogammaglobulinemic and dysgammaglobulinemic states. Nonetheless, ACIP and AAP recommend that asymptomatic children with HIV infection be vaccinated.

Do not vaccinate persons with a history of anaphylactoid or other immediate reactions (eg, hives, swelling of the mouth or throat, difficulty breathing, hypotension, shock) following ingestion of eggs. Skin test persons suspect ed of being hypersensitive to egg protein, using a dilution of the vaccine as the antigen. Refer to the Introduction section. Do not vaccinate persons with adverse reactions to such testing. Persons are apparently not at risk if they have egg allergies that are not anaphylactoid in nature; vaccinate such persons in the usual manner. There is no evidence that persons with allergies to chickens or feathers are at increased risk of reaction to the vaccine.

Relative: Defer immunization during the course of any acute illness.

Elderly: Most persons born in 1956 or earlier are likely to have been infected naturally and generally are considered not susceptible.

Adults: Vaccinate persons born more recently than 1956, unless they have a personal contraindication to vaccination, since they are considered susceptible. Vaccinate persons who may be immune but who lack adequate documentation of immunity as evidenced by physician diagnosis, laboratory evidence of immunity, or adequate immunization with live vaccine on or after the first birthday.

Pregnancy: *Category C.* Contraindicated. Contracting natural measles during pregnancy enhances fetal risk. There are no adequate studies of attenuated measles vaccine in pregnant females. Do not intentionally give measles vaccine to pregnant females, since the possible effects of the vaccine on fetal development are unknown at this time. If postpubertal females are vaccinated, counsel these women to avoid pregnancy for 3 months following vaccination. It is not known if attenuated measles virus or corresponding antibodies cross the placenta. Generally, most IgG passage across the placenta occurs during the third trimester.

Lactation: It is not known if attenuated measles virus or corresponding antibodies are excreted in breast milk. Problems in human mothers or children have not been documented.

Children: Attenuated measles vaccine is safe and effective in persons ≥12 months of age. Younger persons may fail to respond due to circulating residual measles antibodies passively transferred from the child's mother. Revaccinate infants vaccinated when <12 months of age after they reach 15 months of age. There is evidence to suggest that infants immunized when <1 year old may not develop sustained antibody levels when later reimmunized. Weigh the advantage of early protection against the chance for failure to respond adequately on reimmunization. Trivalent MMR vaccine is the preferred agent for children and many adults.

Adverse Reactions: Burning or stinging of short duration at the injection site have occurred. Occasional reactions include moderate fever (38.3° to 39.4°C, 101° to 102.9°F), fever, or rash (commonly appearing between the fifth and twelfth days after vaccination). Less common effects include high fever (>39.4°C; >103°F) or mild lymphadenopathy.

Rarely, erythema multiforme has followed vaccination, as have allergic reactions at the injection site, urticaria, diarrhea, febrile and afebrile convulsions or seizures, thrombocytopenia and purpura, and optic neuritis. Very rarely, encephalitis and encephalopathy have occurred within 30 days after measles vaccination, but no cause-and-effect relationship has been established. The risks of encephalitis and encephalopathy are far greater after natural measles infection than after vaccination. A similar relationship exists between attenuated measles vaccine and subacute sclerosing panencephalitis (SSPE).

Local reactions characterized by swelling, redness and vesiculation at the injection site and systemic reactions (including atypical measles), have occurred in persons who previously received killed measles vaccine. Rarely, more severe reactions requiring hospitalization, including prolonged high fevers, panniculitis and extensive local reactions, have been reported. There have been no published reports of transmission of attenuated measles virus from vaccinees to susceptible contacts.

Children under treatment for tuberculosis have not experienced exacerbation of that disease when immunized with attenuated measles vaccine. No studies have reported the effect of attenuated measles vaccine on untreated tuberculosis in children.

Pharmacologic & Dosing Characteristics

Dosage:

Vaccination: 0.5 ml, for both children and adults, preferably at 12 to 15 months of age. Trivalent MMR vaccine is the preferred product for most vaccinations.

In some other countries, measles vaccine is routinely administered at 9 months of age, even though seroconversion rates are lower than at ages 12 to 15 months. Revaccinate those children who were vaccinated against measles before their first birthday.

Minimum intervals between doses of the same vaccine: 4 weeks (except 6 weeks for OPV). Typically, 6 months should elapse before giving the final dose in a vaccine series. Do not count doses within the minimum interval, because too short an interval may interfere with antibody response and protection from disease. Increasing the interval beyond the recommended timing does not affect the ultimate efficacy of immunization, but waiting does delay achieving adequate protection from infection.

Route & Site: SC, preferably in the outer aspect of the upper arm, with a 25 gauge, $\frac{5}{8}$ inch needle. The 10 dose vial may be used with either syringe or jet injector. Use the 50 dose vial by jet injection only. Do not inject IV.

Documentation Requirements: Federal law requires that (1) the manufacturer and lot number of this vaccine, (2) the date of its administration, and (3) the name, address and title of the person administering the vaccine be documented in the recipient's permanent medical record or in a permanent office log. Certain adverse events must be reported to the VAERS system, 1-800-822-7967.

Efficacy: Induces hemagglutination-inhibiting (HI) antibodies in at least 97% of susceptible recipients. Seroconversion is somewhat less in adults. Disease incidence is typically reduced by 95% in family and classroom cohorts.

Onset: 2 to 3 weeks

Duration: Antibody levels persist ≥13 years in most recipients without substantial decline.

Drug Interactions: Reconstitute measles vaccine with the diluent provided. Addition of a diluent with an antimicrobial preservative may inactivate the attenuated viruses.

Like all live viral vaccines, administration of this vaccine to patients receiving immunosuppressant drugs, including steroids, or radiation may predispose patients to disseminated infections or insufficient response to immunization. They may remain susceptible despite immunization.

To avoid inactivation of the attenuated virus, administer live virus vaccines at least 14 to 30 days before or 6 to 8 weeks after administration of any immune globulin or other blood product. Alternately, check antibody titers or repeat the vaccine dose 3 months after immune globulin administration. Base the interval on the dose of IgG administered: 3 months for 3 to 10 mg/kg, 4 months for 20 mg/kg, 5 months for 40 mg/kg, 6 months for 60 to 100 mg/kg, 7 months for 160 mg/kg, 8 months for 300 to 400 mg/kg, 10 months for 1 g/kg, 11 months for 2 g/kg (CDC, 1994).

To avoid the hypothetical concern over antigenic competition, administer measles vaccine after or ≥1 month before administration of other virus vaccines, except those given simultaneously. Several routine vaccines may safely and effectively be administered simultaneously at separate injection sites (eg, DTP, MMR, OPV or e-IPV, Hib, hepatitis B). National authorities recommend simultaneous immunization at separate sites as indicated by age or health-risk, if return of a vaccine recipient for a subsequent visit is doubtful. Give two live vaccines simultaneously or wait at least 4 weeks between immunizations (does not apply to MMR-OPV or OPV-oral typhoid).

Live virus vaccines may cause delayed-hypersensitivity skin tests (eg, tuberculin, histoplasmin) to appear falsely negative. Evaluate such tests knowingly. The effect may persist for several weeks after vaccination. ACIP and AAP recommend that tuberculin tests be given prior to live-virus vaccination, simultaneously or 6 or more weeks after vaccination.

Concurrent administration of a live-virus vaccine and an interferon product may inhibit antibody response to the vaccine, although this is poorly studied. Avoid concurrent use.

Concurrent immunization with measles vaccine and meningococcal polysaccharide vaccine resulted in a reduced seroconversion rate to meningococci in one study. If possible, separate these two vaccinations by ≥1 month.

Methacholine inhalation challenge may be falsely positive for a few days after influenza, measles or other immunization. This effect appears to mimic the bronchospastic effect associated with acute respiratory infections. The effect has been observed in 44% to 90% of asthmatic patients, but apparently not among normal subjects.

Simultaneous administration of large doses of vitamin A impaired the response to Schwarz-strain measles vaccine in a group of Indonesian infants at 6 months of age (Semba et al, 1995).

Pharmaceutical Characteristics

Concentration: Not less than 1000 $TCID_{50}$ per 0.5 ml dose

Packaging: Single-dose package of separate vials of vaccine powder and diluent, package of 10 single-dose vial sets. Packages available to government agencies: 10 dose multidose vial with 7 ml diluent, 50 dose multidose vial with 30 ml diluent for jet injection only.

Dose Form: Powder for solution

Diluent for Reconstitution: Sterile water for injection without preservative

Storage/Stability: Store at 2° to 8°C (35° to 46°F). Freezing does not harm the vaccine, but may crack diluent vials. Store diluent at room temperature or in the refrigerator. Shipped at 10°C (50°F) or colder. Protect vaccine from light. Vaccine powder can tolerate 7 days at room temperature.

Reconstituted vaccine can tolerate 8 hours in the refrigerator.

Handling: Maintain jet injectors properly. Discard jet-injector vials at the end of each day.

Mumps Virus Vaccine Live

VIRAL VACCINES

NAME:
Mumpsvax

MANUFACTURER:
Merck Vaccine Division, ❦ Merck Frost

Synonym: The disease is also known as parotitis.

Viability: Live, attenuated

Antigenic Form: Whole virus

Antigenic Type: Protein

> Trivalent measles–mumps–rubella (MMR) vaccine is the preferred immunizing agent for most children and many adults.

Use Characteristics

Indications: Selective active immunization against mumps. Prior to international travel, give individuals known to be susceptible to measles, mumps or rubella either a single-antigen vaccine or a polyvalent vaccine, as appropriate. Trivalent measles-mumps-rubella (MMR) vaccine is preferred for persons likely to be susceptible to mumps and rubella.

Almost all children and some adults need >1 dose of MMR vaccine. If single-antigen vaccines are not readily available, give travelers trivalent MMR regardless of their immune status to mumps or rubella.

Contraindications:

Absolute: Pregnant patients and patients with a personal history of a hypersensitivity reaction to this vaccine or any of its components (eg, eggs). Patients receiving immunosuppressive therapy, patients with a blood dyscrasia, leukemia, lymphoma of any type, or other malignant neoplasms affecting the bone marrow or lymphatic systems, patients with primary or acquired immunodeficiency, active untreated tuberculosis, and persons with a family history of congenital or hereditary immunodeficiency, until the immune competence of the potential vaccine recipient is demonstrated.

Do not vaccinate persons who are immunosuppressed in association with AIDS or other clinical manifestations of infection with HIV, cellular immune deficiencies, and hypogammaglobulinemic and dysgammaglobulinemic states. Nonetheless, vaccinate asymptomatic children with HIV infection.

Do not vaccinate persons with a history of anaphylactoid or other immediate reactions (eg, hives, swelling of the mouth and throat, difficulty breathing, hypotension, shock) subsequent to egg ingestion. Skin-test persons suspected of being hypersensitive to egg protein, using a dilution of the vaccine as the antigen. Refer to the Introduction section. Do not vaccinate persons with adverse reactions to such testing. Persons are apparently not at risk if they have egg allergies that are not anaphylactoid in nature; vaccinate such persons in the usual manner. There is no evidence that persons with allergies to chickens or feathers are at increased risk of reaction to the vaccine.

Relative: Defer immunization during the course of any acute illness.

Elderly: Persons born prior to 1956 are generally considered immune and need not be vaccinated.

Adults: Vaccinate persons born more recently than 1956, unless they have a personal contraindication to vaccination, since they are considered susceptible. Vaccinate persons who may be immune but who lack adequate documentation of immunity as evidenced by physician diagnosis, laboratory evidence of immunity, or adequate immunization with live vaccine on or after the first birthday.

Pregnancy: *Category C.* Contraindicated. Although mumps virus can infect the placenta and fetus, there is no good evidence that it causes congenital malformations in humans. Attenuated mumps vaccine virus can infect the placenta, but virus has not been isolated from fetal tissues of susceptible women who were vaccinated and underwent elective abortions. Nonetheless, do not intentionally give attenuated mumps vaccine to pregnant females. If postpubertal females are vaccinated, counsel these women to avoid pregnancy for 3 months following vaccination. Generally, most IgG passage across the placenta occurs during the third trimester.

Lactation: It is not known if attenuated mumps virus or corresponding antibodies are excreted in breast milk.

Problems in humans have not been documented.

Children: Mumps vaccine is safe and effective for children 12 months of age or older. Vaccination is not recommended for children <12 months of age since remaining maternal virus neutralizing antibody may interfere with the immune response. Trivalent MMR vaccine is the preferred agent for children and many adults.

Adverse Reactions:
Burning or stinging of short duration at the injection site have occurred. Occasional reactions include mild fever, mild lymphadenopathy or diarrhea. Fever >39.4°C (>103°F) is uncommon. Rarely, parotitis or orchitis may occur. In most of these cases, prior exposure to natural mumps was established. Infrequently, optic neuritis may follow vaccination. Allergic reactions at the injection site or erythema multiforme occurred rarely. Very rarely, encephalitis, febrile seizures, nerve deafness and other nervous system reactions have occurred in vaccinees, but no cause-and-effect relationship has been established.

There have been no published reports of transmission of attenuated mumps virus from vaccinees to susceptible contacts.

Pharmacologic & Dosing Characteristics

Dosage:

Vaccination: 0.5 ml, for both children at 12 to 15 months of age and adults. Trivalent MMR vaccine is the preferred product for most vaccinations.

Minimum intervals between doses of the same vaccine: 4 weeks (except 6 weeks for OPV). Typically, 6 months should elapse before giving the final dose in a vaccine series. Do not count doses within the minimum interval, because too short an interval may interfere with antibody response and protection from disease. Increasing the interval beyond the recommended timing does not affect the ultimate efficacy of immunization, but waiting does delay achieving adequate protection from infection.

Route & Site: SC, preferably in the outer aspect of the upper arm, with a 25 gauge, $\frac{5}{8}$ inch needle. The 10 dose vial may be used with either syringe or jet injector. Use the 50 dose vial by jet injection only. Do not inject IV.

Documentation Requirements: Federal law requires that (1) the manufacturer and lot number of this vaccine, (2) the date of its administration, and (3) the name, address and title of the person administering the vaccine be documented in the recipient's permanent medical record or in a permanent office log. Certain adverse events must be reported to the VAERS system, 1-800-822-7967.

Efficacy: Induces mumps-neutralizing antibodies in about 97% of susceptible children and 93% of susceptible adults. Mumps vaccine reduced disease incidence by 95% in family and classroom cohorts for at least 20 months.

Onset: 2 to 3 weeks

Duration: Antibody levels persist 15 years or longer in most recipients, with a rate of decline comparable to natural infection.

Drug Interactions: Reconstitute mumps vaccine with the diluent provided. Addition of a diluent with an antimicrobial preservative may inactivate the attenuated vaccine.

Like all live viral vaccines, administration of this vaccine to patients receiving immunosuppressant drugs, including steroids, or radiation may predispose patients to disseminated infections or insufficient response to immunization. They may remain susceptible despite immunization.

To avoid inactivation of the attenuated virus, administer live virus vaccines at least 14 to 30 days before or 6 to 8 weeks after administration of any immune globulin or other blood product. Alternatively, check antibody titers or repeat the vaccine dose 3 months after IG administration. Base the interval on the dose of IgG administered: 3 months for 3 to 10 mg/kg, 4 months for 20 mg/kg, 5 months for 40 mg/kg, 6 months for 60 to 100 mg/kg, 7 months for 160 mg/kg, 8 months for 300 to 400 mg/kg, 10 months for 1 g/kg, 11 months for 2 g/kg (*CDC, 1994*).

To avoid the hypothetical concern over antigenic competition, administer mumps vaccine after or not <1 month before administration of other virus vaccines, except those given simultaneously. Several routine vaccines may safely and effectively be administered simultaneously at separate injection sites (eg, DTP, MMR, OPV or e-IPV, Hib, hepatitis B, influenza). National authorities recommend simultaneous immunization at separate sites as indicated by age or health-risk, if return of a vaccine recipient for a subsequent visit is doubtful.

Live virus vaccines may cause delayed-hypersensitivity skin tests (eg, tuberculin, histoplasmin) to appear falsely negative. The effect may persist for several weeks after vaccination. ACIP and AAP recommend that tuberculin tests be given prior to live-virus vaccination, simultaneously, or 6 or more weeks after vaccination.

Concurrent administration of a live-virus vaccine and an interferon product may inhibit antibody response to the vaccine, although this is poorly studied. Avoid concurrent use.

Pharmaceutical Characteristics

Concentration: Not less than 20,000 TCID$_{50}$ per 0.5 ml dose

Packaging: Single-dose package of separate vials of powder and diluent, package of 10 single-dose vial sets. Packages available to government agencies: 10 dose multidose vial with 7 ml diluent, 50 dose multidose vial with 30 ml diluent for jet injection only

Dose Form: Powder for solution

Diluent for Reconstitution: Sterile water for injection without preservative

Storage/Stability: Store at $2°$ to $8°$C ($35°$ to $46°$F). Freezing does not harm this product, although the diluent vials may crack. Store diluent at room temperature or in the refrigerator. Shipped at $10°$C ($50°$F) or colder. Protect vaccine from light. Vaccine powder can tolerate 5 days at room temperature.

Reconstituted vaccine can tolerate 8 hours in the refrigerator.

Handling: Maintain jet injectors properly to prevent blood-borne diseases. Discard jet-injector vials at the end of each day.

Rubella Virus Vaccine Live

VIRAL VACCINES

NAME:
Meruvax II, Generic

MANUFACTURER:
Meruvax II, Merck Vaccine Division; ♣ Generic, Connaught-Cana-

Synonym: Rubella is also known as the German measles. Do not use this term, to avoid confusion with measles itself

(which is also called rubeola, another source of confusion).

Viability: Live, attenuated
Antigenic Form: Whole virus

Antigenic Type: Protein

Trivalent measles-mumps-rubella (MMR) vaccine is the preferred immunizing agent for most children and many adults.

Use Characteristics

◎ **Indications:** Selective active immunization against rubella. The national rubella immunization program is intended to reduce the occurrence of congenital rubella syndrome (CRS) among offspring of women who contract rubella during pregnancy.

Vaccination is routinely recommended for persons from 12 months of age to puberty. Give previously unimmunized children of susceptible pregnant women attenuated rubella (or preferably MMR) vaccine, since an immunized child is less likely to acquire natural rubella and introduce it into the household. Vaccination of adolescent or adult males is a useful procedure in preventing or controlling outbreaks of rubella in circumscribed populations. Immunization of susceptible nonpregnant adolescent and adult females of childbearing potential is indicated, if precautions to avoid pregnancy are observed. When vaccinating postpubertal females, counsel these women to avoid pregnancy for 3 months following vaccination. Vaccinating susceptible postpubertal females confers individual protection against subsequently acquiring rubella infection during pregnancy, which in turn prevents infection of the fetus and CRS. It may be convenient to vaccinate rubella-susceptible women in the immediate postpartum period.

Prior to international travel, give individuals known to be susceptible to measles, mumps or rubella either a single-antigen vaccine or a polyvalent vaccine, as appropriate. Trivalent measles-mumps-rubella (MMR) vaccine is preferred for persons likely to be susceptible to mumps and rubella. Almost all children and some adults need >1 dose of MMR vaccine. If single-antigen vaccines are not readily available, give travelers trivalent MMR regardless of their immune status to mumps or rubella.

Unlicensed Uses: Intranasal administration may boost antibody titers, although this route is not confirmed as safe and effective by the FDA and is not commonly employed.

STOP **Contraindications:**

Absolute: Pregnant patients, patients with a personal history of a hypersensitivity reaction to this vaccine or any of its components, patients receiving immunosuppressive therapy, patients with a blood dyscrasia, leukemia, lymphoma of any type, or other malignant neoplasms affecting the bone marrow or lymphatic systems, patients with primary or acquired immunodeficiency, active untreated tuberculosis, and persons with a family history of congenital or hereditary immunodeficiency, until the immune competence of the potential vaccine recipient is demonstrated.

Do not vaccinate persons who are immunosuppressed in association with AIDS or other clinical manifestations of infection with HIV, cellular immune deficiencies, and hypogammaglobulinemic and dysgammaglobulinemic states. Nonetheless, vaccinate asymptomatic children with HIV infection.

Relative: Defer immunization during the course of any acute illness.

Elderly: Most persons born in 1956 or earlier are likely to have been infected naturally and generally are considered not susceptible.

Adults: Vaccinate persons born more recently than 1956, unless they have a personal contraindication to vaccination, since they are considered susceptible. Vaccinate persons who may be immune but who lack adequate documentation of immunity as evidenced by physician diagnosis, laboratory evidence of immunity, or adequate immunization with live vaccine on or after the first birthday.

Pregnancy: *Category C.* Contraindicated. Natural rubella infection of the fetus may result in congenital rubella syndrome. There is evidence suggesting transmission of attenuated rubella virus to the fetus, although the vaccine is not known to cause fetal harm when administered to pregnant women. Nonetheless, do not intentionally give attenuated rubella vaccine to pregnant females. If postpubertal females are vaccinated, counsel these women to avoid pregnancy for 3 months following vaccination. It may be convenient to vaccinate rubella-susceptible women in the immediate postpartum period.

In counseling women who are inadvertently vaccinated when pregnant or who become pregnant within 3 months of vaccination, the following information may be useful. In a 10 year survey of >700 pregnant women who received rubella vaccine within 3 months before or after conception (of whom 189 received the current RA27/3 strain), none of the newborns had abnormalities compatible with congenital rubella syndrome.

Generally, most IgG passage across the placenta occurs during the third trimester.

Lactation: Vaccine-strain virus is secreted in milk and may be transmitted to infants in this manner. In the infants with serologic evidence of rubella infection, none exhibited severe disease. However, one exhibited mild clinical illness typical of acquired rubella.

Children: Safe and effective for children ≥12 months of age. Vaccination is not recommended for children <12 months of age, since remaining maternal rubella neutralizing antibody may interfere with the immune response. Trivalent MMR vaccine is the preferred agent for children and many adults.

Adverse Reactions:

Burning or stinging of short duration at the injection site have occurred. Symptoms of the same kind as seen following natural rubella infection may occur after vaccination: Mild regional lymphadenopathy, urticaria, rash, malaise, sore throat, fever, headache, dizziness, nausea, vomiting, diarrhea, polyneuritis, and arthralgia or arthritis (usually transient and rarely chronic). Local pain, induration and erythema may occur at the site of injection. Reactions are usually mild and transient. Moderate fever (38.3° to 39.4°C; 101° to 102.9°F) occurs occasionally, high fever (>39.4°C or 103°F) less commonly.

Erythema multiforme has been reported rarely, as has optic neuritis. Isolated cases of polyneuropathy, including Guillain-Barré syndrome, have been reported after immunization with rubella-containing vaccines. Encephalitis and other nervous-system reactions have occurred very rarely in subjects given this vaccine, but a cause-and-effect relationship has not been established. In view of reported decreases in platelet counts, thrombocytopenic purpura is a theoretical hazard of rubella vaccination.

Chronic arthritis has been associated with natural rubella infection. Only rarely have vaccine recipients developed chronic joint symptoms, but an Institute of Medicine (IOM) report classified the association as consistent with a causal relation. Following vaccination in children, reactions in joints are uncommon (≤3%) and generally of brief duration. In adult women, incidence rates for arthritis and arthralgia are generally higher (12% to 20%) and the reactions tend to be more marked and of longer duration. Symptoms may persist for months or, on rare occasions, for years. In adolescent girls, the reactions appear to be intermediate in incidence between those seen in children and in adult women. Even in older women (35 to 45 years of age), these reactions are generally well tolerated and rarely interfere with normal activities. Myalgia and paresthesia have been reported rarely. Advise postpubertal females of the frequent occurrence of generally self-limited arthralgia or arthritis beginning 2 to 4 weeks after vaccination.

Excretion of small amounts of attenuated rubella virus from the nose or throat has occurred in the majority of susceptible individuals 7 to 28 days after vaccination. There is no firm evidence that such virus is transmitted to susceptible persons in contact with vaccinees. Transmission through close personal contact, while accepted as a theoretical possibility, is not regarded as a significant risk. However, transmission of attenuated rubella virus to infants through breast milk has been documented.

Pharmacologic & Dosing Characteristics

Dosage:

Vaccination: 0.5 ml, for both children, at 12 to 15 months of age and adults. Trivalent MMR vaccine is the preferred product for most vaccinations. A booster dose is recommended under certaincircumstances.

Minimum intervals between doses of

the same vaccine: 4 weeks (except 6 weeks for OPV). Typically, 6 months should elapse before giving the final dose in a vaccine series. Do not count doses within the minimum interval, because too short an interval may interfere with antibody response and protection from disease. Increasing the interval beyond the recommended timing does not affect the ultimate efficacy of immunization, but wating does delay achieving adequate protection from infection.

Route & Site: SC, preferably in the outer aspect of the upper arm, with a 25 gauge, $\frac{5}{8}$ inch needle. The 10 dose vial may be used with either syringe or jet injector. Use the 50 dose vial by jet injection only. Do not inject IV.

Documentation Requirements: Federal law requires that (1) the manufacturer and lot number of this vaccine, (2) the date of its administration, and (3) the name, address and title of the person administering the vaccine be documented in the recipient's permanent medical record or in a permanent office log. Certain adverse events must be reported to the VAERS system, 1-800-822-7967.

Efficacy: Induces hemagglutination-inhibiting (HI) antibodies in at least 97% of susceptible children. Seroconversion is somewhat less in adults. Disease incidence is typically reduced by 95% in family and classroom cohorts.

Onset: 2 to 6 weeks

Duration: Antibody levels persist 10 years or longer in most recipients.

Drug Interactions: Reconstitute rubella vaccine with the diluent provided. Addition of a diluent with an antimicrobial preservative may inactivate the attenuated vaccine.

Like all live viral vaccines, administration of this vaccine to patients receiving immunosuppressant drugs, including steroids, or radiation may predispose patients to disseminated infections or insufficient response to immunization. They may remain susceptible despite immunization.

To avoid inactivation of the attenuated virus, administer live virus vaccines at least 14 to 30 days before or 6 to 8 weeks after administration of any immune globulin or other blood product. Alternatively, check antibody titers or repeat the vaccine dose 3 months after immune globulin administration. Base the interval on the dose if IgG administered: 3 months for 3 to 10 mg/kg, 4 months for 20 mg/kg, 5 months for 40 mg/kg, 6 months for 60 to 100 mg/kg, 7 months for 160 mg/kg, 8 months for 300 to 400 mg/kg, 10 months for 1 g/kg, 11 months for 2 g/kg (CDC, 1994).

To avoid hypothetical concerns over antigenic competition, administer rubella vaccine after or ≥ 1 month before other virus vaccines, except those given simultaneously. Several routine vaccines may safely and effectively be administered simultaneously at separate injection sites (eg, DTP, MMR, OPV or e-IPV, Hib, hepatitis B). National authorities recommend simultaneous immunization at separate sites as indicated by age or health-risk, if return of a vaccine recipient for a subsequent visit is doubtful.

Live virus vaccines may cause delayed-hypersensitivity skin tests (eg, tuberculin, histoplasmin) to appear falsely negative. Evaluate such tests knowingly. The effect may persist for several weeks after vaccination. ACIP and AAP recommend that tuberculin tests be given prior to live-virus vaccination, simultaneously, or 6 or more weeks after vaccination.

Concurrent administration of a live-virus vaccine and an interferon product may inhibit antibody response to the vaccine, although this is poorly studied. Avoid concurrent use.

Anti-Rh$_o$ (D) immune globulin does not appear to impair rubella vaccine efficacy. Susceptible postpartum women who received blood products or anti-Rh$_o$ (D) immune globulin may receive attenuated rubella vaccine prior to discharge, provided that a repeat HI titer is drawn 6 to 8 weeks after vaccination to assure seroconversion.

Pharmaceutical Characteristics

Concentration: Not less than 1000 TCID$_{50}$ per 0.5 ml dose

Packaging: Single-dose package of separate vials of powder and diluent, package of 10 single-dose vial sets. Packages available to government agencies: 10 dose multidose vial with 7 ml diluent, 50 dose vial with 30 ml diluent for jet injection only.

Dose Form: Powder for solution

Diluent for Reconstitution: Sterile water for injection without preservative

Storage/Stability: Store at 2° to 8°C (35° to 46°F). Freezing does not harm the vaccine, but may crack diluent vials. Store diluent at room temperature or in the refrigerator. Shipped at ≤10°C (50°F). Protect vaccine from light. Contact manufacturer regarding prolonged exposure to room temperature or elevated temperatures. Reconstituted vaccine can tolerate 8 hours in the refrigerator.

Handling: Maintain jet injectors properly to prevent blood-borne diseases. Discard jet-injector vials at the end of each day.

Poliovirus Vaccine Inactivated

NAME:
IPOL, ☫ Imovax Poli

MANUFACTURER:
IPOL, Pasteur Mérieux Sérum & Vaccines in Lyon, France, and distributed by Connaught Laboratories in US and Canada; ☫ *Imovax Poli,* Connaught

Synonyms: IPV, enhanced-potency IPV, e-IPV, ep-IPV, Salk vaccine

Comparison: e-IPV is more potent and more consistently immunogenic than previous IPV formulations, which may still be available in other countries. e-IPV and OPV are generically different. OPV was long recommended for routine immunization of infants and children in the US. Now, e-IPV is still used for vaccination of adults and of immunocompromised persons and their contacts. e-IPV is preferred for adult immunization, because adults are slightly more likely to develop OPV-induced poliomyelitis than children.

Viability: Inactivated

Antigenic Form: Whole viruses

Antigenic Type: Protein

Use Characteristics

◎ Indications: For induction of active immunity of infants, children and adults against poliovirus, to protect against poliomyelitis. e-IPV is recommended for routine use as the first two immunizing doses in infants and children. OPV is now recommended for the third and fourth doses. The combined IPV-OPV regimen is intended to reduce further the already rare occurence of OPV-associated paralytic poliomyelitis.

Immunization of adults residing in the continental US is not usually necessary because of the extremely low probability of exposure. Vaccinate adults traveling to regions where poliomyelitis is endemic or epidemic (eg, developing countries), healthcare workers in close contact with patients who may be excreting polioviruses, laboratory workers handling specimens that may contain polioviruses, and members of communities or specific population groups with disease caused by wild polioviruses.

Offer e-IPV to individuals who have declined OPV or in whom OPV is contraindicated. Immunization with e-IPV may be indicated for unimmunized parents and those in other special situations where protection may be needed. In a household with an immunocompromised member or among other close contacts, or in a household with an unimmunized adult, use only e-IPV for all those requiring poliovirus immunization.

If <4 weeks remain before protection is needed, a single dose of OPV is recommended, with the remaining vaccine doses given later if the person remains at increased risk.

Previous clinical poliomyelitis (usually due to only a single poliovirus type) or incomplete immunization with OPV are not contraindications to completing the primary series of immunization with e-IPV.

Unlicensed Uses: Alternative immunization schedules for children using both OPV and e-IPV have been shown to be safe and immunogenic.

Contraindications:
Absolute: Patients with a history of hypersensitivity to any component of the vaccine. If anaphylaxis or anaphylactic shock occurs within 24 hours of administration, give no further doses.

Relative: Defer immunization during the course of any acute illness.

Elderly: No specific information is available about geriatric use of e-IPV.

Pregnancy: *Category C.* Use only if clearly needed. It is not specifically known if e-IPV or corresponding antibodies cross the placenta. Generally, most IgG passage across the placenta occurs during the third trimester.

Lactation: It is not known if e-IPV or corresponding antibodies cross into human breast milk. Problems in humans have not been documented and are unlikely.

Children: e-IPV is safe and effective in children as young as 6 weeks of age.

Adverse Reactions:
No paralytic reactions to e-IPV are known to have occurred since a 1955 manufacturing accident in which live polioviruses escaped inactivation. e-IPV administration may result in erythema, induration and pain at the injection site (13%). Temperatures $\geq 39°C$ ($\geq 102°F$) were reported in 38% of e-IPV vaccinees.

Pharmacologic & Dosing Characteristics

Dosage:
Children: The national policy is to give two doses of e-IPV, followed by one primary dose of OPV and a booster dose of OPV. Typically, this would include e-IPV doses at 2 and 4 months of age and OPV doses at 6 to 12 and 12 to 18 months of age. Separate the first 2 doses by at least 4 weeks, but preferably 8 weeks; they are commonly given at 2 and 4 months of age. Give the third dose at least 2 months after the second dose, commonly at 6 to 12 months of age. Give the second OPV dose at least 4 and preferably 8 weeks after the earlier OPV dose. If only e-IPV is used, the primary series consists of three 0.5 ml doses of poliovirus vaccine; an additional booster dose is given several years later.

Adults: For unvaccinated adults at increased risk of exposure to poliovirus, give a primary series of e-IPV: 2 doses given at a 1 to 2 month intervals, with a third dose given 6 to 12 months later. If <3 months, but >2 months, remain before protection is needed, give 3 doses of e-IPV at least 1 month apart. Likewise, if only 1 or 2 months remain, give 2 doses of e-IPV 1 month apart. If <4 weeks remain, give a single dose of either OPV or e-IPV.

Give adults at increased risk of exposure who have had at least 1 dose of OPV, <3 doses of conventional e-IPV (available before 1988), or a combination of conventional e-IPV and OPV totaling <3 doses at least one dose of OPV of e-IPV. Give any additional doses needed to complete a primary series if time permits.

Give adults who have completed a primary series with any poliovirus vaccine and who are at increased risk of exposure to poliovirus a single dose of either OPV or e-IPV.

Minimum intervals between doses of the same vaccine: 4 weeks (except 6 weeks for OPV). Typically, 6 months should elapse before giving the final dose in a vaccine series. Do not count doses within the minimum interval, because too short an interval may interfere with antibody response and protection from disease. Increasing the interval beyond the recommended timing does not affect the ultimate efficacy of immunization, but waiting does delay achieving adequate protection from infection.

Route & Site: SC, in the deltoid region. In infants and children, the preferred site is the anterolateral thigh.

Documentation Requirements: Federal law requires that (1) the manufacturer and lot number of this vaccine, (2) the date of its administration and (3) the name, address and title of the person administering the vaccine be documented in the recipient's permanent medical record or in a permanent office log. Certain adverse events must be reported to the VAERS system, 1-800-822-7967.

Efficacy: 97.5% to 100% seroconversion to each type after 2 doses. This formulation is more potent and more consistently immunogenic than previous IPV formulations.

Onset: Antibodies develop within 1 to 2 weeks following several doses.

Duration: Many years

Drug Interactions: Like all inactivated vaccines, administration of e-IPV to persons receiving immunosuppressant drugs, including high-dose corticosteroids, or radiation therapy may result in an insufficient response to immunization. They may remain susceptible despite immunization.

Inactivated vaccines are not generally affected by circulating antibodies or administration of exogenous antibodies. Vaccination may occur at any time before or after antibody administration.

Several routine pediatric vaccines may safely and effectively be administered simultaneously at separate injection sites (eg, DTP, MMR, OPV or e-IPV, Hib, hepatitis A, hepatitis B, influenza). National authorities recommend simultaneous immunization at separate sites as indicated by age or health risk, if return of a vaccine recipient for a subsequent visit is doubtful.

A Canadian DTP vaccine evoked a higher pertussis antibody response given with e-IPV or OPV than did a tetravalent, parenteral DTP-IPV vaccine from the same manufacturer or DTP and IPV given as a separate injection (*Baker et al, 1992*).

Pharmaceutical Characteristics

Concentration: 40, 8 and 32 D-Antigen units per 0.5 ml dose of poliovirus types 1, 2 and 3, respectively. The D antigen is one of two major antigenic components of polioviruses.

Packaging: One 0.5 ml single-dose syringe with 25-gauge, $\frac{5}{8}$ inch needle; package of 10 syringes.

Dose Form: Suspension (even though the product appears clear)

Solvent: Phosphate-buffered saline

Storage/Stability: Store at 2° to 8°C (35° to 46°F). Discard if frozen. Contact manufacturer regarding prolonged exposure to room temperature or elevated temperatures. Shipped by second-day courier in insulated containers with coolant packs.

Poliovirus Vaccine Live Oral Trivalent
VIRAL VACCINES

NAME:
Orimune, Generic

MANUFACTURER:
Orimune, Wyeth-Lederle Vaccines & Pediatrics; ♣ Generic, Connaught-Canada

Synonyms: OPV, TOPV, Sabin vaccine

Comparison: e-IPV and OPV are generically different. OPV was long recommended for routine immunization of infants and children in the US. Now, e-IPV is recommended for the first two infant doses, followed by two doses of OPV. e-IPV is still used for vaccination of adults and of immunocompromised persons and their contacts. e-IPV is preferrred for adult immunization because adults are slightly more likely to develop OPV-induced poliomyelitis than children.

Viability: Live, attenuated

Antigenic Form: Whole viruses

Antigenic Type: Protein

Use Characteristics

Indications: For induction of active immunity against infections caused by poliovirus types 1, 2 and 3, to prevent poliomyelitis. e-IPV is recommended for routine use as the first two immunizing doses in infants and children. OPV is now recommended for the third and fourth doses. The combined IPV-OPV regimen is intended to reduce further the already rare occurence of OPV-associated paralytic poliomyelitis. OPV is also recommended for control of outbreaks of epidemic poliomyelitis.

Protection of adults: Immunization of adults residing in the continental US is not usually necessary because of the extremely low probability of exposure. Primary immunization with e-IPV is recommended whenever feasible for unimmunized adults subject to increased risk of exposure, such as by travel to or contact with epidemic or endemic areas (eg, developing countries) and for those employed in medical and sanitation facilities. If <4 weeks remain before protection is needed, a single dose of OPV is recommended, with the remaining vaccine doses given later if the person remains at increased risk. Immunization with e-IPV may be indicated for unimmunized parents and those in other special situations where protection may be needed. In a household with an immunocompromised member or among other close contacts, or in a household with an unimmunized adult, use only e-IPV for all those requiring poliovirus immunization.

Contraindications:
Absolute: Do not administer OPV to any person with immunosuppression, or to any household member of an immunodeficient person. This includes those with combined immunodeficiency, hypogammaglobulinemia, agammaglobulinemia, thymic

abnormalities, leukemia, lymphoma, generalized malignancy, lowered resistance to infection from therapy with corticosteroids, alkylating drugs, antimetabolites or radiation. Advise vaccine recipients to avoid such persons for at least 6 to 8 weeks.

To preclude vaccine-associated disease, do not give OPV to a member of a household in which there is a family history of immunodeficiency until the immune status of the intended recipient and other children in the family is determined to be normal. e-IPV is preferred for immunizing all persons in the circumstances described above. Give adults in such households 3 doses of e-IPV a month apart before the children receive OPV; the children may receive their first dose at the same time the adults receive their third dose of e-IPV.

Relative: Defer immunization in those experiencing any acute illness and in those with any advanced debilitated condition or persistent vomiting or diarrhea.

Elderly: No specific information is available about geriatric use of OPV. e-IPV is generally preferred for immunization of susceptible adults.

Adults: e-IPV is generally preferred for immunization of susceptible adults.

Pregnancy: *Category C.* Use only if clearly needed. Use OPV in pregnancy if exposure is imminent and immediate protection is needed.

Lactation: Breastfeeding does not generally interfere with successful immunization of infants, despite IgA antibody secretion in breast milk.

In certain tropical epidemic areas where vaccination may be recommended for the infant at birth, the manufacturer suggests that immunization be withheld until the child is 3 days old. Advise women to abstain from breastfeeding for 2 to 3 hours before and after vaccination of their infants, to permit establishment of viruses in the gut. Because successful immunization is likely in newborn infants, complete the OPV series following the neonatal dose when the infant reaches 2 months of age.

Children: OPV was long recommended for routine immunization of infants and children in the US. Now, e-IPV is recommended for the first two infant doses, followed by two doses of OPV.

Adverse Reactions:

Vaccine-associated paralysis occurs with a frequency of 1 case per 2.6 million OPV vaccine doses distributed. Of 105 cases of paralytic poliomyelitis known from 1973 through 1984 (when 274.1 million OPV doses were distributed), 35 cases occurred in vaccine recipients, 50 in household and nonhousehold contacts of vaccinees, 14 in immunodeficient recipients or contacts and 6 occurred in persons with no history of vaccine exposure. First doses are more likely to result in a case of paralysis than subsequent doses (1 case per 520,000 first doses vs 1 case per 12.3 million subsequent doses).

Since 1980, all reported domestic cases of paralytic polio have apparently been caused by OPV. Of 85 paralytic cases from 1980 to 1989, 80 involved vaccine-associated disease and 5 were cases of imported disease.

OPV does not cause any common side effects.

Pharmacologic & Dosing Characteristics

Dosage:

Primary Immunizing Series: A primary series consists of three 0.5 ml doses of poliovirus vaccine; an additional booster dose is given several years later. The national policy is to give two doses of e-IPV, followed by one primary dose of OPV and a booster dose of OPV, although a specific recommended schedule has not yet been issued. Separate the first two doses by at least 4 weeks, but preferably 8 weeks; they are commonly given at 2 and 4 months of age. Give the third dose at least 4 months after the second dose, commonly at 6 to 18 months of age. Give all children who received a primary series of e-IPV or a combination of e-IPV and OPV a booster dose of OPV or e-IPV before entering school, unless the third dose of the primary series was administered on or after the fourth birthday.

The earlier schedule consisted of three 0.5 ml doses of OPV, optimally starting at 6 to 12 weeks of age. Give the second dose not <6 and preferably 8 weeks later, commonly at 4 months of age. Give the third dose 2 to 12 months after the second dose, commonly at 6 to 18 months of age. An optional additional dose of OPV may be given at 6 months of age in areas where poliomyelitis disease or risk is endemic.

Give older children (up to 18 years of age) 2 OPV doses, not <6 and preferably 8 weeks apart, followed by a third dose, 6 to 12 months after the second dose.

On entering elementary school, give all children who have completed the primary series a single follow-up dose of OPV. All others should complete the primary series. This fourth dose is not required in those who received the third primary dose on or after their fourth birthday.

The multiple doses in the primary series are not administered as boosters, but to ensure that immunity to all three types of virus has been achieved.

In some other countries, the first dose of OPV is routinely administered at birth or prior to 2 weeks of age. Do not count these doses in providing the three-dose primary vaccine series.

If a substantial amount of OPV is spit out, regurgitated or vomited shortly after administration (ie, within 5 to 10 min), another dose may be administered at the same visit. If the repeat dose is not retained, neither dose should be counted and the vaccine should be readministered at the next visit.

Minimum intervals between doses of the same vaccine: 4 weeks (except 6 weeks for OPV). Typically, 6 months should elapse before giving the final dose in a vaccine series. Do not count doses within the minimum interval, because too short an interval may interfere with antibody response and protection from disease. Increasing the interval beyond the recommended timing does not affect the ultimate efficacy of immunization, but waiting does delay achieving adequate protection from infection.

Route & Site: Oral; not for injection.

Documentation Requirements: Federal law requires that (1) the manufacturer and lot number of this vaccine, (2) the date of its administration and (3) the name, address and title of the per son administering the vaccine be documented in the recipient's permanent medical record or in a permanent office log. Certain adverse events must be reported to the VAERS system, 1-800-822-7967.

Efficacy: Greater than 95% of children studied 5 years after immunization with OPV had protective antibodies against all three types of poliovirus. Type-specific neutralizing antibodies will be induced in at least 90% of susceptible persons.

OPV had been preferred over e-IPV for routine immunization of children, because OPV induces intestinal immunity, is simple to administer, was well accepted by patients, results in immunization of some contacts of vaccinated persons and had a record of having essentially eliminated disease associated with wild poliovirus in the US. National policy has shifted to a combined regimen of e-IPV ond OPV, in an effort to reduce the already rare likelihood of OPV-associated paralytic poliomyelitis.

Onset: Antibodies develop within 1 to 2 weeks after several doses.

Duration: Many years

Drug Interactions: Immune globulin (IG) does not appear to interfere with development of immunity following OPV. However, it may be prudent not to administer OPV shortly after IG administration unless unavoidable, such as unexpected travel to or contact with epidemic or endemic areas or persons. If OPV is given with or shortly after IG, the OPV dose should probably be repeated 3 months later, if immunity is still needed.

Like all live viral vaccines, administration to patients or contacts of patients receiving immunosuppressant drugs, including steroids, or radiation may predispose patients to disseminated infections or insufficient response to immunization. They may remain susceptible despite immunization.

Several routine pediatric vaccines may safely and effectively be administered simultaneously at separate injection sites (eg, DTP, MMR, OPV or e-IPV, Hib, hepatitis A, hepatitis B, influenza, varicella). National authorities recommend simultaneous immunization at separate sites as indicated by age or health risk, if return of a vaccine recipient for a subsequent visit is doubtful. Simultaneous immunization with cholera vaccine reduced the seroconversion rate to oral poliovirus type 1 vaccine in one study. Separate these vaccinations by 1 month if possible. Interval between giving two live vaccines: give them simultaneously or wait at least 4 weeks between immunizations (does not apply to MMR-OPV or OPV-oral typhoid).

A Canadian DTP vaccine evoked a higher pertussis antibody response given with e-IPV or OPV than did a tetravalent, parenteral DTP-IPV vaccine from the same manufacturer or DTP and IPV given as separate injections (*Baker et al, 1992*).

No evidence of interaction between simultaneous administration of OPV and oral live typhoid (Ty2la) vaccine has been documented. If both drugs are needed (eg, prior to international travel), both vaccines may be administered simultaneously or at any interval between each other.

Simultaneous immunization with OPV and an experimental oral rotavirus vaccine reduced the seroconversion rate to rotavirus, possibly through antigenic or viral competition (Giamman-co et al, 1988). Separate such vaccinations by 1 month if possible. It is not clear if this interaction would also occur with different rotaviral strains.

Concentration: Contains the following infectivity titers: Type 1 virus—$10^{5.4-6.4}$, Type 2 virus—$10^{4.5-5.5}$, Type 3 virus—$10^{5.2-6.2}$. Comparable to 800,000, 100,000 and 500,000 viral particles, respectively.

Packaging: 0.5 ml single-dose plastic disposable pipettes: Box of ten 0.5 ml pipettes, box of fifty 0.5 ml pipettes

Dose Form: Frozen suspension. This drug may remain in the liquid state at temperatures as cold as $-14°C$ $(+7°F)$, because of its sorbitol content.

Storage/Stability: Store in a freezer. After thawing, use vaccine within 30 days. Vaccine is not stable at room temperature. Do not expose to >10 freeze-thaw cycles, with none exceeding $8°C$ $(46°F)$. If the cumulative period of thaw is >24 hours, use the vaccine within 30 days, during which time it must be stored between $2°$ to $8°C$ $(36°$ to $46°F)$. Shipped at $-18°C$ $(0°F)$ or colder in insulated containers with dry ice.

	Poliovirus Vaccine Comparisons	
	IPOL	*Orimune*
Manufacturer	Mérieux/Connaught	Wyeth-Lederle
Synonyms	IPV, e-IPV, ep-IPV, Salk vaccine	OPV, Sabin vaccine
Packaging	Prefilled syringes	Pipette for oral administration
Indications	Adults; immunocompromised persons and their household contacts, including HIV-infected persons; first two doses in routine immunization of infants; first two doses in routine immunization of infants	Third and fourth doses in routine immunization of infants, children and some adults
Routine storage	Refrigerate	Freeze
Route	Subcutaneous	Oral
Efficacy	95% to 100%	95% to 100%
Viability	Inactivated	Live, attenuated
Ability to induce poliomyelitis	No risk	1 case per 2.6 million OPV doses distributed

Rabies Vaccine
VIRAL VACCINES

NAME:
Rabies Vaccine (Human Diploid Cell): *Imovax Rabies* and *Imovax Rabies ID;* Rabies Vaccine Adsorbed: Generic; Rabies Vaccine (Vero cell): Generic

MANUFACTURERS:
Rabies Vaccine (Human Diploid Cell): *Imovax Rabies* and *Imovax Rabies ID* manufactured by Institut Mérieux in France, distributed by Connaught Laboratories; Rabies Vaccine Adsorbed: Generic manufactured and distributed by Michigan Department of Public Health. Also distributed by SmithKline Beecham Pharmaceuticals. Rabies Vaccine (Vero cell): Generic manufactured by Connaught Laboratories [marketing pending];
* *Imovax Rabies,* Connaught

Synonyms:

Connaught: human diploid-cell vaccine, HDCV. *Michigan/SKB:* RVA. The disease is also called hydrophobia, related to a fear of swallowing among its victims.

Comparison: IM dosage forms are generically equivalent and are considered interchangeable during an individual patient's vaccination series. Michigan's rabies vaccine has not been studied for safety and efficacy by the intradermal (ID) route.

Viability: Inactivated
Antigenic Form: Whole virus

Antigenic Type: Protein

Use Characteristics

Indications: Induction of active immunity against rabies virus, either before or after viral exposure.

Pre-Exposure Immunization: Vaccinate persons with greater than usual risk of exposure to rabies virus by reason of occupation or avocation, including veterinarians, certain laboratory workers, animal handlers, forest rangers, spelunkers and persons staying >1 month in other countries (eg, India) where rabies is a constant threat (see tables at end of monograph).

Post-Exposure Prophylaxis: If a bite from a carrier animal is unprovoked, the animal is not apprehended, and rabies is present in that species in the area, administer RIG and vaccine as indicated in tables at end of monograph. Consider vaccine recipients adequately immunized if they previously completed pre- or post-exposure prophylaxis with any current rabies vaccine or have a documented adequate antibody response to duck-embryo rabies vaccine (DEV).

Contraindications:

Absolute: There are essentially no absolute contraindications to rabies vaccination when used for post-exposure prophylaxis.

Relative: No antirabies treatment is indicated unless the skin is broken or a mucosal surface has been contaminated with the animal's saliva. Rabies vaccine may theoretically be contraindicated in persons who have had life-threatening allergic reactions to rabies vaccine or any of its components. But carefully consider a patient's risk of developing rabies before deciding to discontinue vaccination. Local or mild post-vaccination reactions are not a contraindication to continuing immunization.

Give persons who experience immune-complex-like (or serum-sickness-like) hypersensitivity reactions during pre-exposure prophylaxis no further doses of rabies vaccine unless they are exposed to rabies or they are likely to be unapparently or unavoidably exposed to rabies virus and have unsatisfactory antibody titers.

Elderly: No specific information is available about geriatric use of rabies vaccine.

Pregnancy: *Category C.* Use is not contraindicated, but use only if clearly needed. It is not known if rabies vaccine or corresponding antibodies cross the placenta. Generally, most IgG passage across the placenta occurs during the third trimester.

Lactation: It is not known if rabies vaccine or corresponding antibodies cross into breast milk. Problems in humans have not been documented.

Children: Pediatric and adult doses are the same. Safety and efficacy are established in children. Safe and effective use of the Michigan/SKB vaccine is established for persons ≥6 years of age.

Adverse Reactions:

Diploid: Transient pain, erythema, swelling or itching at the injection site (25%). Treat such reactions with simple analgesics.

Mild systemic reactions (20%): Headache, nausea, abdominal pain, muscle aches and dizziness. In general, intradermal administration results in fewer adverse reactions, except for a slight increase in transient local reactions. Serum-sickness-like reactions occur in 6% of those receiving intradermal booster doses, occurring 2 to 21 days after injection. These reactions may be due to albumin in the vaccine formula rendered allergenic by beta-propiolactone during the manufacturing process.

Michigan/SKB: Transient pain, redness and swelling at the injection site (65% to 70%). In a few cases, these effects persist 48 hours and may be successfully treated with simple analgesics. Mild, transient constitutional reactions (8% to 10%): Headache, nausea, slight fever or fatigue. Serum-sickness-like reaction (<1%): Between 7 and 14 days after booster vaccination; this low is perhaps due to lack of albumin in the vaccine formula.

Pharmacologic & Dosing Characteristics

Dosage:

Pre-Exposure Prophylaxis: Vaccine doses on days 0, 7 and 21 to 28, and then every 2 to 5 years based on antibody titers. Give 1 ml IM (either manufacturer) or 0.1 ml intradermally (diploid only).

Post-Exposure Prophylaxis: Do not inject post-exposure vaccine intradermally.

Give rabies immune globulin (RIG, 20 IU/kg, refer to specific monograph in the Immune Globulins section) as soon after exposure as possible, followed by IM vaccine doses (either manufacturer) on days 0, 3, 7, 14 and 28.

For patients who have previously received pre-exposure prophylaxis, give 1 ml of either vaccine IM only on days 0 and 3. Do not give RIG.

Route & Site: The deltoid area is the only acceptable site for post-exposure vaccination of adults and older children. For younger children, use the outer aspect of the thigh. Never administer rabies vaccine in the gluteal area.

Travelers to endemic areas may receive vaccine by the intradermal route if the 3-dose series can be completed 30 days or longer before departure; otherwise give the vaccine IM.

Diploid: IM in deltoid muscle or ID. Use only the IM route for post-exposure prophylaxis. ID injections given in the lateral aspect of the upper arm are less likely to result in adverse reactions, compared with ID injection in the forearm.

Michigan/SKB: IM only, in deltoid muscle. Do not inject ID. Vaccinate children in the anterolateral aspect of the thigh muscle.

Efficacy: Essentially 100%, when administered according to ACIP recommendations.

Onset: After IM injection, antibodies appear in 7 days and peak within 30 to 60 days. Adequate titers usually develop within 2 weeks after the third pre-exposure dose. Antibody kinetics after ID injection are presumably comparable.

Duration: Antibodies persist at least 1 year.

Drug Interactions: Like all inactivated vaccines, administration of rabies vaccine to persons receiving immunosuppressant drugs, including high-dose corticosteroids, or radiation therapy may result in an insufficient response to immunization. They may remain susceptible despite immunization.

Do not give immunosuppressive agents during post-exposure therapy, unless essential for treatment of other conditions. Exercise caution especially with corticosteroids used to treat life-threatening neuroparalytic reactions, as they may inhibit the development of active immunity to rabies. It may be helpful to test steroid-treated patients for development of antirabies antibodies.

Simultaneous administration of RIG may slightly delay the antibody response to rabies vaccine, through partial antigen-antibody antagonism. Because of this possibility, follow CDC recommendations exactly and give no more than the recommended dose of RIG.

Long-term therapy with chloroquine may suppress the immune response to low-dose HDCV administered ID. Complete pre-exposure rabies vaccination 1 to 2 months before chloroquine administration begins. If this is not feasible, perform serologic tests several weeks after vaccination to determine the magnitude of the recipient's antibody response.

Rabies immunogenicity was not impaired by simultaneous vaccination with yellow fever, OPV, MMR, DT, cholera, meningococcal and hepatitis B vaccines in one study (Bernard et al, 1985).

As with other drugs administered by IM injection, give rabies vaccine with caution to persons receiving anticoagulant therapy.

Pharmaceutical Characteristics

Concentration:

IM: Not less than 2.5 IU/ml

ID: 0.25 IU/0.1 ml

Packaging:

Diploid: IM: Single-dose package containing vial of powder, syringe with transfer needle of unspecified gauge and length, 1 ml diluent, and IM administration needle of unspecified gauge and length

ID: Single-dose package containing vial of powder, syringe with transfer needle of unspecified gauge and length, 1 ml diluent, and ID administration needle of unspecified gauge and length; use caution to add only 0.1 ml diluent, according to package directions

Michigan/SKB: Single-dose 1 ml vial

Dosage Form:

Diploid: Powder for suspension

Michigan/SKB: Suspension

Solvent: *Michigan/SKB:* Phosphate-buffered sodium chloride

Diluent for Reconstitution: *Diploid:* Sterile water for injection. Gently swirl until completely dissolved. The ID package contains more diluent than needed, to permit withdrawal of diluent without introduction of air.

Storage/Stability: Store at 2° to 8°C (35° to 46°F). Discard if frozen.

Diploid: Powder can presumably tolerate 30 days at room temperature. Lots produced by the same process for distribution in Europe can tolerate one month at 37°C (98.6°F). Contact the manufacturer regarding exposure to freezing temperatures. Use vaccine immediately after reconstitution. Shipping data not provided.

Michigan/SKB: Contact manufacturer regarding prolonged exposure to room temperature or elevated temperatures. Shipped by the distributor in insulated containers with temperature monitors.

Rabies Vaccine Comparisons

	Imovax Rabies	Generic
Manufacturer	Mérieux/Connaught	Michigan/SKB
Cell culture	MRC-5 human diploid cell culture	Dipliod fetal rhesus lung-2-cell culture
Strain	PM-1503-3M	Kissling/MDPH strain
Dose form	Powder for suspension	Suspension
Indications and route	Pre-expsoure prophylaxis (IM or ID) Post-exposure prophylaxis (IM only)	Pre-exposure prophylaxis (IM only) Post-exposure prophylazxis (IM only)
Packaging	1 ml IM package or 0.1 ml ID package	1 ml IM package only
Incidence of serum-sickness-like reaction	6%	<1%

Treatment Schedule for Pre-Exposure Rabies Prophylaxis

Type of vaccination	Route	Regimen
Primary	IM	1 ml in the deltoid area on days 0, 7 and 21 or 28 (either diploid or RVA).
	ID	0.1 ml on days 0, 7 and 21 ro 28 (diploid only).
Booster	IM	One 1 ml dose in the deltoid area (either diploid or RVA).
	ID	One 0.1 ml dose (diploid only).

Treatment Schedule for Post-Exposure Rabies Prophylaxis

Vaccination status	Treatment[1]
Not previously vaccinated	Local wound cleansing: All post-exposure treatment should begin with immediate thorough cleansing of each wound with soap and water. Rabies Immune Globulin: Give 20 IU/kg body weight. If anatomically feasible, infiltrate up to one-half the dose around the wound(s) and inject the balance IM in the gluteal area. Do not give RIG through the same syringe or into the same anatomical site as rabies vaccine. Beacuse RIG may partially supress active induction of antirabies antibody, give no more than the recommended dose. Rabies Vaccine: Give 1 ml IM in the deltoid area on days 0, 3, 7, 14 and 28.
Previously vaccinated[2]	Local wound cleansing: All post-exposure treatments begin with immediate thorough cleansing of each wound with soap and water. Do not administer RIG. Rabies vaccine: Give 1 ml IM in the deltoid area on days 0 and 3.

[1]These regimens apply to all age groups, including children.
[2]Any person with a history of pre- or post-exposure vaccination with diploid or RVA; or with both a history of prior vaccination with any other type of rabies vaccine and a documented history of antibody response to that vaccination.

Vaccinia (Smallpox) Vaccine, Dried, Calf-lymph Type

NAME:
Dryvax, 🍁 Generic

MANUFACTURERS:
Dryvax, Wyeth-Ayerst Laboratories-US, Connaught-Canada. Currently available only from the Centers for Disease Control and Prevention or the Canadian Laboratory Centres for Disease Control on a limited basis. 🍁 Generic, Connaught

Synonyms: Vaccinia vaccine, vaccinia virus, vaccine virus, cowpox virus, Jennerian vaccine. Although this product is classically called smallpox vaccine, this term is a misnomer since it contains no smallpox (variola) virus.

Viability: Live, attenuated

Antigenic Form: Whole virus

Antigenic Type: Protein

Indications: Induction of active immunity against vaccinia and smallpox (variola major and variola minor) in laboratory workers directly involved with smallpox or closely related orthopox viruses (eg, monkeypox, cowpox).

For induction of active immunity against vaccinia among healthcare workers involved with clinical trials of recombinant vaccinia viruses. Such workers might be exposed to vaccinia while changing dressings or other cutaneous exposure.

For induction of active immunity against vaccinia and smallpox among military recruits. Vaccination typically occurs during basic training to protect against a perceived biological warfare threat.

Unlabeled Uses: Vaccinia virus can be genetically engineered to express foreign DNA. Such recombinant vaccinia viruses can encode protein antigens and are being investigated as tools to induce protection against one or more other infectious agents.

Contraindications:

Absolute: Do not vaccinate persons of any age with eczema, other exfoliative skin conditions, atopic dermatitis, impetigo, varicella zoster, wounds or burns, and household contacts of such persons, because of an increased risk of eczema vaccinatum. Do not vaccinate persons receiving therapy with radiation, ACTH, corticosteroids, or other immunosuppressive drugs, nor persons with disorders of immune globulin synthesis, leukemia, lymphomas, or other malignant neoplasms affecting the bone marrow or lymphatic systems. Do not vaccinate persons hypersensitive to any of the components of this vaccine. Exposure of HIV-infected persons to smallpox had led to disseminated vaccinia infection (Redfield et al, 1987). Do not give to HIV-infected persons or those residing in a household with an HIV-infected person.

Relative: Defer vaccination during the course of an acute illness.

Elderly: No specific information is available about geriatric use of vaccinia (smallpox) vaccine.

Pregnancy: *Category C.* Contraindicated. On rare occasions, usually after primary vaccination, vaccinia virus has caused fetal infection. Fetal vaccinia usually results in stillbirth or death of the infant shortly after delivery. This vaccine is not known to cause congenital malformations. It is not known if corresponding antibodies cross the placenta. Generally, most IgG passage across the placenta occurs during the third trimester.

Lactation: It is not known if vaccinia virus or corresponding antibodies are excreted in breast milk. Problems in humans have not been documented.

Children: Contraindicated. Need is based on occupational exposure only.

Adverse Reactions:
A fever is common after vaccination. Up to 70% of children have 1 or more days of temperature $\geq 37.8°C$ $(100°F)$ from 4 to 14 days after primary vaccination and 15% to 20% have temperatures $\geq 38.9°C$ $(102°F)$. After revaccination, 35% of children develop temperatures $\geq 37.8°C$ $(100°F)$ and 5% have temperatures $\geq 38.9°C$ $(102°F)$. Fever is less common among adults than children after both primary vaccination and revaccination.

Erythematous or urticarial rashes may occur 10 days after primary vaccination. Such vaccinees are usually afebrile and the rash resolves spontaneously within 2 to 4 days. Rarely, bullous erythema multiforme (Stevens-Johnson syndrome) may occur.

Accidental infection at another site (usually as a result of autoinoculation) is the most frequent complication of vaccination, accounting for about half of all complications of primary vaccination and revaccination. The most common sites involved are the face, eyelid, nose, mouth, genitalia and rectum. Most lesions heal without specific therapy, but vaccinia immune globulin (VIG) may be useful for cases of ocular implantation.

General vaccinia among persons without underlying illnesses is characterized by a vesicular rash of varying extent. The rash is generally self-limited and requires little or no therapy, except among persons whose conditions appear to be toxic or who have serious underlying illness. More severe complications of vaccination include eczema vaccinatum, progressive vaccinia and postvaccinial encephalitis. These complications occur at least 10 times more often among primary vaccinees than among revaccinees and also more frequently among infants than among older children and adults.

Encephalomyelitis, encephalopathy, transverse myelitis, acute infectious polyneuritis, vaccinia necrosum and secondary pyogenic infections at the site of vaccination have also been reported following vaccination. Death is rare (1 to 2 deaths per million primary vaccinations, 1 death per 10 million revaccinations), most frequently resulting from postvaccinal encephalitis or progressive vaccinia.

Vaccinia may be transmitted from a vaccine recipient to a close contact (27 infections per million vaccinations). Over 60% of contact transmission results in uncomplicated inadvertent inoculation. About 30% of contact transmission results in eczema vaccinatum, which may be fatal. Eczema vaccinatum may be more severe among contacts than vaccinees, possibly because of simultaneous multiple inoculations at several sites. Contact transmission rarely results in postvaccinal encephalitis or vaccinia necrosum.

Consultation: Advice on the diagnosis and management of vaccinia infection and vaccination complications is available from CDC. Telephone 404-639-1870 during the day and 404-639-3311 during evenings and weekends.

Pharmacologic & Dosing Characteristics

Dosage: Shake product well before withdrawing each dose.

Apply 2 or 3 pressures or punctures for primary vaccination.

Cutaneous Response to Vaccination: A papule typically develops at the site of vaccination 2 to 5 days after administration to a non-immune person. The papule becomes vesicular, then pustular, and reaches its maximum size in 8 to 10 days. The pustule dries and forms a scab, which separates within 14 to 21 days after vaccination, leaving a typical scar. Primary vaccination can produce swelling and tenderness of regional lymph nodes, beginning 3 to 10 days after vaccination and persisting for 2 to 4 weeks after the skin lesion

has healed. Maximum viral shedding occurs 4 to 14 days following vaccination, but vaccinia can be recovered from the site of vaccination until the scab separates from the skin.

If no vesicle is observed, repeat vaccination with another batch of vaccine.

Route & Site: Percutaneous, using a bifurcated needle, traditionally at an upper deltoid site. This procedure is also called scarification. A residual scar indicates prior vaccination.

Cover the vaccination site at all times with a porous bandage until the scab detaches and the underlying skin heals. Do not use an occlusive bandage. Keep the site dry. While bathing, cover the site with an impermeable bandage. The most important measure to prevent inadvertent implantation and contact transmission is thorough handwashing after changing bandages or after any contact with the vaccination site.

Efficacy: After percutaneous administration, >95% of persons receiving their first vaccinia (smallpox) vaccination will develop neutralizing or hemagglutination-inhibition antibody at a titer ≥1:10.

Neutralizing antibody titers ≥1:10 are found among 75% of persons for 10 years after receiving 2 doses and up to 30 years after receiving 3 doses.

Onset: Antibody appears in 4 to 5 days, peaks within 4 weeks

Duration: 3 to 30 years

Drug Interactions: Since vaccinia (smallpox) vaccine consists of live viruses, reconstitute it with a diluent that does not contain preservatives. Preservatives may inactivate constituent viruses and render the vaccine ineffective.

The product insert recommends intervals of 2 days to 2 weeks between live-virus vaccinations. The product labeling accepts simultaneous immunization with poliovirus, measles, vaccinia (smallpox) and yellow fever vaccines, if each is indicated and a 30 day interval between vaccinations is not feasible. Some researchers have failed to find any impairment of effect of either vaccine at various intervals from 3 to 28 days.

Vaccinia immune globulin (VIG) is the antidote to disseminated vaccinia infection resulting from vaccinia (smallpox) vaccine. Refer to VIG monograph in the Immune Globulins section.

Like all live viral vaccines, administration to patients receiving immunosuppressant drugs, including steroids, or radiation may predispose patients to disseminated infections or insufficient response to immunization. They may remain susceptible despite immunization.

Simultaneous administration of vaccinia (smallpox) vaccine and indomethacin caused an exaggerated cutaneous response in one isolated case. Avoid concurrent use. It is not known if this effect occurs with other nonsteroidal anti-inflammatory drugs.

Concurrent administration of exogenous interferon products may inhibit viral replication and thus inhibit antibody response to the vaccine. Avoid concurrent use.

As a general rule, to avoid inactivation of the attenuated virus, administer live virus vaccines at least 14 to 30 days before or 6 to 8 weeks after administration of any immune globulin or other blood product. Alternately, check antibody titers or repeat the vaccine dose 3 months after IG administration.

Pharmaceutical Characteristics

Concentration: Contains 10^8 pock-forming units per ml. An administered dose contains an estimated 2.5×10^5 pock-forming units.

Packaging: Package containing vial and diluent sufficient for 100 vaccinations, with sufficient bifurcated needles

Dose Form: Powder for suspension

Diluent for Reconstitution: 50% glycerin in sterile water: 0.15 ml per 25 vaccination vial, 0.25 ml per 100-vaccination vial.

Storage/Stability: Store at $2°$ to $8°C$ ($35°$ to $46°F$). Keep in coldest part of refrigerator or in freezer, colder than $-18°C$ ($0°F$) if possible.

Freezing will not harm this product. Ship at $0°C$ ($32°F$) or colder.

Vaccine powder can tolerate 10 days at room temperature.

Reconstituted vaccine can tolerate 3 months in a refrigerator.

Varicella Virus Vaccine Live

VIRAL VACCINES

NAME:
Varivax

MANUFACTURERS:
Merck Vaccine Division, licensed from the Research Foundation for Microbial Disease of Osaka University (Biken).

Synonyms: Varicella virus infection is also known as chickenpox, herpes zoster and shingles.

Viability: Live, attenuated

Antigenic Form: Whole virus

Antigenic Type: Protein

Use Characteristics

Indications: Induction of active immunity against infections caused by varicella-zoster virus in people ≥12 months of age.

Unlabeled Uses: Research in progress is assessing the role of varicella vaccine in preventing or reducing the severity of herpes zoster ("shingles") in adults and the elderly.

Contraindications:

Absolute: A history of hypersensitivity to any component of the vaccine, including gelatin. A history of anaphylactoid reaction to neomycin. Patients with a blood dyscrasia, leukemia, lymphomas of any type, or other malignant neoplasms affecting the bone marrow or lymphatic systems. People receiving immunosuppressive therapy, because they are more susceptible to infections than healthy people; vaccination with live attenuated varicella vaccine can result in a more extensive vaccine-associated rash or disseminated disease in people on immunosuppressant doses of corticosteroids (2 mg/kg prednisone or equivalent). People with primary and acquired immunodeficiency states, including those who are immunosuppressed in association with AIDS or other clinical manifestations of infection with human immunodeficiency virus; cellular immune deficiencies; and hypogammaglobulinemic and dysgammaglobulinemic states. Active untreated tuberculosis. Pregnancy.

Relative: A family history of congenital or hereditary immunodeficiency, until the immune competence of the potential vaccine recipient is evaluated. Any febrile respiratory illness or other active febrile infection.

Elderly: Varicella vaccine can boost immunity to varicella-zoster virus in the elderly and may prevent or attenuate herpes zoster ("zoster" or "shingles") in that group (Levin et al, 1992).

Adults: Varicella vaccine is safe and effective in adults. Vaccination is recommended for susceptible people in close contact with others at high risk for serious complications (eg, health care workers and family contacts). Consider vaccinating susceptible people in the following settings:

• People who live or work in environments where varicella transmission is likely (eg, teachers of young children, day-care employees, residents and staff in institutional settings).

• People who live or work in environments in which transmission can occur (eg, college students, inmates and staff of corrrectional institutions, military personnel).

• Nonpregnant women of childbearing age, to reduce the risk of viral transmission to the fetus.

• International travelers, expecially if the traveler expects to have close personal contact with local populations.

Pregnancy: *Category C.* It is not known if attenuated varicella virus or corresponding antibodies cross the placenta. Generally, most IgG passage across the placenta occurs during the third trimester. The possible effects of the vaccine on fetal development are unknown at this time. However, natural varicella is known to sometimes cause fetal harm. If vaccination of postpubertal females is undertaken, pregnancy should be avoided for 1 month following each vaccination. To assess any effects of *Varivax* on fetal development, clinicians are encouraged to register any patient vaccinated within 3 months before pregnancy or any time during pregnancy by calling 1-800-986-8999.

Lactation: It is not known if attenuated varicella virus or corresponding antibodies cross into human breast milk. Problems in humans have not been documented. Varicella vaccination may be considered for a nursing mother.

Children: Safe and effective in immunocompetent children ≥12 months of age. Safety and efficacy of varicella vaccine in children <12 months old have not been established. There is a 17% transmission rate of disease from vaccinated leukemic children to healthy seronegative individuals if the vaccinated leukemic child develops a rash. Children and adolescents with acute lymphoblastic leukemia (ALL) in remission can receive the vaccine under an investigational protocol.

Adverse Reactions:

In clinical trials, varicella vaccine was given to 11,102 healthy children, adolescents and adults. The vaccine was generally well tolerated.

In a double-blind placebo-controlled study among 914 healthy children and adolescents who were serologically confirmed to be susceptible to varicella, the only adverse reactions that occurred at a significantly greater rate in vaccine recipients than in placebo recipients were pain and redness at the injection site.

In clinical trials involving healthy children monitored for up to 42 days after a single dose of varicella vaccine, the frequency of fever, injection-site complaints or rashes were reported as follows:

Fever ≥39°C (102°F) oral (14.7%; this rate was measured over a 6-week interval, without any control group to compare it with);

Injection-site complaints, including pain/soreness, swelling or erythema, rash, pruritis, hematoma, induration, stiffness (19.3%; peaking 0 to 2 days after vaccination);

Varicella-like rash at the injection site (3.4%; peaking after 8 to 19 days; median number of lesions, 2);

Generalized varicella-like rash (3.8%; median number of lesions, 5; peaking after 5 to 26 days).

In addition, the following most frequently (≥1%) reported adverse experiences, without regard to causality, are listed in decreasing order of frequency: Upper respiratory illness, cough, irritability/nervousness, fatigue, disturbed sleep, diarrhea, loss of appetite, vomiting, otitis, diaper rash/contact rash, headache, teething, malaise, abdominal pain, other rash, nausea, eye complaints, chills, lymphadenopathy, myalgia, lower respiratory illness, allergic reactions (including allergic rash, hives), stiff neck, heat rash/prickly heat, arthralgia, eczema/dry skin/dermatitis, constipation, itching. Pneumonitis and febrile seizures have occurred rarely (<1%) in children; a causal relationship has not been established.

A chickenpox rash develops in 40% of vaccinated leukemic children, but usually consists of <10 lesions.

In clinical trials involving healthy adolescents, the majority of whom received two doses of varicella vaccine and were monitored for up to 42 days after any dose, the frequency of fever, injection-site complaints or rashes were reported as follows: Fever ≥37.7°C (100°F) oral (9.5% to 10.2%); injection-site complaints, including soreness, erythema, swelling, rash, pruritis, pyrexia, hematoma, induration, numbness (24.4% to 32.5%; peaking 0 to 2 days after vaccination); varicella-like rash at the injection site (3% after the first dose; peaking after 6 to 20 days; 1% after the second dose, peaking after 0 to 6 days; median number of lesions,

2); generalized varicella-like rash (5.5% after the first dose, peaking after 7 to 21 days; 0.9% after the second dose; median number of lesions, 5).

In addition, the following most frequently (≥1%) reported adverse experiences, without regard to causality, are listed in decreasing order of frequency: Upper respiratory illness, headache, fatigue, cough, myalgia, disturbed sleep, nausea, malaise, diarrhea, stiff neck, irritability/nervousness, lymphadenopathy, chills, eye complaints, abdominal pain, loss of appetite, arthralgia, otitis, itching, vomiting, other rashes, constipation, lower respiratory illness, allergic reactions (including allergic rash, hives), contact rash, cold/cankersore.

After vaccine licensing, cases of encephalitis, ataxia and erythema multiforme were reported within 6 weeks after varicella vaccination. Three cases of anaphylaxis within 10 minutes of vaccination were reported in the first 12 months of widespread vaccine availability. A casual relationship has not been determined between vaccination and these events.

Herpes Zoster ("shingles"): Overall, 9454 healthy children (1 to 12 years of age) and 1648 adolescents and adults (≥13 years of age) have been vaccinated with Oka/Merck live attenuated varicella vaccine in clinical trials. Eight cases of herpes zoster have been reported in children during 44,994 person-years of follow-up in clinical trials, resulting in a calculated incidence of at least 18 cases per 100,000 person-years. The completeness of this reporting has not been determined. This rate is considerably less than a rate of 77 per 100,000 person-years in a separate study of healthy unvaccinated children after natural infection. One case of herpes zoster has been reported in the adolescent and adult age group during 7826 person-years of follow-up in clinical trials, resulting in a calculated incidence of 12.8 cases per 100,000 person years. All nine cases were mild and without sequelae. Two cultures (from one child and one adult) obtained from vesicles were positive wild-type varicella-zoster virus as confirmed by restriction endonuclease analysis. The long-term effect of varicella vaccine on the incidence of herpes zoster, particularly in those vaccinees exposed to natural varicella, is unknown at present.

Pharmacologic & Dosing Characteristics

 Dosage: *Children (1 to 12 years of age):* A single 0.5 ml dose

Adults and adolescents (≥13 years of age): A single 0.5 ml dose, followed by a second 0.5 ml dose 4 to 8 weeks later.

Route and Site: SC. When some children inadvertently received varicella vaccine IM, seroconversion rates were similar to the SC route. Persistence of antibody and efficacy after IM injection is unknown.

The outer aspect of the upper arm (deltoid) is the preferred site of injection, although the anterolateral thigh may be used.

Documentation Requirements: Prudent long-term record-keeping is appropriate.

Efficacy: A seroconversion rate ≥95% after a single dose was seen in healthy children. The rate in adolescents and adults is about 75% to 94% after the

first dose. A second dose of varicella vaccine produces virtually 100% seroconversion. Seroconversion was defined as acquisition of any detectable varicella antibodies (gpELISA value >0.3). This is a highly sensitive assay which is not commercially available.

In trials of several formulations of varicella vaccine, at doses ranging from 1,000 to 17,000 PFU, the majority of subjects who received varicella vaccine and were exposed to wild-type virus were either completely protected from chickenpox or developed a milder form of the disease. The protective efficacy of varicella vaccine was evaluated in three different ways: 1) By comparing chickenpox rates in vaccinees versus historical controls, 2) by assessment of protection from disease following household exposure and 3) by a placebo-controlled, double-blind clinical trial.

In one trial of 4142 children, 2.1% to 3.6% of vaccinees per year reported chickenpox (called breakthrough cases). This represents a 57% to 77% decrease from the total number of cases expected based on attack rates in children aged 1 to 9 years over this same period (8.3% to 9.1%). In those who developed breakthrough chickenpox after vaccination, the majority experienced mild disease (median number of lesions <50). In one study, 47% (27/58) of breakthrough cases had <50 lesions, compared with 8% (7/92) in unvaccinated individuals; 7% (4/58) of breakthrough cases had >300 lesions, compared with 50% (46/92) in unvaccinated individuals. In studies of vaccinated children who contracted chickenpox after a household exposure, 57% (31/54) of the cases reported <50 lesions and 1.9% (1/54) reported

>300 lesions with an oral temperature >37.8°C (100°F).

In later studies of the current vaccine, 1164 children received 2900 to 9000 PFU of attenuated virus per dose and have been followed for up to 3 years after a single dose. From 0.2% to 1% of vaccinees per year reported breakthrough chickenpox for up to 3 years after vaccination. This represents a 93% decrease from the number of cases expected. In those who developed breakthrough chickenpox after vaccination, the majority experienced mild disease.

Among a subset of vaccinees who were actively followed, 259 were exposed to an individual with chickenpox in a household setting. There were no reports of breakthrough chickenpox in 80% of exposed children; 20% reported a mild form of chickenpox. This represents a 77% reduction in the expected number of cases when compared to the historical 87% attack rate of varicella following household exposure in unvaccinated individuals.

Although no placebo-controlled trial was carried out with varicella vaccine using the current vaccine formula, a placebo-controlled trial was conducted using a formulation containing 17,000 PFU per dose. In this trial, a single dose of varicella vaccine protected 96% to 100% of children 1 to 14 years of age against chickenpox over a 2-year period.

Although no placebo-controlled trial was carried out in adolescents and adults, efficacy was determined by evaluation of protection when vaccinees received two doses of varicella vaccine 4 or 8 weeks apart and were subsequently exposed to chickenpox in a household setting. In up to 2 years of active follow-up, 17 of 64 (27%) vaccinees reported breakthrough chickenpox following household exposure; of the 17 cases, 12 (71%) reported <50lesions, 5 reported 50 to 300 lesions, and none reported >300 lesions with an oral temperature >100°F. In combined clinical studies of adolescents and adults (n=1019) who received two doses of varicella vaccine and later developed breakthrough chicken pox (42 of 1019), 25 of 42 (60%) reported <50 lesions, 16 (38%) reported 50 to 300 lesions and 1 of 42 (2%) reported >300 lesions and an oral temperature >100°F. In combined clinical studies of adolescents (n=1019) who received doses of varicella vaccine and later developed breakthrough chickenpox (42 of 1019), 25 of 42 (60%) reported <50 lesions, 16 (38%) reported 50 to 300 lesions and 1 of 42 (2%) reported >300 lesions and an oral temperature >100°F.

The attack rate among unvaccinated adults exposed to a single contact in a household has not been previously studied. When compared with the previously reported attack rate of natural varicella of 87% following household exposure among unvaccinated children, this represents an approximate 70% reduction in the expected number of cases in the household setting.

Onset: 97% of healthy children had seroconverted when assessed 4 to 6 weeks after vaccination.

Duration: The duration of protection of *Varivax* is not precisely known at present and the need for booster doses is not fully defined. This vaccine provides 70% to 90% protection against infection and 95% protection against severe disease for 7 to 10 years after vaccination.

A boost in antibody levels has been observed in vaccinees following exposure to natural varicella, as well as after a booster dose of *Varivax* given 4 to 6 years after vaccination. In a highly vaccinated population, immunity for some people may wane due to lack of exposure to natural varicella as a result of shifting epidemiology. Post-marketing surveillance studies are ongoing to evaluate the need and timing for booster vaccination.

Studies in vaccinees examining chickenpox breakthrough rates over 5 years showed the lowest rates (0.2% to 2.9%) in the first 2 years after vaccination, and somewhat higher but stable rates in the third through fifth year. The severity of reported breakthrough chickenpox, as measured by number of lesions and maximum temperature, appeared not to increase with time since vaccination.

In clinical studies involving healthy children who received one dose of vaccine, detectable varicella antibodies (gpELISA >0.3) were present in 98.8% at 1 year, 98.9% at 2 years, 97.5% at 3 years and 99.5% at 4 years after vaccination. Antibody levels were present at least 1 year in 97.2% of healthy adolescents and adults who received two doses of live varicella vaccine separated by 4 to 8 weeks. A boost in antibody levels has been observed in vaccinees following exposure to natural varicella. This could account for the apparent long-term persistence of antibody levels after vaccination in these studies. The duration of protection from varicella obtained using *Varivax* vaccine in the absence of wild-type boosting is unknown. *Varivax* also induces cell-mediated immune responses in vaccinees. The relative contributions of humoral immunity and cell-mediated immunity to protection from chickenpox are unknown.

Drug Interactions: Since varicella vaccine consists of live viruses, reconstitute it with a diluent that does not contain preservatives. Preservatives may inactivate constituent viruses and render the vaccine ineffective.

Like all live viral vaccines, administration to patients receiving immunosuppressant drugs, including steroids or radiation, may predispose patients to disseminated infections or insufficient response to immunization. They may remain susceptible despite immunization. Immunosuppressive doses of corticosteriods are generally considered to be 20 mg/day or 2 mg/kg/day of prednisone, or an equivalent dose of other systemic steroids. Inhaled or topical corticosteroids are not immunosuppressive, nor are some alternate-day or short courses of systemic steroids. Otherwise, wait 1 to 3 months or more after discontinuing steroids before giving varicella vaccine. Withhold steroids for 2 to 3 weeks after vaccination, if possible.

Varivax can be given at the same time as MMR vaccine. Otherwise, give the vacine ≥30 days apart. To assess any interaction between *Varivax* and *M-M-R II* (Merck's measles-mumps-rubella vaccine), children were given them either concomitantly at separate sites or 6 weeks apart. Seroconversion rates and antibody levels were comparable between the two groups at about 6 weeks after vaccination to each of the virus vaccine components. No differences were noted in adverse reactions reported.

Limited data from an experimental product containing varicella vaccine suggest that varicella vaccine can be given simultaneously with diphtheria, tetanus, acellular pertussis (DTaP) vaccine and *PedvaxHIB* (Merck's Hib vaccine) using separate sites and syringes. However, there are no data relating to simultaneous administration of varicella vaccine with DTP or oral poliovirus vaccine (OPV). In one study, children received an investigational vaccine (a formulation combining measles, mumps, rubella and varicella in one syringe) at the same time as booster doses of DTaP and OPV, or received *M-M-R II* with booster doses of DTP and OPV, followed by varicella vaccine 6 weeks later. Six weeks after vaccination, seroconversion rates for measles, mumps, rubella and varicella and the percentage of vaccinees whose titers were boosted for diphtheria, tetanus, pertussis and polio were comparable between the two groups. But anti-varicella levels were slightly, perhaps insignificantly, decreased when the investigational vaccine containing varicella was administered concomitantly with DTaP. No clinically significant differences were noted in adverse reactions between the two groups.

In another study, one group of children received an investigational vaccine (a formulation combining measles, mumps, rubella and varicella in one syringe) at the same time as a booster dose of *PedvaxHIB*. Another group received *M-M-R II* and a booster dose of *PedvaxHIB* followed by varicella vaccine 6 weeks later. Six weeks after vaccination, seroconversion rates for measles, mumps, rubella and varicella and geometric mean titers for *PedvaxHIB* were comparable between the two groups, but anti-varicella levels were decreased when the investigational vaccine containing varicella was

given with *PedvaxHIB*. No clinically significant differences in adverse reactions were seen.

To avoid inactivation of the attenuated virus, give varicella vaccine at least 14 to 30 days before, or 5 months after, giving any immune globulin or other blood product. After giving varicella vaccine, any immune globulin, including VZIG, should not be given for 2 months thereafter, unless its use outweighs the benefits of vaccination. Alternately, check antibody titers or repeat the vaccine dose 5 months after IG administration.

Acyclovir and perhaps other antiviral drugs antagonize disseminated varicella infection, which may rarely be induced in vaccine recipients.

No data are yet available about possible suppression of tuberculin skin tests by varicella vaccine virus. Live virus vaccines may cause delayed-hypersensitivity skin tests (eg, tuberculin, histoplasmin) to appear falsely negative. Evaluate such tests knowingly. The effect may persist several weeks after vaccination. ACIP and AAP recommend that tuberculin tests be given prior to live-virus vaccination, simultaneously with it, or 6 or more weeks after vaccination.

Salicylates: Reye's syndrome has occurred in children and adolescents following natural varicella infection. The majority of these cases had received salicylates. Caution varicella vaccine recipients, parents and guardians not to use salicylates in vaccine recipients for 6 weeks after vaccination. There were no reports of Reye's syndrome in varicella vaccine recipients during clinical trials.

Patient Information: Ask patients, parents or guardians about reactions to previous doses of varicella vaccine or a similar product.

Pharmaceutical Characteristics

Concentration: At least 1350 plaque-forming units (PFU) per 0.5 ml dose 30 minutes after reconstitution at room temperature (20° to 25°C; 68° to 77°F).

Packaging: A single-dose vial of freeze-dried vaccine with a box of 10 vials of diluent (package B). A box of 10 single-dose vials of freeze-dried vaccine with a box of 10 vials of diluent (package B).

Dose Form: Lyophilized powder for suspension

Diluent for Reconstitution: Sterile water for injection without preservative

Storage/Stability: Keep powdered vaccine frozen, at an average temperature of −15°C (+5°F) or colder. Storage in a frost-free freezer with an average temperature of −15°C (+5°F) or colder is acceptable. Before reconstitution, protect from light. Store the diluent separately at room temperature or in a refrigerator. During shipment, to ensure that there is no loss of potency, the vaccine must be maintained at a temperature of −20°C (−4°F) or colder. Shipped in insulated containers with coolants. Minimal potency can be maintained if the vaccine powder is stored continuously for ≤72 hours at 2° to 8°C (36° to 46°F). Discard vaccine stored at 2° to 8°C if not used within 72 hours of beginning storage at 2° to 8°C. For information regarding stability at temperatures other than those recommended for storage, call 1-800-9-VARIVAX.

Administer the vaccine immediately after reconstitution to minimize loss of potency. Discard if reconstituted vaccine is not used within 30 minutes. Do not freeze reconstituted vaccine.

Handling: To reconstitute the vaccine, first withdraw 0.7 ml of diluent into a syringe. Inject all the diluent in the syringe into the vial of freeze-dried vaccine and gently agitate to mix thoroughly. Withdraw the entire contents into a syringe, change the needle and inject the total volume (about 0.5 ml).

Yellow Fever Vaccine
VIRAL VACCINES

NAME:
YF-Vax

MANUFACTURERS:
Connaught Laboratories. Distribution is limited to designated Yellow Fever Vaccination Centers authorized to issue certificates of yellow-fever vaccination. Contact health departments for locations of local centers. ♣ Connaught

Synonyms: Yellow fever is also known as fiebre amarilla and yellow jack, for the flag of quarantine that flew over infected sailing vessels.

Viability: Live, attenuated

Antigenic Form: Whole virus

Antigenic Type: Protein

Use Characteristics

Indications: Induction of active immunity against yellow-fever virus, primarily among travelers to yellow-fever endemic areas (especially sub-Saharan Africa and Central and northern South America).

Contraindications:
Absolute: Patients with a history of a hypersensitivity reaction to this vaccine or any of its components. Patients with any form of immunodeficiency.

Relative: Defer immunization during the course of any acute illness.

Elderly: No specific information is available about geriatric use of yellow-fever vaccine.

Pregnancy: *Category* C. Avoid use unless travel to high-risk area is unavoidable. Generally, most IgG passage across the placenta occurs during the third trimester. Yellow fever vaccine virus crossed the placenta to one newborn among 41 mothers unknow-ingly vaccinated during pregnancy (Tsai et al, 1993). The child appeared unaffected by infection, but yellow-fever virus is known to be neurotropic. Avoid vaccination during pregnancy if at all possible.

Lactation: It is not known if yellow-fever virus or corresponding antibodies are excreted in breast milk. Problems in humans have not been documented.

Children: The same dose is used for children as for adults. Do not administer to infants <6 months of age unless travel to high-risk area is unavoidable, to avoid a risk of encephalitis. Vaccinate pregnant women and infants 6 to 9 months of age only if they must travel and they cannot avoid mosquito bites. Vaccinate infants 4 to 6 months of age only if the risk of infection is high. Use the same dose for children and adults. Do not vaccinate infants <4 months of age. They are especially vulnerable to swelling of the brain after vaccination.

Adverse Reactions:
About 10% of recipients may experience fever or malaise following immunization, usually appearing 7 to 14 days after administration. In rare instances, encephalitis has developed in very young infants. This usually has not been severe and recovery has ordinarily occurred without sequelae. One death was reported. Anaphylaxis may occur.

Pharmacologic & Dosing Characteristics

Dosage: 0.5 ml
For a test of hypersensitivity, inject 0.02 ml to 0.03 ml intradermally on the volar surface of the forearm. Inject a negative control test of an equivalent volume of 0.9% sodium chloride at an analogous site. Even this low dose of vaccine may induce some limited immunity.

Route: SC

Efficacy: Essentially 100%

Onset: 7 to 10 days

Duration: 10 years or longer

Drug Interactions: Since yellow-fever vaccine consists of live viruses, reconstitute it with a diluent that does not contain preservatives. Preservatives may inactivate constituent viruses and render the vaccine ineffective.

Like all live viral vaccines, administration to patients receiving immunosuppressant drugs, including steroids, or radiation may predispose patients to disseminated infections or insufficient response to immunization. They may remain susceptible despite immunization.

Concurrent cholera and yellow fever vaccination impairs the immune response to each vaccine. Separate these vaccinations by ≥3 weeks, if possible, or administer them on the same day if separation is not feasible.

Concurrent vaccination against hepatitis B and yellow fever viruses in one study reduced the antibody titer expected from yellow-fever vaccine. Separate these vaccinations by 1 month, if possible.

Yellow-fever vaccine does not interact with American-produced immune globulins, although it may be prudent to maintain an interval of several weeks between these drugs if time permits.

Concurrent administration of chloroquine to yellow-fever vaccine recipients does not affect antibody response.

Patient Information: Advise vaccinated persons to take personal precautions to reduce exposure to mosquito bites. Travelers should stay in screened or air-conditioned rooms, use insecticidal space sprays as necessary, and use mosquito repellents and protective clothing to avoid mosquito bites. Mosquitoes are most active at twilight hours and in the evening.

Pharmaceutical Characteristics

Concentration: Not less than 5.04 $\log_{10}$ plaque-forming units per 0.5 ml, not less than 2000 mouse LD_{50} units; 75% suspension of embryo particles by weight.

Packaging: Five single-dose vials with accompanying 1 ml diluents, 5 dose vial with an unspecified volume of diluent, 20 dose vial with an unspecified volume of diluent; a 100 dose vial with an unspecified volume of diluent is available on a contract basis only.

Dose Form: Powder for suspension

Diluent for Reconstitution: 0.9% sodium chloride without preservative. Add diluent slowly. Allow to stand 1 to 2 minutes, then swirl gently until uniformly suspended. To avoid foaming and protein degradation, do not shake. Do not dilute further.

Storage/Stability: Store in freezer at −30°C to +5°C (−22°F to 41°F), preferably <0°C (32°F). Shipped at −18°C (0°F) or lower, with dry ice. Do not accept shipment if no dry ice remains upon arrival. Elevated-temperature studies suggest a potency half-life of 14 days at 35°C to 37°C (95°F to 99°F) and 3.3 to 4.5 days at 45°C to 47°C (113°F to 117°F).

After reconstitution, potency persists for only 1 hour.

Immune Globulins

Broad-Spectrum Immune Globulins

Immune Globulin Intramuscular (Human)

Immune Globulin Intravenous (Human)

Anti-Infective Immune Globulins

Cytomegalovirus Immune
Globulin Intravenous (Human)

Hepatitis B Immune Globulin (Human)

Respiratory Syncytial Virus (RSV)
Immune Globulin (Human)

Rabies Immune Globulin (Human)

Vaccinia Immune Globulin (Human)

Varicella-Zoster Immune Globulin

Immune Globulin Intramuscular (Human)

BROAD-SPECTRUM IMMUNE GLOBULINS

NAMES:

Gammar IM, Generic

MANUFACTURERS:

Gammar IM, Armour Pharmaceutical Company; Generic, Massachusetts Public Health Biological; Michigan Department of Public Health; New York Blood Center

Synonyms: IG, IGIM, IMIG, gamma globulin, GG, Cohn globulin; formerly called immune serum globulin, ISG. Human normal immunoglobulin (HNIG) is the comparable term used in the United Kingdom. Gamma globulin is a misnomer, originally based on electrophoretic mobility. IgG and IgA primarily exist as gamma globulins, although some are beta globulins. To further confound the issue, most IgM and IgD molecules are beta globulins, although some are gamma globulins. Nonetheless, the usual therapeutic meaning of the term gamma globulin refers to IgG.

Comparison: Therapeutically equivalent

Viability: Inactive, passive, transient

Antigenic Form: Human immunoglobulin, unmodified

Antigenic Type: Protein, IgG antibody, polyclonal, 20% to 30% polymeric

Use Characteristics

Indications: For passive prevention of or modification of hepatitis A, especially if given before or soon after exposure.

For passive prevention of or modification of measles infection in susceptible persons exposed <6 days previously, especially household contacts <1 year of age, in whom the risk of measles complications is highest.

For IgG-replacement therapy in certain persons with hypo-or agammaglobulinemia. Prophylactic therapy, especially against infections due to encapsulated bacteria, is effective in Bruton-type, sex-linked congenital agammaglobulinemia, agammaglobulinemia and severe combined immunodeficiency.

For passive prevention of varicella in immunocompromised patients if varicella-zoster immune globulin (VZIG) is not available and IGIM can be given promptly.

For reduction of the likelihood of fetal damage in susceptible women exposed to rubella in the first trimester of pregnancy and who will not consider a therapeutic abortion. This mode of therapy is of questionable value.

The ACIP (1993) explicitly recommends immune globulin (IV or IM, as appropriate) administration to symptomatic HIV-infected persons and other severely immunocompromised persons exposed to measles, regardless of immunization status. Operationally defined, severe immunosuppression may result from congenital immunodeficiency, HIV infection, leukemia, lymphoma, aplastic anemia, generalized malignancy, therapy with alkylating agents, antimetabolites, radiation or large, sustained doses of corticosteroids.

Contraindications:

Absolute: Patients with isolated immunoglobulin A (IgA) deficiency, since circulating IgE antibodies that specifically neutralize IgA may react with IgA in this product and induce an anaphylactoid reaction.

Relative: Patients with thrombocytopenia or other coagulation disorders, in view of the IM route of administration. Give IGIM with caution to patients with a history of systemic allergic reactions following the administration of human IG preparations.

Elderly: Generally safe and effective.

Pregnancy: *Category* C. Use only if clearly needed. Intact IgG crosses the placenta from the maternal circulation increasingly after 30 weeks gestation.

Lactation: It is not known if IGIM antibodies are excreted in breast milk. Problems in humans have not been documented.

Children: Generally safe and effective.

Adverse Reactions: Local pain and tenderness at the injection site, urticaria, and angioedema may occur. Anaphylactic reactions, although rare, have been reported following injection of this product.

Pharmacologic & Dosing Characteristics

Dosage:

Hepatitis A: 0.02 ml/kg for household and institutional contacts of persons infected with hepatitis A. Give travelers to hepatitis A-endemic areas (eg, developing countries with inadequate sanitation systems) who will stay <3 months 0.02 ml/kg. Give travelers staying 3 months or longer 0.06 ml/kg, with booster doses every 4 to 6 months throughout their stay.

Measles (Rubeola): 0.25 ml/kg to prevent or modify measles in susceptible persons exposed <6 days previously. Give susceptible immunocompromised children 0.5 ml/kg (maximum dose: 15 ml).

Immunoglobulin Deficiency: IGIM may prevent serious infections in patients if circulating IgG levels are maintained around 200 mg/100 ml plasma. Give 0.66 ml/kg (at least 100 mg/kg) every 3 to 4 weeks. A larger initial dose (eg, 1.2 ml/kg) is often given at the onset of therapy. Fast metabolizers may require more frequent injections.

Varicella: If VZIG is unavailable, give 0.6 to 1.2 ml/kg IGIM.

Rubella: IGIM 0.55 ml/kg may benefit the offspring of women who will not consider a therapeutic abortion.

Route & Site:

IM, preferably in the upper, outer quadrant of the gluteal region. Divide doses >10 ml and inject into several muscle sites to reduce local pain and discomfort.

Do not inject IGIM intravenously, because its high proportion of aggregates may cause serious adverse reactions (eg, activation of the complement cascade).

Additional Doses:

Additional doses may be warranted if disease exposure continues and no other prophylactic alternatives are available (eg, hepatitis A).

Efficacy:

Hepatitis A: IGIM is 80% to 95% effective in preventing hepatitis A, depending on the temporal relation between administration and exposure and on the severity of exposure.

Measles: IGIM reduces the risk of clinical evidence of measles by an estimated 50%. A lower incidence of measles encephalitis has also been associated with use of IGIM.

Varicella: IGIM reduces severity of disease, as measured by temperature and the number of pox.

Onset: IgG titers peak 2 to 5 days after IM injection.

Duration: Mean IgG half-life in circulation of persons with normal IgG levels is 23 days.

Drug Interactions: IGIM may diminish the antibody response to attenuated measles, mumps and rubella vaccines through antigen-antibody antagonism. As a general rule, administer live virus vaccines 14 to 30 days before or 6 to 12 weeks after IGIM. Alternately, administer live virus vaccines during this interval if corresponding antibody titers are measured 3 months after IGIM administration. Siber et al (1993) recommend basing the interval on the dose of IgG administered.

IGM does not appear to interfere with development of immunity following oral poliovirus or yellow fever vaccination. However, it may be prudent not to administer these vaccines shortly after IGIM administration. Exceptions include unexpected travel to or contact with epidemic or endemic areas or persons. If OPV is given with or shortly after IG, repeat the OPV dose 3 months later if immunization is still indicated.

It is not known if IGIM interferes with the efficacy of other attenuated vaccines (eg, adenovirus, BCG, typhoid, vaccinia). It may be prudent not to administer these vaccines shortly after IGIM administration unless such a procedure is unavoidable.

As with other drugs administered by IM injection, give IGIM with caution to persons receiving anticoagulant therapy.

Pharmaceutical Characteristics

Concentration: 15% to 18% protein, ≥90% IgG

Packaging:

Armour: 2 ml multidose vial, 10 ml multidose vial.

Massachusetts: Data not provided, excess production is distributed outside the State of Massachusetts.

Michigan: 2 ml multidose vial.

New York: Data not provided.

Dose Form: Solution

Storage/Stability: Store at 2° to 8°C (36° to 46° F). Discard if frozen.

Armour: Product can tolerate 72 hours at room temperature, not exceeding 30°C (86°F). Shipped via overnight courier in insulated containers. Refrigerate upon receipt.

Massachusetts, Michigan, New York: Contact manufacturer regarding prolonged exposure to room temperature or elevated temperatures. Shipping data not provided.

Immune Globulin Intravenous (Human)
BROAD-SPECTRUM IMMUNE GLOBULINS

NAME:

Venoglobulin-I, Venoglobulin-S, Polygam S/D, Gammar-P IV, Gamimune N, Gammagard S/D, Iveegam, Sandoglobulin

MANUFACTURER:

Venoglobulin-I, Venoglobulin-S, Alpha Therapeutic Corporation; *Polygam S/D,* American Red Cross (ARC) Blood Services; prepared with ARC's plasma using Hyland's process and facilities; *Gammar-P IV,* Armour Pharmaceutical Company; *Gamimune N,* Bayer Corporation; *Gammagard S/D,* Hyland Division of Baxter Healthcare Corporation; *Iveegam,* Immuno-U.S,; *Sandoglobulin,* Swiss Red Cross, distributed by Sandoz Pharmaceuticals Corporation

Synonyms: IGIV, IVIG, IVIgG, IVGG. The N suffix in *Gamimune N* refers to its native character. The I and S suffixes in *Venoglobulin* names refer to intact nature and solution form. The S/D suffix in *Polygam* and *Gammagard* refers to solvent-detergent treatment. The -P suffix to the *Gammar* name refers to pasteurization.

Viability: Inactive, passive, transient

Antigenic Form: Human immunoglobulin, unmodified. The Fc portion of the IgG molecule remains functionally intact.

Comparison: For most purposes, the various IGIV products are therapeutically equivalent in function. There are obvious differences in concentration, method of infusion, storage and other variables. In a very small subset of patients with anti-IgA antibodies, the quantity of IgA in the IGIV product must be minimized.

Antigenic Type: Protein, IgG antibody, polyclonal, primarily monomeric, permitting IV administration.

Use Characteristics

Indications: The various brands of IGIV have been licensed for one or more of the following uses. FDA-licensed indications for each brand appear in the table at the end of the monograph. IGIV is especially useful when high levels or rapid elevation of circulating antibodies are desired or

when IM injections are contraindicated, such as in patients with limited muscle mass or with a bleeding tendency.

IGIV is indicated for treatment of primary immunodeficiency states with severe impairment of antibody-forming capacity, such as congenital hypo- or agammaglobulinemia, common variable immunodeficiency, X-linked immunodeficiency with hyper IgM, transient hypogammaglobulinemia of infancy, IgG subclass deficiency with or without IgA deficiency, antibody deficiency with near-normal immunoglobulin levels, severe combined immunodeficiency, X-linked lymphoproliferative syndrome, ataxia-telangiectasia and Wiskott-Aldrich syndrome.

B-cell Chronic Lymphocytic Leukemia (CLL): For passive prevention of bacterial infections in patients with hypogammaglobulinemia or recurrent bacterial infections associated with CLL.

Immune Thrombocytopenic Purpura (ITP, formerly called idiopathic thrombocytopenic purpura): For treatment of ITP, in situations that require a rapid rise in platelet count, such as prior to surgery, in control of excessive bleeding, or as a measure to defer splenectomy. It is presently not possible to predict which ITP patients will respond to IGIV therapy, although the increase in platelet counts in children seems to be better than in adults. Childhood ITP may resolve spontaneously without treatment.

Kawasaki Syndrome: For use in combination with aspirin in the treatment of Kawasaki disease, within 10 days of onset of disease, to prevent the development of coronary artery abnormalities (eg, dilation, aneurysm, ectasia) that could lead to myocardial infarction.

Children with AIDS: Treatment of HIV-infected children can decrease the frequency of bacterial infections, increase the time free from serious bacterial infections and decrease the frequency of hospitalizations in children with AIDS. A double-blind, placebo controlled trial among 394 HIV-infected children 1 month to 12 years of age was conducted, using Miles' *Gamimune N* 400 mg/kg monthly. The rate of bacterial infections fell from 56.7 infections per 100 patient-years among placebo recipients to 33.1 infections using IGIV, a 40% drop. Similarly, the frequency of hospitalizations fell by 36%.

Bone-Marrow Transplant Patients: IGIV is safe and effective in reducing the incidence and severity of infections and graft-vs-host disease in bone-marrow transplant recipients >20 years old. A controlled clinical trial was conducted using Miles' *Gamimune N* 500 mg/kg weekly, reduced to monthly infusions 100 days after transplant. Among 384 patients, the frequency of GvHD was reduced from 51% in the control group to 34% in the treated group of patients >20 years of age. Mortality after 100 days was unaffected by IGIV. Little or no benefit was apparent among younger patients.

Unlabeled Uses: An expert panel convened by the University Hospital Consortium (UHC) determined that there is documented evidence of efficacy for only three indications not currently recognized by the FDA (Ratko et al, 1995). These include posttransfusion purpura and Guillain-Barré syndrome or chronic inflammatory demyelinating polyneuropathy (as an alternative to plasma exchange). Use might be warranted for select patients with certain other conditions for whom other interventions have been unsuccessful or intolerable: Patients with autoimmune hemolytic anemia, parvovirus B19 infection and severe anemia, multiple myeloma, immune-mediated neutropenia, neonatal alloimmune thrombocytopenia, thrombocytopenia refractory to platelet transfusions, acute decompensation in severe myasthenia gravis, severe active dermatomyositis or polymyositis, systemic lupus erythematosus, systemic vasculitic syndromes, West or Lennox-Gastaut forms of pediatric intractable epilepsy, in CMV-seronegative recipients of CMV-seropositive organs, low-birth-weight infants (<1500 g) or hypogammaglobulinemic infants. The UHC panel found no convincing evidence of efficacy for routine IGIV use in 35 other indications suggested in case reports or other preliminary publications, including some described in the following paragraph.

IGIV is being investigated in the prevention or treatment of the following diseases: HIV infection, autoimmune diseases (eg, rhesus hemolytic disease, factor VIII deficiencies, bullous pemphigoid, rheumatoid arthritis, Sjögren's syndrome, type I diabetes mellitus), IgG4 subclass deficiencies, intractable epilepsy (possibly due to IgG2 subclass deficiency), cystic fibrosis, trauma, thermal injury (eg, severe burns), cytomegalovirus infection, neuromuscular disorders, prophylaxis of infections associated with bone-marrow transplantation, and GI protection (ie, oral administration).

A study of IGIV therapy to prevent neonatal sepsis (Baker et al, 1992) demonstrated significant reduction in time to first nosocomial infection and length of hospital stays. Nonetheless, Siber (1992) has expressed reservations about IGIV use in this manner.

Oral administration of IGIV may provide some local protection of the GI tract from bacterial, viral and fungal infections. IGIV given orally reduced the duration of rotaviral diarrhea, viral

excretion and hospitalization in a placebo controlled trial (Guarino et al, 1994). IgG is not extensively absorbed from the GI tract. Native IgA predominates in the GI tract, with smaller amounts of IgM and IgG. Oral immune globulin supplements should be considered investigational. In one experiment of an oral dose of radiolabeled IgG, 50% of the recovered radioactivity was found in the stool in an immunologically active form, while the balance was excreted in the urine (Losonsky et al, 1985). A trial of an oral IgA-IgG preparation shows promise (Eibl et al, 1988).

 Contraindications:

Absolute: None

Relative: IGIV is contraindicated in persons with a history of anaphylactic or severe systemic response to human IM or IV immune globulin products. IGIV products are generally contraindicated in persons with IgA deficiency, some 17% to 40% of whom have circulating anti-IgA antibodies. Nonetheless, *Iveegam, Gammagard, Polygam,* and perhaps other formulations may successfully be given to some of these patients with due caution.

Elderly: No specific information is available about geriatric use of IGIV.

Pregnancy: *Category C.* Use only if clearly needed. Intact IgG crosses the placenta from the maternal circulation increasingly after 30 weeks gestation. In cases of maternal ITP, where IGIV was administered to the mother prior to delivery, the platelet response and clinical effect were similar in mother and neonate.

Lactation: It is not known if IGIV antibodies are excreted in breast milk.

Problems in humans have not been documented.

Children: Generally safe and effective.

Adverse Reactions: Most adverse reactions are mild, transient systemic reactions: Anxiety, back pain, chills, headache, muscle pain, arthralgia, pruritus, malaise, joint pain, fever, nausea, vomiting, abdominal cramps, flushing, tightness of the chest, palpitations, diaphoresis, hypotension, hypertension, dizziness, pallor, cyanosis, dyspnea and wheezing. Rash occurs rarely. Immediate anaphylactic and hypersensitivity reactions have been observed in exceptional cases.

Some of the infusion-related adverse effects (eg, temperature, chills, nausea, vomiting) may be due to reaction between administered antibodies and free antigens in the blood and tissues of recipients. When free antigen is fully bound, further administration of IGIV usually does not cause subsequent untoward side effects. These reactions may recur if the time interval since the last IGIV treatment is >8 weeks or if a different brand of IGIV is used.

A detailed case of maltose-induced hyponatremia was reported following infusion of IGIV in 10% maltose (*Gamimune N 5%*; Palevsky et al, 1993). The authors attribute maltose accumulation to the patient's acute renal failure.

Non-A/non-B hepatitis (hepatitis C) has occurred rarely following IGIV administration, most often in other countries. A hepatitis C outbreak in the US was linked to IGIV products that did not include a specific viral inactivation step. All current IGIV products include one or more virucidal processing steps. One outbreak of IGIV-associated hepatitis B occurred in India, possibly due to inadequate quality-control procedures.

Blood-group antibodies in the donor population may be transferred to IGIV recipients; in isolated cases this has been associated with confusion regarding the recipient's blood type and rarely hemolysis. In one case, blood-group antigens may have been transferred to an IGIV recipient (Lucas et al, 1987).

An aseptic meningitis syndrome (AMS) has been reported infrequently in association with IGIV. AMS usually begins within several hours to 2 days after IGIV treatment. AMS includes symptoms and signs such as severe headache, nuchal rigidity, drowsiness, fever, photophobia, painful eye movements, nausea and vomiting. CSF studies frequently show pleocytosis up to several thousand cells per mm^3, mostly granulocytes, and protein levels elevated up to several hundred mg/dl. Give patients with such symptoms and signs a thorough neurological examination, including CSF studies, to rule out other causes of meningitis. AMS occurs more frequently in association with high does (>2 g/kg) IGIV therapy. Stopping the IGIV has resulted in remission of AMS within several days without sequelae.

Several reports of acute renal failure have been published among patients who received IGIV, particularly those with compromised renal function.

Pharmacologic & Dosing Characteristics

Handling: All forms: Avoid foaming. To prevent denaturation of antibody proteins, swirl to facilitate dissolution;

do not shake. Discard any unused portions. If large doses will be administered, several containers may be pooled into an empty sterile IV solution container using aseptic technique. Bring IGIV solutions to room temperature before infusion.

Individual IgG molecules measure <0.002 micron in diameter. American Red Cross, Hyland and Immuno recommend use of a 15-micron in-line filter to preclude infusion of aggregates. Filtering of *Sandoglobulin, Venoglobulin-S* or *Gammar-P IV* is acceptable but not required. Pore diameters 15 microns or wider are less likely to slow down infusion rates, especially at higher concentrations. Sterilizing filters (eg, 0.2 microns) may be used.

Recommendations to record lot numbers and manufacturers of all serum-based products are becoming common.

Dosage: No consensus exists on whether IGIV dosage should be based on actual, ideal or adjusted body mass (Kasperek & Wetmore, 1990).

Immunoglobulin Replacement Therapy: As the initial dose, give 100 to 400 mg/kg (4 to 8 ml/kg) per month, repeated every 3 to 4 weeks. If the clinical response is inadequate or the level of serum IgG achieved is insufficient, increase the periodic dose to 300 to 400 mg/kg (6 to 8 ml/kg) monthly or repeat the same dose at shorter intervals. Monthly doses up to 800 mg/kg or more have been used.

B-Cell Chronic Lymphocytic Leuke- mia (CLL): 400 mg/kg is the recommended dose, given every 3 to 4 weeks.

Immune Thrombocytopenia Purpura, acute: For induction therapy, 400 to 2000 mg/kg of body weight daily for 1 to 7 consecutive days. Various protocols have used 400 mg/kg daily for 5 days, 1 g/kg/day for 1 or 2 days or daily for 3 doses on alternate days, or 2 g/kg/day for 2 to 7 consecutive days.

IGIV therapy in patients who respond to induction therapy with a platelet count of 30,000 to 50,000 cells/mm^3 may be discontinued after 2 to 7 daily doses. The extent and rapidity of platelet recovery for induction therapy and degree of success for maintenance therapy in clinical trials were independent of dose.

Immune Thrombocytopenic Purpura, chronic: After induction therapy in adults and children, if the platelet count falls to <30,000 cells/mm^3 or the patient manifests clinically significant bleeding, give 400 to 2000 mg/kg as a single infusion every 2 weeks, or more frequently as needed to maintain the platelet count >30,000 cells/mm^3 in children and >20,000 cells/mm^3 in adults.

Kawasaki Syndrome: Within 10 days of onset of disease, treatment with either a single dose of 2 g/kg body mass given over a 10 hour period or 400 mg/kg body mass on 4 consecutive days. Give concurrent aspirin therapy, at a dose such as 100 mg/kg/day through the fourteenth day of illness, then 3 to 5 mg/kg/day thereafter for a period of 5 weeks.

Children With Aids: Fewer bacterial infections were observed in children infected with HIV-1 who received 400 mg/kg every 28 days.

Bone-Marrow Transplant Patients: Give 500 mg/kg 7 and 2 days before transplantation (or at the time conditioning therapy for transplantation begins), then weekly through day 90 after transplant. Administer through a central line while it is in place, thereafter through a peripheral vein.

Route:

IV infusion. In general, begin infusions at a rate of 0.01 ml/kg/min (0.6 ml/kg/hr), increasing to 0.02 ml/kg/min (1.2 ml/kg/hr) after 15 to 30 minutes. Most patients tolerate a gradual increase to 0.03 to 0.08 ml/kg/min (1.8 to 4.8 ml/kg/hr). For a typical 70 kg person, this is equivalent to 2 to 4 ml/min (120 to 240 ml/hr). If adverse reactions develop, slowing the infusion rate will usually eliminate the reaction. Specific recommended rates of infusion appear in the table at the end of the monograph. Sandoglobulin has been infused as fast as 30 mg/kg/min in one study (Schiff et al, 1991).

Efficacy: Immunoglobulin deficiency: IGIV therapy reduces the incidence of infection.

CLL: IGIV therapy reduces the incidence of bacterial infections to about 50% of the incidence without IGIV administration. The median time to the first bacterial infection was increased from 192 days in the control group to >365 days in the IGIV-treated group.

ITP, acute: In various studies, 64% to 100% of IGIV recipients attained platelet counts ≥100,000 cells/ml within 7 days, and were considered full treatment successes.

ITP, chronic: From 67% to 86% of IGIV recipients responded satisfactorily to maintenance therapy.

Kawasaki Syndrome: IGIV in conjunction with aspirin therapy can reduce the incidence of coronary artery abnormalities by 65% to 78%, compared to treatment with aspirin alone.

Onset: Rapid

Duration: In general, the mean half-life in normal persons is 18 to 25 days, although there is tremendous inter-subject variability. Fever or infection may decrease antibody half-life because of increased catabolism or consumption, respectively. In ITP the increase in platelets usually lasts from several days to several weeks, although it may rarely persist for a year or longer. The half-life in a group of burn patients ranged from 47 to 154 days. Reported half-lives appear in the table at the end of the monograph.

Drug Interactions: IGIV may diminish the antibody response to attenuated measles, mumps and rubella vaccines through antigen-antibody antagonism. As a general rule, administer live virus vaccines 14 to 30 days before or 6 to 12 weeks after IGIV. For varicella vaccine, wait 5 months. For a vaccine containing measles virus, wait 8 months after standard 400 mg/kg IGIV therapy. After high-dose IGIV therapy for ITP or Kawasaki disease, wait 8 to 11 months. Alternately, administer live virus vaccines during this interval if antiviral antibody titers are measured 3 months after IGIV administration.

IGIV is unlikely to interfere with development of immunity following oral poliovirus or yellow fever vaccination. However, it may be prudent not to administer these vaccines shortly after IGIV administration. Exceptions include unexpected travel to or contact with epidemic or endemic areas or persons. If OPV is given with or shortly after IGIV, repeat the OPV dose 3 months later if immunization is still indicated.

It is not known if IGIV interferes with the efficacy of other attenuated vaccines (eg, adenovirus, BCG, typhoid, vaccinia). It may be prudent not to administer these vaccines shortly after IGIV administration unless unavoidable.

Pharmaceutical Characteristics

Concentration: *Alpha-powder:* 5% (50 mg/ml) solution when reconstituted according to directions, containing not <97% IgG, not <95% in the monomer and dimer form. Use of a more concentrated 10% solution was reported (Ippoliti et al, 1991).

Alpha-solution: 5% (50 mg/ml) or 10% (100 mg/ml) solution, typically containing >99% IgG in monomeric or dimeric form.

Armour: 5% (50 mg/ml) solution of IgG when reconstituted as directed, containing at least 98% IgG, at least 98.5% in monomeric or dimeric form, with a total IgG concentration of 4.5% to 5.5%.

Bayer: ≥98% IgG, and ≥90% in monomeric form; 5% form: 4.5% to 5.5% (45 to 55 mg/ml) solution; 10% form: 9% to 11% (90 to 110 mg/ml) solution.

Hyland: 5% (50 mg/ml) solution when reconstituted according to directions, containing not <90% IgG, 95% monomeric. The powder can also be reconstituted to a 10% solution.

Immuno: 4.5% to 5.5% (45 to 55mg/ml) IgG solution, when reconstituted according to directions, nearly 100% IgG, 93.8% monomeric (7S), with a total protein concentration of 52 to 58 mg/ml.

Red Cross: 5% (50 mg/ml) solution when reconstituted according to directions, containing not <90% IgG, 98% monomeric and dimeric. The powder can also be reconstituted to a 10% solution.

Sandoz: 3%, 6%, 9% or 12% solution, depending on quantity of diluent added, when reconstituted according to directions, containing not <96% IgG, 92% monomeric (7S), with the remainder dimeric and a small portion polymeric. Fragments <10% (mean, 6%), aggregates <3% (mean, <1%).

Native human IgG subclass distributions typically follow this pattern: IgG_1—60% to 70%, IgG_2—23% to 29%, IgG_3—4% to 8%, IgG_4—2% to 6%. Product-specific subclass distributions appear in the table at the end of the monograph.

Packaging:

Alpha-powder: 500 mg single-dose vial with reconstitution kit including 10 ml diluent, 2.5 g single-dose vial with reconstitution kit including 50 ml diluent, 5 g single-dose vial with reconstitution kit including 100 ml diluent, 10 g single-dose vial with reconstitution kit including 192 ml diluent. Each reconstitution kit includes a double-ended transfer device.

Alpha-solution: All packages include IV administration set.

5% form: 2.5 g/50 ml single-dose vial, 5 g/100 ml single-dose vial, 10 g/200 ml single-dose vial.

10% form: 5 g/50 ml single-dose vial, 10 g/100 ml single-dose vial, 20 g/200 ml single dose vial.

Armour: 1 g single-dose vial with 20 ml diluent, 2.5 g single-dose vial with 50 ml diluent, 5 g single-dose vial with 100 ml diluent, six 5 g single-dose vials without diluent, 10 g single-dose vial with 200 ml diluent and administration set. Each diluent package includes a sterile, vented transfer spike for reconstitution.

Bayer: 5% form: 500 mg/10 ml single-dose vial, 2.5 g/50 ml single-dose vial, 5 g/100 ml single-dose vial, 12.5 g/250 ml single-dose vial with administration set.

10% form: 5 g/50 ml single-dose vial, 10 g/100 ml single-dose vial, 20 g/200 ml single-dose vial.

Hyland: 500 mg single-dose vial with 10 ml diluent, 2.5 g single-dose vial with 50 ml diluent, 5 g single-dose vial with 100 ml diluent, 10 g single-dose vial with 200 ml diluent. The 2.5, 5 and 10 g packages include an administration set with integral airway and a 15-micron filter.

Immuno: 500 mg single-dose vial with 10 ml diluent, 1 g single-dose vial with 20 ml diluent, 2.5 g single-dose vial with 50 ml diluent, 5 g single-dose vial with 100 ml diluent. All packages include a double-ended spike transfer device and a 15-micron filter needle. The 2.5 g and 5 g packages feature an infusion-size bottle and infusion sets.

Red Cross: 2.5 g single-dose vial with 50 ml diluent, 5 g single-dose vial with 96 ml diluent, 10 g single-dose vial with 192 ml diluent. Each package contains an administration set with integral airway and a 15-micron filter.

Sandoz: 1 g single-dose vial with 33 ml diluent, 3 g single-dose vial with 100 ml diluent, ten 3 g vials without diluent, 6 g single-dose vial with 200 ml diluent, ten 6 g vials without diluent.

Dose Form: See tables at the end of the monograph.

Diluents for Reconstitution:

Sandoz: Reconstitute with 0.9% sodium chloride that accompanies each package. Alternately, use 5% dextrose (D5W) or sterile water for injection (SWFI) as the diluent. Dissolves in generally <10 minutes. Add no other products to the final solution, especially protein-denaturing agents. Little data on specific physical or chemical incompatibilities with other infused drugs have been published.

All Others: Sterile water for injection, without bacteriostatic agents or other preservatives. Add no other products to the final solution, especially protein-denaturing agents. Little data on specific drug interactions or incompatibilities have been published.

Alpha (Venoglobulin-I), Hyland & Red Cross: Adjusting the volume of fluid for reconstitution permits preparation of 5% or 10% solutions.

Diluent for Infusion

Alpha-powder: 0.9% sodium chloride. Do not infuse into 5% dextrose or other acidic fluids.

Alpha-solution: 0.9% sodium chloride or 5% dextrose

Armour: 0.9% sodium chloride or 5% dextrose

Bayer: 5% dextrose

Hyland: 0.9% sodium chloride

Immuno: 0.9% sodium chloride or isotonic sugar (eg, 5% dextrose, 5% or 10% levulose [ie, fructose])

Red Cross: 0.9% sodium chloride

Sandoz: 0.9% sodium chloride, 5% dextrose, 5% dextrose with 0.2% sodium chloride, preferably acid or neutral fluids, pH not >7.4

Storage/Stability:

See the table at the end of the mono-graph. Freezing may break diluent bot-tles, but will not affect the potency of powdered IGIV products. Discard solu-tion forms of IGIV if frozen. Infuse IGIV at room temperature.

Admixtures with other drugs have not been evaluated. Administer IGIV sepa-rately from other drugs or medications the patient receives. Delay in adminis-tration may be safer following recon-stitution in a laminar-air flow hood (to reduce risk of bacterial contamina-tion), if the solution was refrigerated before use.

No manufacturer data is available on stability in plastic containers. The Fc portion of IgG molecules will adhere to plastic in milligram quantities, but no clinical problems have been docu-mented (Sandoz, 1991).

Alpha-powder: During reconstitution do not warm above $37°C$ ($99°F$). Shipped at ambient temperature.

Alpha-solution: 5%: Do not warm above $25°C$ ($77°F$). Shipped at ambient tem-perature.

10%: Product will tolerate up to $30°C$ ($86°F$) for up to 4 days during shipment.

Armour: Contact manufacturer regard-ing prolonged exposure to elevated temperatures. The powder can tolerate freezing. Discard frozen diluent, because diluent expansion can damage its container. Shipped at ambient tem-perature.

Bayer: Both forms can tolerate 7 days at temperatures up to $25°C$ ($77°F$). Shipped in insulated containers with coolant packs.

Hyland: Contact manufacturer regarding prolonged exposure to elevated tem-peratures. Shipped at ambient temper-ature. *Gammagard* is physically compat-ible with a variety of concentrations of dextrose and parenteral nutrition solu-tions (Lindsay et al, 1994).

Immuno: Product can tolerate 5 days at room temperature. Shipped in insulat-ed containers with coolant packs.

Red Cross: Contact manufacturer regard-ing prolonged exposure to elevated temperatures. Shipped at ambient tem-perature.

Sandoz: Do not warm above $37°C$ ($99°F$). Do not freeze *Sandoglobulin* solution. Shipped at ambient temperature.

IGIV Comparisons

	Polygam S/D	Venoglobulin-I	Venoglobulin-S	Gammar-P IV	Gammagard S/D	Gamimune N	Iveegam	Sandoglobulin
Distributor	American Red Cross	Alpha (Powder)	Alpha (Solution)	Centeon	Baxter/Hyland	Bayer	Immuno-US	Sandoz
Pharmaceutical Characteristics								
Concentration	5% (10%)	5% (10%)	5%, 10%	5%	5% (10%)	5%, 10%	5%	3%, 6%, 9%, 12%
Package sizes	2.5 g, 5 g, 10 g	500 mg, 2.5 g, 5 g, 10 g	5%: 2.5 g, 5 g, 10 g 10%: 5 g, 10 g, 20 g	1 g, 2.5 g, 5 g, 10 g	500 mg, 2.5 g, 5 g, 10 g	5%: 500 mg, 2.5 g, 5 g, 12.5 g 10%: 5 g, 10 g, 20 g	500 mg, 1 g, 2.5 g, 5 g	1 g, 3 g, 6 g
Dose form	powder	powder	solution	powder	powder	solution	powder	powder
Diluent for reconstitution	SWFI	SWFI	n/a	SWFI	SWFI	n/a	SWFI	0.9% NaCl, D5W, SWFI
Diluent for infusion	0.9% NaCl	0.9% NaCl	0.9% NaCl or D5W	0.9% NaCl or D5W	0.9% NaCl	D5W	0.9% NaCl or D5W	0.9% NaCl, D5W, D5-0.2% NaCl
IgA content	<3.7 mcg/ml	24-38 mcg/ml	5%: 15 mcg/ml 10%: 20-50 mcg/ml	25-50 mcg/ml	<3.7 mcg/ml	5%: <270 mcg/ml 10%: DNP	<2 mcg/ml	<970 mcg/ml
Normal storage	≤25°C (≤77°F)	≤30°C (≤86°F)	5%: <30°C 10%: 2°-8°C	≤30°C (≤86°F)	≤25°C (≤77°F)	2°-8°C (36°-46°F)	2°-8°C (36°-46°F)	≤30°C (≤86°F)
Stability after reconstitution	Begin use within 2 hours	Use immediately	n/a	Use within 3 hours	Begin use within 2 hours	n/a	Use promptly	Begin use within 6-24 hours
Pharmacologic & Dosing Characteristics								
Infusion rates: Initial	0.5 ml/kg/hr	0.6-1.2 ml/kg/hr x 30 min	0.6-1.2 ml/kg/hr x 30 min	0.6 ml/kg/hr x 15-30 min	0.5 ml/kg/hr	0.6-1.2 ml/kg/hr x 30 min	60 ml/hr	3% <1 ml/min, increased gradually
Eventual	5%: 4 ml/kg/hr 10%: 8 ml/kg/hr	2.4 ml/kg/hr	5%: 2.4-4.8 ml/kg/ hr 10%: 3 ml/kg/hr	1.2-3.6 ml/kg/hr	5%: 4 ml/kg/hr 10%: 8 ml/kg/hr	4.8 ml/kg/hr	120 ml/hr	

Abbreviations: SWFI–Sterile water for injection
n/a–not applicable   DNP–data not provided

Cytomegalovirus Immune Globulin Intravenous (Human)

ANTI-INFECTIVE IMMUNE GLOBULINS

NAME:
CytoGam

MANUFACTURER:
Massachusetts Public Health Biologic Laboratories (PHBL), distributed by MedImmune

SYNONYMS:
CMV-IG, CMV-IVIG

Viability: Inactive, passive, transient

Antigenic Form: Human immunoglobulin, unmodified

Antigenic Type: Protein, IgG antibody, polyclonal, primarily monomeric

Use Characteristics

Indications: For attenuation of primary cytomegalovirus (CMV) disease associated with kidney transplantation, specifically for CMV-seronegative recipients of kidneys from CMV-seropositive donors.

Unlabeled Uses: For prevention or attenuation of primary cytomegalovirus (CMV) disease in immunosuppressed recipients of organ transplants (eg, bone marrow, liver). Also used in immunocompromised patients with CMV pneumonia or to prevent CMV disease.

Contraindications:

Absolute: None.

Relative: Patients with a history of a severe reaction associated with administration of IM or IV human immune globulin products.

Persons with selective immunoglobulin A deficiency have the potential for developing anti-IgA antibodies and could have anaphylactic reactions to subsequent administration of blood products (including immune globulin preparations) that contain IgA.

Elderly: No specific information is available about geriatric use of CMV-IGIV. Problems have not been documented and are unlikely.

Pregnancy: *Category* C. Use only if clearly needed. It is not specifically known if RSV antibodies cross the placenta. Intact IgG crosses the placenta from the maternal circulation increasingly after 30 weeks gestation. Problems in humans have not been documented and are unlikely.

Lactation: It is not known if anti-CMV antibodies are excreted in breast milk. Problems in humans have not been documented and are unlikely.

Children: CMV-IGIV is generally safe and effective in children.

Adverse Reactions: Flushing, chills, muscle cramps, back pain, fever, nausea, vomiting and wheezing were the most common adverse reactions (<5% of infusions), usually related to infusion rates. Hypotension has not been reported. Severe reactions such as angioedema and anaphylactic shock might theoretically occur rarely. Consider slowing the rate immediately or interrupting the infusion, according to the patient's response.

RSV-IGIV is made from human plasma. Like other plasma products, it carries the possibility for transmission of blood-borne pathogenic agents. The risk of transmission of recognized blood-borne viruses is considered to be low because of screening of plasma donors, an added viral inactivation step and removal properties in the Cohn-Oncley cold-ethanol precipitation procedure used for purification of immune globulin products. Because new blood-borne agents may yet emerge, some of which may not be inactivated or eliminated by the manufacturing process or by solvent-detergent treatment, give RSV-IGIV only if a benefit is expected.

Pharmacologic & Dosing Characteristics

Handling: Do not shake; avoid foaming to prevent protein degradation.

Dosage: Preoperative prophylaxis is preferred, otherwise administer within 72 hours after transplant. Give 150 mg/kg. At 2, 4, 6 and 8 weeks after transplant give 100 mg/kg. At 12 and 16 weeks after transplant give 50 mg/kg.

Route: IV infusion, starting at 15 mg/kg/hr, then progressing to 30 and then to 60 mg/kg/hr if no reaction occurs. Use an IV infusion pump for administration. In-line filters are not necessary, but may be used. The maximum recommended rate of infusion is 75 mg/kg/hr. If any reaction occurs, slow or stop the infusion until the reaction abates. Use epinephrine or an anti-

histamine to treat allergic symptoms.

Efficacy: In one clinical trial, the incidence of virologically confirmed CMV-associated syndromes in renal-transplant recipients at risk for primary CMV disease was reduced from 60% in 35 control patients to 21% among 24 CMV-IGIV recipients (p <0.01). Marked leukopenia fell from 37% in controls to 4% in recipients (p <0.01). Fungal or parasitic superinfections were not seen in recipients, but occurred in 20% of controls (p=0.05). Serious CMV disease dropped from 46% to 13%. The incidence of CMV pneumonia also fell, from 17% of controls to 4% among recipients, but this difference was not statistically significant. No effect on rates of viral isolation or seroconversion was seen, although the rate of viremia was less in CMV-IGIV recipients.

In a later nonrandomized trial in 36 renal-transplant recipients, the rate of virologically confirmed CMV-associated syndrome fell to 36% of recipients. The rates of CMV-associated pneumonia, CMV-associated hepatitis and concomitant fungal or parasitic superinfection were similar to those observed in the earlier trial.

Onset: Rapid

Duration: Mean half-life: 21 days, shorter in transplant recipients, where half-lives have been measured as 8 days immediately after transplant, or 13 to 15 days if given ≥60 days after transplant.

Drug Interactions: CMV-IGIV may diminish the antibody response to attenuated measles, mumps and rubella vaccines through antigen-antibody antagonism. For a vaccine containing measles virus, wait 6 months after giving CMV-IGIV. For varicella vaccine, wait 5 months after CMV-IGIV. Alternately, administer live virus vaccines during this interval if corresponding antibody titers are measured 3 months after CMV-IGIV administration. Revaccinate if necessary.

IGIM does not appear to interfere with development of immunity following oral poliovirus (OPV) or yellow-fever vaccination. However, it may be prudent not to administer these vaccines shortly after CMV-IGIV administration. Exceptions include unexpected travel to or contact with epidemic or endemic areas or persons. If OPV is given with or shortly after CMV-IGIV, repeat the OPV dose 3 months later if protection is still needed.

It is not known if CMV-IGIV interferes with the efficacy of other attenuated vaccines (eg, adenovirus, BCG, typhoid, vaccinia). It may be prudent not to administer these vaccines shortly after CMV-IGIV administration unless unavoidable.

Responses to inactivated vaccines are not substantially affected by IGIVs. Consider giving a booster dose of routine childhood vaccines 3 or 4 months after the last dose of RSV-IG, to ensure immunity to diphtheria, tetanus, pertussis, *Haemophilus influenzae* type b and poliovirus.

Pharmaceutical Characteristics

Concentration: 40 to 60 mg Ig per ml, primarily IgG

Packaging: Vial containing 2250 to 2750 mg/50 ml.

Dose Form: Solution

Diluent for Infusion: Administer directly or piggyback into 0.9% sodium chloride or into 2.5%, 5%, 10% or 20% dextrose in water (with or without sodium chloride added). Do not dilute the CMV-IGIV primary IV fluid >1:2 (ie, 50 ml CMV-IGIV with ≤100 ml infusion fluid).

Storage/Stability: Store at $2°$ to $8°$C ($36°$ to $46°$F). Contact manufacturer regarding prolonged exposure to room temperature or elevated or freezing temperatures. Shipping data not provided.

Begin infusion within 6 hours and complete within 12 hours after entering the vial. Do not mix CMV-IGIV with other drugs.

NAME:
H-BIG, HyperHep, Hep-B-Gam-magee

MANUFACTURER:

H-BIg, Abbott Laboratories, distributed by North American Biologicals, Inc. (NABI); *HyperHep*, Bayer Corporation; *Hep-B-Gam-magee*, Merck Vaccine Division

Synonym: HBIG

Comparison: Therapeutically equivalent

Viability: Inactive, passive, transient

Antigenic Form: Human immunoglobulin, unmodified

Antigenic Type: Protein, IgG antibody (anti-HBsAb) to hepatitis B surface antigen (HBsAg), polyclonal, primarily monomeric

Use Characteristics

Indications: For passive, transient, post-exposure prevention of hepatitis B infection. Such exposures may include parenteral exposure (eg, needle-stick, human bites that penetrate the skin), mucous-membrane contact (eg, accidental splashes), sexual contact or oral ingestion (eg, pipetting accidents) of HBsAg-positive materials such as blood, plasma or serum.

For passive, transient post-exposure prophylaxis of hepatitis B in infants born to HBsAg-positive mothers. Such infants are at risk of being infected with hepatitis B virus and becoming chronic carriers. The risk is especially great if the mother is HBeAg-positive. HBIG is most effective when used within 7 days of exposure, or 14 days in the case of sexual contact.

Unlabeled Uses: HBIG continues to be evaluated for efficacy in other situations that involve nonparenteral exposure to hepatitis B, such as in dialysis patients, among hospital workers and close contacts of HBsAg-positive persons.

Hepatitis B vaccination is appropriate for persons expected to receive human alpha₁-proteinase inhibitor (*Prolastin*, Bayer). If insufficient time is available for development of adequate antibody responses to active vaccination, give a single dose of hepatitis B immune globulin with the initial dose of vaccine. *Prolastin* is produced from heat-treated, pooled human plasma that may contain the causative agents of hepatitis and other viral diseases. Manufacturing procedures at plasma collection centers, plasma testing laboratories and fractionation facilities are designed to reduce the risk of transmitting viral infection, but that risk cannot be totally eliminated.

HBIG has been given in utero to fetuses of HBsAg-positive mothers during cordocentesis (Yurdakök M, Beksaç S, 1994).

Contraindications:
Absolute: None.

Relative: Use caution in persons with a history of prior systemic allergic reactions following administration of human immune globulin products. Persons with selective immunoglobulin A deficiency have the potential for developing anti-IgA antibodies and could have anaphylactic reactions to subsequent administration of blood products (including immune globulin preparations) that contain IgA.

Elderly: No specific information is available about geriatric use of HBIG. Problems have not been documented and are unlikely.

Pregnancy: *Category C.* Use is not contraindicated. Use only if clearly needed. Clinical experience suggests that there are no known adverse effects on the fetus from immune globulins per se. Intact IgG crosses the placenta from the maternal circulation increasingly after 30 weeks gestation.

Lactation: It is not known if anti-HBs antibodies are excreted in human breast milk. Problems in humans have not been documented and are unlikely.

Children: Safe and effective in newborns, infants and children.

Adverse Reactions: Pain and tenderness at injection site, urticaria or angioedema may occur. Anaphylaxis occurs rarely.

Pharmacologic & Dosing Characteristics

Dosage: *Adults and Children:* 0.06 ml/kg (usually 3 to 5 ml). Equivalent to 10 mg IgG/kg.

Give as soon as possible after exposure, preferably within 7 days. In the case of sexual contact, give within 14 days. Repeat 28 to 30 days after exposure.

If the exposed person failed to respond to a primary vaccine series, give the person either a single dose of HBIG and another dose of vaccine as soon as possible after exposure, or two 0.06 ml/kg doses of HBIG, 1 dose as soon as possible and a second dose 1 month later.

Newborns Born of HBsAg-Positive Mothers: 0.5 ml. Give first HBIG dose as soon as possible, preferably ≤12 hours after birth. Also give appropriate volume of either hepatitis B vaccine formulation within 7 days after birth. If the first dose of vaccine is delayed as long as 3 months, give a repeat HBIG dose of 0.5 ml at 3 months of age. If hepatitis B vaccine is declined, repeat HBIG at 3 and 6 months of age.

Route & Site: IM only, preferably in gluteal or deltoid region in adults and children. The anterolateral thigh is preferred in newborns. Do not inject IV.

Additional Doses: In adults, repeat HBIG 28 to 30 days after the first HBIG dose, if vaccine is declined. In infants of HBsAg-positive mothers, if hepatitis B vaccine is declined, give HBIG at birth and at 3 and 6 months of age.

Efficacy: HBIG reduces disease incidence by 75% among sexual partners of HBsAg-positive people. In infants of HBsAg-positive mothers, combined use of HBIG and vaccine protects 98% or more from infection.

After accidental percutaneous exposures (eg, needle-sticks) involving HBsAg, the incidence of both clinical and subclinical hepatitis B during the following 6 months was 0.7% in a group treated with HBIG and 6.1% in a group treated with IGIM. After 6 months, 32% of the IGIM group demonstrated anti-HBs antibodies, compared to 6% among the HBIG group (Seeff, 1975).

Onset: Antibodies appear within 1 to 6 days after IM administration and peak in 3 to 11 days.

Duration: Mean half-life: 17 to 25 days (range, 6 to 35). Clinical protection persists 2 months or longer.

Drug Interactions: There is no significant interaction between simultaneous administration of HBIG and hepatitis B vaccine if administered at separate sites.

HBIG may diminish the antibody response to attenuated measles, mumps, rubella or varicella vaccines through antigen-antibody antagonism. As a general rule, administer live virus vaccines 14 to 30 days before or 6 to 12 weeks after immune globulin administration. Alternately, administer live virus vaccines during this interval if corresponding antibody titers are measured 3 months after HBIG administration. Revaccinate if necessary.

IGIM does not appear to interfere with development of immunity following oral poliovirus or yellow fever vaccination. However, it may be prudent not to administer these vaccines shortly after HBIG administration. Exceptions include unexpected travel to or contact with epidemic or endemic areas or persons. If OPV is given with or shortly after HBIG, repeat the OPV dose 3 months later if immunization is still indicated.

It is not known if HBIG interferes with the efficacy of other attenuated vaccines (eg, adenovirus, BCG, typhoid, vaccinia). It may be prudent not to administer these vaccines shortly after HBIG administration unless unavoidable.

As with other drugs administered by IM injection, give HBIG with caution to people receiving anticoagulant therapy.

Pharmaceutical Characteristics

Concentration: Not less than 80% monomeric IgG form

Bayer: 15% to 18% protein

Merck: 10% to 18% protein

NABI: 15% to 18% protein

Packaging:

Bayer: 0.5 ml neonatal single-dose syringe with 22 gauge, 1.5 inch needle, 1 ml multidose vial, 5 ml multidose vial.

Merck: 5 ml multidose vial.

NABI: 0.5 ml neonatal single-dose syringe with needle of unspecified gauge and length, 1 ml multidose vial, 5 ml multidose vial.

Dose Form: Solution

Storage/Stability: Store at $2°$ to $8°C$ ($36°$ to $46°F$). Discard if frozen.

Bayer: Product can tolerate 30 days at $30°C$ ($86°F$). Shipping data not provided.

Merck: Contact manufacturer regarding prolonged exposure to room temperature or elevated temperatures. Shipping data not provided.

NABI: Product can tolerate 21 days at room temperature. Shipping data not provided.

Guide to Post-Exposure Prophylaxis for Hepatitis B

Type of exposure	Immunoprophylaxis
Perinatal	HBIG and vaccine
Infant (<12 months of age) – acute case in primary caregiver	HBIG and vaccine
Sexual – exposed to acute case	HBIG with or without vaccine
Sexual – exposed to chronic carrier	Vaccine
Household contact – exposed to acute case	None unless known exposure
Household contact – exposed to acute case, known exposure	HBIG with or without vaccine
Household contact – exposed to chronic carrier	Vaccine
Inadvertent – percutaneous or permucosal exposure	Vaccine with or without HBIG

Recommendations for Hepatitis B Prophylaxis Following Percutaneous or Permucosal Exposure

	Treatment of exposed person when source is found to be:		
	HBsAg-positive	HBsAg-negative	Source not tested or unknown
Unvaccinated	HBIG x 1[1], then initiate vaccine[2]	Initiate vaccine[2]	Initiate vaccine[2]
Previously Vaccinated: Known responder	Test exposed person for anti-HBs antibody 1. If adequate[3], no treatment. 2. If inadequate, give vaccine booster dose.	No treatment	No treatment
Known nonresponder	HBIG x 2[1] or HBIG x 1 plus 1 vaccine dose.	No treatment	If known high-risk source, may treat as if source were HBsAg-positive.
Response unknown	Test exposed person for anti-HBs antibody 1. If adequate[3], no treatment. 2. If inadequate, HBIG x 1[1] plus vaccine booster dose.	No treatment	Test exposed person for anti-HBs antibody 1. If adequate[3], no treatment. 2. If inadequate, HBIG x 1[1] plus vaccine booster dose.

[1]HBIG dose: 0.06 ml/kg IM.
[2]Hepatitis B vaccine dose–Refer to vaccine monograph for appropriate age-specific doses of each marketed vaccine.
[3]Adequate anti-HBs is ≥10 SRU by RIA or positive by EIA.

Hepatitis B Post-Exposure Treatment Schedule

	HBIG		Hepatitis B Vaccine	
Exposure	Dose	Recommended timing	Dose	Recommended timing
Perinatal	0.5 ml IM	Within 12 hours of birth	3 doses[1]	Within 12 hours of birth[2]
Sexual	0.06 ml/kg IM	Single dose within 14 days of last sexual contact	3 doses[1]	First dose at time of HBIG treatment[2]

[1]Standard dose. Refer to hepatitis B vaccine monograph for appropriate age-specific doses for each marketed vaccine brand.

[2]The first vaccine dose can be given at the same time as the HBIG dose, but at a different site. Give subsequent doses as recommended for the specific vaccine.

Respiratory Syncytial Virus (RSV) Immune Globulin (Human)

ANTI-INFECTIVE IMMUNE GLOBULINS

NAME:
RespiGam

MANUFACTURER:
Manufactured by **Massachusetts Public Health Biologic Laboratories, under license from Massachusetts Health Resource Institute. Distributed by MedImmune and comarketed by Wyeth-Lederle Vaccines & Pediatrics.**

Synonyms: RSV-IG. Early proprietary names included *Respivir* and *Hypermune RSV.*

Viability: Inactive, passive, transient

Antigenic Form: Human immunoglobulin, unmodified

Antigenic Type: Protein, IgG antibody, polyclonal, monomeric

Use Characteristics

 Indications: For the prevention of serious lower respiratory tract infection caused by respiratory syncytial virus (RSV) in children <24 months of age with bronchopulmonary dysplasia (BPD) or a history of premature birth (≤ 35 weeks gestation). RSV-IG is safe and effective in reducing the incidence and duration of RSV hospitalization and the severity of RSV illness in these high-risk infants.

Contraindications:
Absolute: None.

Relative: Patients with a history of a severe prior reaction associated with administration of RSV-IG or other human antibody preparations. Patients with selective IgA deficiency have the potential for developing antibodies to IgA and could have ana-phylactic or allergic reactions to subsequent administration of blood products that contain IgA, including RSV-IG.

Elderly: No specific information is available about geriatric use of RSV-IG. Problems have not been documented and are unlikely.

Pregnancy: *Category* C. Use only if clearly needed. It is not specifically known if RSV antibodies cross the placenta. Intact IgG crosses the placenta increasingly after 30 weeks gestation. Problems in humans have not been documented and are unlikely.

Lactation: It is not known if RSV-IG crosses into human breast milk. Problems in humans have not been documented and are unlikely.

Children: Safety and efficacy in children are described below in the Efficacy section.

Adverse Reactions: RSV-IG is generally well tolerated. In the Prophylaxis of RSV in Elevated-Risk Neonates (PREVENT) trial of RSV-IG in children with BPD or prematurity, there was no statistically significant difference in the proportion of children in the RSV-IG and placebo groups who reported adverse events. Further, the distribution of severity of adverse events was not significantly different between the two groups. Respiratory distress occurred in 2% of children receiving RSV-IG, compared to <1% of control children. Patients in the RSV-IG group reported a slightly higher incidence of fever (6%), compared with the placebo group (2%). Rash occurred in 2% of placebo recipients and in 1% of RSV-IG recipients.

The incidence of serious adverse events potentially related to the study drug was equivalent in both treatment groups, with 2% of children in each group reporting such events. The rate of serious adverse events is similar to rates reported for other IGIVs. Infrequent adverse reactions (<1%) were reported in the PREVENT trial as potentially related to the use of RSV-IG, including edema, pallor, hypotension, heart murmur, gagging, cyan- osis, sleepiness, cough, rhinorrhea, eczema, cold and clammy skin and conjunctival hemorrhage. Adverse events occurring only in the placebo group are not listed.

Reactions similar to those reported with other IGIVs may occur with RSV-IG. These include dizziness, flushing, blood pressure changes, anxiety, palpitations, chest tightness, dyspnea, abdominal cramps, pruritus, myalgia or arthralgia. Such reactions are often related to the rate of infusion; immediate allergic, anaphylactic or hypersensitivity reactions may be observed.

In the NIAID trial in children with BPD, CHD or prematurity, adverse reactions were reported in 3% of all RSV-IG infusions. Five of 150 children were considered to have had mild fluid overload associated with infusion. The remaining adverse reactions consisted of mild decreases in oxygen saturation (5%) and fever (3%). In the CARDIAC study of 429 children with CHD, children with CHD with right to left shunts appeared to have an increased frequency of cardiac surgery and had a greater frequency of severe and life-threatening adverse events associated with cardiac surgery.

Infants with underlying lung disease may be sensitive to extra fluid volume. Infusion of RSV-IG, particularly in children with BPD, may precipitate symptoms of fluid overload. Overall, 8.4% of participants (1% premature and 13% BPD) received new or extra diuretics during the period 24 hours before through 48 hours after at least one of their infusions in the PREVENT trial. The reason for this use was not recorded (eg, prophylaxis, treatment or part of routine care during a clinical visit). RSV-IG-related fluid overload was reported in 3 patients (1.2%) and RSV-IG-related respiratory distress was reported in 4 patients (1.6%); all had underlying BPD. With the exception of one child with respiratory distress (part of an acute allergic reaction) for whom RSV-IG was discontinued, these children were managed with diuretics or modification of the infusion rate and went on to receive subsequent infusions. Complications related to fluid volume were recorded as a reason for incomplete or prolonged infusion in 2% of children receiving RSV-IG (2.5% BPD and 1.1% premature) and in 1.5% of children receiving placebo in the PREVENT trial. Do not infuse RSV-IG into children with clinically apparent fluid overload.

Severe reactions, such as anaphylaxis or angioneurotic edema, have been reported in association with IV antibodies even in patients not known to be sensitive to human antibodies or blood products. Serious allergic reaction was noted in 2 patients in the PREVENT trial. These reactions were manifest as an acute episode of cyanosis, mottling and fever in one patient and respiratory distress in the other. The rate of allergic reaction appears to be low and consistent with rates observed for other IGIV products. If hypotension, anaphylaxis or severe allergic reaction occurs, discontinue infusion and administer epinephrinc 1:1000 as required.

Although equivalent proportions of children in the RSV-IG and control groups in the CARDIAC trial had adverse events, a larger number of RSV-IG recipients had severe or life-threatening adverse events. These events were most frequently observed in infants with CHD with right to left shunts who underwent cardiac surgery.

Except for hypersensitivity reactions, adverse reactions to IGIVs may be related to the rate of administration. Careful adherence to the infusion rate is important. Although systemic allergic reactions are rare, have epinephrine and diphenhydramine available for treatment of acute allergic symptoms. Rare occurrences of aseptic meningitis syndrome (AMS) have been reported in association with IGIV treatment. AMS usually begins within several hours to two days following IGIV treatment and is characterized by symptoms and signs including severe headache, drowsiness, fever, photophobia, painful eye movements, muscle rigidity and nausea and vomiting. Cerebrospinal fluid studies generally demonstrate pleocytosis, predominantly granulocytic, and elevated protein levels. Thoroughly evaluate patients exhibiting such symptoms and signs to rule out other causes of meningitis. AMS may occur more frequently in association with high dose (2 g/kg) IGIV treatment. Discontinuation of IGIV treatment has resulted in remission of AMS within several days without sequelae.

RSV-IG is made from human plasma. Like other plasma products, it carries the possibility for transmission of blood-borne pathogenic agents. The risk of transmission of recognized blood-borne viruses is considered to be low because of screening of plasma donors, an added viral inactivation step and removal properties in the Cohn-Oncley cold-ethanol precipitation procedure used for purification of immune globulin products. Because new blood-borne agents may yet emerge, some of which may not be inactivated or eliminated by the manufacturing process or by solvent-detergent treatment, give RSV-IG only if a benefit is expected.

Pharmacologic & Dosing Characteristics

Dosage: Do not shake; avoid foaming to prevent protein degradation. The maximum recommended total dosage per monthly IV infusion is 750 mg/kg. Give the first RSV-IG dose before the beginning of the RSV season. Give subsequent doses monthly throughout the RSV season to maintain protection. In the northern hemisphere, the RSV season typically begins in November and runs through April. Treat children from early November through April, unless RSV activity begins earlier or persists later in a community. Also consider factors such as other clinical illness, how well the child has grown and risk of exposure from siblings or daycare.

Route & Site: IV infusion. Begin infusions at 1.5 ml/kg/hr for the first 15 minutes. Use an infusion pump. If the patient's clinical condition permits, the rate may be increased to 3 mg/kg/hr for the next 15 minutes. After these 30 minutes, the rate may be increased to 6 ml/kg/hr. Do not exceed this rate of administration. Monitor the patient carefully during and after each rate change. In especially ill children with BPD, slower rates of infusion may be appropriate.

Give RSV-IG cautiously. During administration, monitor the patient's vital signs frequently: Before infusion, before each rate increase and at 30 minute intervals until 30 minutes after the infusion is complete. Observe the patient for increases in heart rate, respiratory rate, retractions and rales. A loop diuretic such as furosemide or bumetanide should be available for management of fluid overload.

Efficacy: In randomized, controlled studies of RSV disease prophylaxis, monthly doses of 750 mg/kg of RSV-IG reduced the incidence of RSV hospitalization in high-risk children. Children with BPD may be at high risk for serious RSV disease up to 60 months of age. Children born prematurely may be at high risk for serious RSV disease during the first year of life.

In the pivotal randomized, placebo controlled, double-blind PREVENT study, RSV-IG was evaluated in the prevention of RSV disease in infants and children with BPD ≤24 months of age or premature birth (≤35 weeks gestation) ≤6 months of age at study entry. The age of premature infants at the end of the study ranged from 4.8 to 11.4 months. In this trial, 510 patients were randomized to receive monthly infusions in November through April of either 750 mg/kg (15 ml/kg) RSV-IG or 15 ml/kg albumin 1% as a control. Results appear in the following table:

The PREVENT trial was not designed to enroll sufficient subjects to detect treatment differences among subsets of patients. Reductions in RSV hospitalization ranged from 17% to 58% in subgroups defined by gender, age > or < 6 months at entry, and diagnosis. The largest reductions occurred in children >6 months of age, all of whom had BPD. The smallest observed reduction occurred among children <6 months of age. This subgroup also had a low incidence of RSV hospitalization, which limited the ability to measure the treatment effect. As a result, the effect of RSV-IG in premature infants without BPD could not be definitively shown in this study. Analyses using body mass as a categorical variable revealed that children with entry weight <4.3 kg (the median) had a 49% lower rate of RSV hospitalization.

A randomized, uncontrolled, single-blind study sponsored by NIAID assessed the safety and effectiveness of RSV-IG in the prophylaxis of RSV disease in 274 infants and children at high risk of RSV disease due to chronic pulmonary disease (primarily BPD), congenital heart disease (CHD) or premature birth (≤35 weeks gestation). Compared with 90 control children, 92 children randomized to receive 750 mg/kg RSV-IG showed a 57% reduction in incidence of RSV hospitalization, a 59% reduction in total days of RSV hospitalization per 100 children, a 97% reduction in RSV ICU days per 100 children and a 100% reduction in mechanical ventilation per 100 children.

Onset: Rapid

Duration: The mean half-life of serum RSV neutralizing antibodies after RSV-IG infusion is 22 to 28 days.

Drug Interactions: Antibodies may interfere with the immune response to live virus vaccines, such as mumps, rubella, varicella and particularly measles. If these vaccines are given during or within 10 months after RSV-IG infusion, reimmunization is recommended, if needed.

IGIM does not appear to interfere with development of immunity following oral poliovirus or yellow fever vaccination. However, it may be prudent not to administer these vaccines shortly after RSV-IG administration unless

unavoidable. If OPV is given with or shortly after RSV-IG, repeat the OPV dose 3 months later, if immunization is still indicated.

It is not known if RSV-IG interferes with the efficacy of other attenuated vaccines (eg, adenovirus, BCG, typhoid, vaccinia). It may be prudent not to administer these vaccines shortly after RSV-IG administration unless unavoidable.

Responses to inactivated vaccines are not substantially affected by IGIVs. Consider giving a booster dose of routine childhood vaccines 3 or 4 months after the last dose of RSV-IG, to ensure immunity to diphtheria, tetanus, pertussis, *Haemophilus influenzae* type b and poliovirus.

Pharmaceutical Characteristics

Concentration: 40 to 60 mg immunoglobulin per ml, primarily IgG

Packaging: 50 ml vial containing 2,500 ± 500 mg RSV-IG

Dose Form: Solution

Diluent for Infusion: Predilution of RSV-IG before infusion is not recommended. RSV-IG may be piggy-backed into a pre-existing IV line if that line contains one of the following dextrose solutions (with or without sodium chloride): 2.5%, 5%, 10% or 20% dextrose in water. Do not dilute more than 1:2 with any other of the above-named solutions (eg, 50 ml RSV-IG with ≤100 ml infusion fluid). While filters are not necessary, an in-line filter with a pore size >15 micrometers may be used.

Storage/Stability: Store at 2° to 8°C (36° to 46°F). Do not freeze. Contact manufacturer regarding prolonged exposure to room temperature or elevated or freezing temperatures. Shipping data not provided.

Begin infusion within 6 hours and complete the infusion within 12 hours after piercing container seal. Do not mix RSV-IG with other drugs.

Rabies Immune Globulin (Human)
ANTI-INFECTIVE IMMUNE GLOBULINS

NAME:
Imogam Rabies, Hyperab

MANUFACTURER:
Imogam Rabies, Manufactured by Institut Mérieux, distributed by Connaught Laboratories; *Hyperab,* Cutter Biological, Miles Pharmaceutical Division

Synonyms: RIG. Rabies disease is also called hydrophobia.

Comparison: Therapeutically equivalent

Viability: Inactive, passive, transient

Antigenic Form: Human immunoglobulin, unmodified

Antigenic Type: Protein, IgG antibody, polyclonal, up to 20% polymeric

Use Characteristics

Indications: For passive, transient post-exposure prevention of rabies infection. Administer as soon as possible after exposure, up to 8 days after first vaccine dose. Give RIG to all persons suspected of exposure to rabies with one exception: Persons who have been completely immunized with rabies vaccine and are known to have an adequate antibody titer should receive post-exposure vaccine booster doses only, not RIG.

Contraindications:
Absolute: Successful pre-exposure vaccine prophylaxis.

Relative: Use caution in persons with a history of systemic allergic reactions following administration of human immune globulin products.

Persons with selective immunoglobulin A deficiency have the potential for developing anti-IgA antibodies and could have anaphylactic reactions to subsequent administration of blood products (including immune globulin preparations) that contain IgA.

Elderly: No specific information is available about geriatric use of RIG.

Pregnancy: *Category* C. Use is not contraindicated. Use only if clearly needed. Intact IgG crosses the placenta from the maternal circulation increasingly after 30 weeks gestation.

Lactation: It is not known if antirabies antibodies are excreted in breast milk. Problems in humans have not been documented.

Children: RIG is generally safe and effective in children.

Adverse Reactions: Local tenderness, soreness or stiffness at the injection site, and mild temperature elevations may persist for several hours. Sensitization to repeated injections has occurred occasionally in immunoglobulin-deficient recipients. Angioedema, urticaria, skin rash, nephrotic syndrome and anaphylactic shock have been reported rarely.

Pharmacologic & Dosing Characteristics

Dosage: Immediate and thorough washing of all bite wounds and scratches with soap and water is perhaps the most effective measure for preventing rabies. Give RIG 20 IU/kg (0.133 ml/kg) as soon as possible after exposure, preferably with the first dose of vaccine. Use up to half the dose to infiltrate the wound site, if the nature and location of the wound site permits. Administer the balance of the dose IM at a different site and in a different extremity from the vaccine.

Route & Site: IM, preferably in gluteal muscle (upper, outer quadrant only) or deltoid muscle.

Additional Doses: No RIG booster doses are needed. Repeating the RIG dose may interfere with development of active immunity from rabies vaccine. Follow rabies vaccination schedules exactly.

Efficacy: Nearly perfect; efficacy demonstrated in a group of persons attacked by a rabid wolf in Iran in 1955.

Onset: Adequate levels of antibody appear in serum within 24 hours and peak within 2 to 13 days. Since rabies vaccine takes approximately 1 week to induce active immunity, the importance of RIG cannot be overemphasized.

Duration: The mean serum half-life of rabies antibody is 24 days, consistent with the 21-day half-life expected of IgG.

Drug Interactions: Simultaneous administration of rabies immune globulin may slightly delay the antibody response to rabies vaccine through partial antigen-antibody antagonism. Because of this tendency, follow CDC recommendations exactly and give no more than the recommended dose of RIG.

RIG may diminish the antibody response to attenuated measles, mumps and rubella vaccines through antigen-antibody antagonism. As a general rule, administer live virus vaccines 14 to 30 days before or 6 to 12 weeks after immune globulin administration. Alternately, administer live virus vaccines during this interval if corresponding antibody titers are measured 3 months after RIG administration.

IMIG does not appear to interfere with development of immunity following oral poliovirus or yellow fever vaccination. However, it may be prudent not to administer these vaccines shortly after RIG administration.

Exceptions include unexpected travel to or contact with epidemic or endemic areas or persons. If OPV is given with or shortly after RIG, repeat the OPV dose 3 months later if immunization is still indicated.

It is not known if RIG interferes with the efficacy of other attenuated vaccines (eg, adenovirus, BCG, typhoid, vaccinia). It may be prudent not to administer these vaccines shortly after RIG administration unless unavoidable.

As with other drugs administered by IM injection, give RIG with caution to persons receiving anticoagulant therapy.

Pharmaceutical Characteristics

Concentration: 150 IU units per ml, 10% to 18% IgG, ≥80% monomeric

Bayer: 2 ml single-dose vial, 10 ml single-dose vial.

Connaught: 2 ml single-dose vial, 10 ml single-dose vial.

Solution

Store at 2° to 8°C (36° to 46°F); discard if frozen.

Bayer: Product can tolerate 30 days at 30°C (86°F). Shipping data not provided.

Connaught: Product can tolerate 4 days at room temperature. Shipped in insulated containers with coolant packs.

Vaccinia Immune Globulin (Human)
ANTI-INFECTIVE IMMUNE GLOBULINS

NAME:
Generic

MANUFACTURER:
Manufactured by Alpha Therapeutic Corporation or Hyland Division of Baxter Healthcare, distributed by the Centers for Disease Control & Prevention.

Synonyms: VIG. Vaccinia is also called cowpox, but is distinct from both variola (smallpox) virus and varicella (chickenpox) virus.

Viability: Inactive, passive, transient

Antigenic Form: Human immunoglobulin, unmodified

Antigenic Type: Protein, IgG antibody, polyclonal, polymeric

Use Characteristics

Indications: For passive, transient prevention of or modification of aberrant infections induced by vaccinia (smallpox) vaccine, the vaccinia virus, such as eczema vaccinatum, some cases of progressive vaccinia, and possibly ocular vaccinia. These might arise from:

(1) Accidental implantation of vaccinia virus in eyes, mouth or other areas where vaccinia infection would constitute a special hazard, or (2) Accidental vaccinia exposure among children who have extensive skin lesions such as eczema, burns, impetigo or varicella.

VIG is recommended for treatment of severe generalized vaccinia if the patient has a toxic condition or a serious underlying disease.

VIG may also be effective for use in postvaccinal complications, such as vaccinia necrosum, vaccinia infections of the mouth and vaccinia infections in the presence of other skin lesions such as burns, impetigo, varicella-zoster or poison ivy.

Contraindications:

Absolute: Patients with vaccinal keratitis, because such use in rabbits caused increased scarring.

Relative: Use caution in persons with a history of systemic allergic reactions following administration of human immune globulin products.

Persons with selective immunoglobulin A deficiency have the potential for developing anti-IgA antibodies and could have anaphylactic reactions to subsequent administration of blood products (including immune globulin preparations) that contain IgA.

Elderly: No specific information is available about geriatric use of VIG. Problems are unlikely.

Pregnancy: *Category* C. Use not contraindicated. Intact IgG crosses the placenta from the maternal circulation increasingly after 30 weeks gestation.

Lactation: It is not known if antivaccinia antibodies are excreted in breast milk. Problems in humans have not been documented.

Children: VIG is presumably safe and effective in children.

Adverse Reactions: Occasional-ly, local tenderness and stiffness occur, persisting from a few hours to 1 to 2 days following VIG injection. A few instances of allergic or anaphylactoid systemic reactions have been reported.

Pharmacological & Dosing Characteristics

Dosage: 0.3 ml/kg, given within 24 hours of exposure to vaccinia virus. For treatment of postvaccinal complications, give 0.6 ml/kg as soon as possible after symptoms appear, repeat depending on severity of symptoms and response to treatment.

Route & Site: IM, preferably in the buttock or anterolateral aspect of the thigh. When the VIG dose exceeds 10 ml, divide the dose and inject it at two or more sites to reduce the trauma of injection. Divided doses may be administered over 24 to 36 hours. Do not administer IV.

Consultation: Obtain advice on the diagnosis and management of vaccinia and vaccination complications from CDC. Telephone 404-639-1870 during the day or 404-639-3311 during evenings and weekends.

Additional Doses: For postvaccinal complications, repeat VIG based on severity of symptoms and response to treatment. This usually involves doses at intervals of 2 to 3 days, until no new lesions appear, implying the beginning of recovery.

Efficacy: Widely considered to be effective. After autoinoculation, 27 of 28 VIG recipients in one study did well. Among persons with eczema vaccinatum, mortality was 7% among VIG recipients, compared with 30% to 40% mortality expected with supportive care alone.

Onset: Prompt

Duration: Mean half-life: 21 days

Drug Interactions: VIG is effective and indicated as an antidote to adverse effects of vaccinia (smallpox) vaccine, through specific antagonism of viral replication.

VIG may diminish the antibody response to attenuated measles, mumps and rubella vaccines through antigen-antibody antagonism. As a general rule, administer live virus vaccines 14 to 30 days before or 6 to 12 weeks after immune globulin administration. Alternately, administer live virus vaccines during this interval if corresponding antibody titers are measured 3 months after VIG administration.

IMIG does not appear to interfere with development of immunity following oral poliovirus or yellow fever vaccination. However, it may be prudent not to administer these vaccines shortly after VIG administration.

Exceptions include unexpected travel to or contact with epidemic or endemic areas or persons. If OPV is given with or shortly after VIG, repeat the OPV dose 3 months later, if immunization is still indicated.

It is not known if VIG interferes with the efficacy of other attenuated vaccines (eg, adenovirus, BCG, typhoid). It may be prudent not to administer these vaccines shortly after VIG administration unless unavoidable.

As with other drugs administered by IM injection, give VIG with caution to persons receiving anticoagulant therapy.

Pharmaceutical Characteristics

Concentration: 15% to 18% protein, not <90% IgG

Packaging: 5 ml vial

Dose Form: Solution

Storage/Stability: Store at $2°$ to $8°C$ ($36°$ to $46°F$); do not freeze.

Contact manufacturer regarding prolonged exposure to room temperature or elevated or freezing temperatures. Shipping data not provided.

Varicella-Zoster Immune Globulin (Human)
ANTI-INFECTIVE IMMUNE GLOBULINS

NAME:
Generic

MANUFACTURER:
Massachusetts Public Health Biologic Laboratories (PHBL) from plasma supplied by the American Red Cross

Synonyms: VZIG. Varicella-zoster infection is also called chickenpox, herpes zoster and shingles.

Viability: Inactive, passive, transient

Antigenic Form: Human immunoglobulin, unmodified

Antigenic Type: Protein, IgG antibody, polyclonal, polymeric

Use Characteristics

Indications: For passive, transient prevention of varicella-zoster infection in exposed, susceptible individuals who are at greater risk of complications from varicella than healthy children. High-risk groups include immunocompromised children, newborns of mothers who develop varicella shortly before or after delivery, premature infants, immunocompromised adults and healthy susceptible adults, and may also include susceptible high-risk infants <12 months of age. Give VZIG to newborns whose mothers develop chickenpox within 5 days before or within 48 hours after delivery.

The risk of postnatally acquired varicella in the premature infant is unknown; it may be prudent to administer VZIG to exposed premature infants of 28 weeks gestation or older if the mother has a negative or uncertain history of varicella. Premature infants <28 weeks gestation or birth weight <1000 grams may receive VZIG regardless of maternal history since they may not yet have acquired transplacental maternal antibody.

VZIG may be warranted for full-term infants <1 year of age on an individual basis.

Expect greatest effectiveness when VZIG is given within 96 hours of exposure. Treatment after 96 hours is of uncertain value.

Contraindications:

Absolute: There is no indication for prophylactic use of VZIG in immunodeficient children or adults with a history of varicella unless the patient has undergone bone-marrow transplantation.

Relative: Use caution in those with a history of systemic allergic reactions following administration of human immune globulin products.

Persons with selective immunoglobulin A deficiency have the potential for developing anti-IgA antibodies and could have anaphylactic reactions to subsequent administration of blood products (including immune globulin preparations) that contain IgA.

Elderly: No specific information is available about geriatric use of VZIG.

Pregnancy: *Category C.* VZIG administration does little to prevent viremia, fetal infection or congenital varicella syndrome.

Therefore, the primary indication for VZIG in pregnant women is for prevention of complications of varicella in a susceptible adult patient, rather than for prevention of intrauterine infection. Intact IgG crosses the placenta from the maternal circulation increasingly after 30 weeks gestation.

Lactation: It is not known if antivaricella-zoster antibodies are excreted in breast milk. Problems in humans have not been documented.

Children: VZIG is generally safe and effective in neonates, infants and children.

Adverse Reactions: The most frequent adverse reaction to VZIG is local discomfort at the injection site. Pain, redness or swelling occurs at the injection site in about 1% of patients. Less frequent adverse reactions: GI symptoms, malaise, headache, rash and respiratory symptoms (0.2%). Severe reactions such as angioedema and anaphylactic shock are rare (0.1%).

Pharmacologic & Dosing Characteristics:

Dosage: Optimally, give VZIG within 96 hours of exposure, based on the body weight of the patient: 0 to 10 kg-125 units; 10.1 to 20 kg-250 units; 20.1 to 30 kg-375 units; 30.1 to 40 kg-500 units; >40 kg-625 units. Higher doses may be necessary in immunocompromised adults. The 125 u/10 kg rate is equivalent to 20 mg IgG/kg.

Route & Site: IM, preferably in the buttock or anterolateral aspect of the thigh. Do not inject IV.

Additional Doses: The duration of protection with VZIG is unknown; therefore, consider giving additional doses of VZIG when high-risk patients have subsequent exposures to varicella-zoster.

Efficacy: Lack of VZIG treatment of immunodeficient children has been associated with death (7%), pneumonia (25%), encephalitis (5%) and disease involving >100 pox (87%). Clinical studies with VZIG have reduced the frequency of death (1%), pneumonia (6%), encephalitis (0%) and widespread pox (27%). Although controlled clinical trials in susceptible neonates, infants and healthy adults have not been done to date, VZIG will probably also attenuate VZV in these groups.

Onset: Prompt

Duration: Duration of protection is unknown. Mean half-life: 21 days.

Drug Interactions: Although the interaction is not completely described, VZIG is likely to impair the efficacy of attenuated varicella-zoster vaccine, possibly through antigen-antibody antagonism.

Similarly VZIG may diminish the antibody response to attenuated measles, mumps and rubella vaccines through antigen-antibody antagonism. As a general rule, administer live virus vaccines 14 to 30 days before or 6 to 12 weeks after immune globulin administration. Alternately, administer live virus vaccines during this interval if corresponding antibody titers are measured 3 months after VZIG administration. IGIM does not appear to interfere with development of immunity following oral poliovirus or yellow fever vaccination. However, it may be prudent not to administer these vaccines shortly after VZIG administration.

Exceptions include unexpected travel to or contact with epidemic or endemic areas or persons. If OPV is given with or shortly after VZIG, repeat the OPV dose 3 months later if immunization is still indicated.

It is not known if VZIG interferes with the efficacy of other attenuated vaccines (eg, adenovirus, BCG, typhoid, vaccinia). It may be prudent not to administer these vaccines shortly after VZIG administration unless unavoidable.

As with other drugs administered by IM injection, give VZIG with caution to persons receiving anticoagulant therapy.

Laboratory Interference: VZIG will produce false-positive tests for immunity to varicella-zoster virus for approximately 2 months after receiving VZIG.

Pharmaceutical Characteristics

Concentration: ≥125 units in ≤2 ml, 10% to 18% protein, ≥99% IgG.

Packaging: At least 125 units in ≤2 ml; at least 625 units in ≤10 ml

Dose Form: Solution

Storage/Stability: Store at 2° to 8°C (35° to 46°F). Do not freeze. Product can tolerate 24 hours at room temperature. Contact manufacturer regarding prolonged exposure to elevated or freezing temperatures. Shipped in insulated containers with coolant packs by overnight courier.

Hypersensitivity Agents

Mycobacterial Antigens

Old Tuberculin (OT) Multipuncture Devices

Tuberculin Purified Protein
Derivative Solution

Tuberculin Purified Protein
Derivative (Multipuncture Device)

Tuberculin Summary

Pulmonary Mycotic Delayed Antigens

Coccidioidin

Histoplasmin

Ubiquitous Delayed Antigens

Mumps Skin Test Antigen

Candida Albicans Skin Test Antigen

Multiple Skin-test Antigen Device

Rational Anergy Test Panels

Old Tuberculin (OT) Multipuncture Devices
MYCOBACTERIAL ANTIGENS

NAME:
Mono-Vacc Test (O.T.); *Tuberculin, Old; Tine Test, Tine Test OT*

MANUFACTURERS:
Mono-Vacc Test (O.T.), Connaught Laboratories, ✤ Connaught; *Tuberculin, Old; Tine Test,* Wyeth-Lederle Vaccines & Pediatrics; ✤ *Tine Test OT,* Wyeth-Ayerst

Synonyms: OT, Tine Test, tuberculin skin test (TST). Tine Test is the registered trademark of Wyeth-Lederle's multipuncture device. This device is also used to deliver other immunodiagnostic skin-test reagents.

Comparison: The various old tuberculin products are generically equivalent, but differ from purified protein derivative (PPD) products. Intradermal PPD is more sensitive and more specific than any tuberculin delivered by multi-puncture devices.

Viability: Inactivated

Antigenic Form: Culture extract

Antigenic Type: Protein. Skin tests assess delayed (type IV) hypersensitivity.

Use Characteristics

(◉) **Indications:** For detection of delayed hypersensitivity to *Mycobacterium tuberculosis*. Multiple-puncture devices are screening tools that aid in determining the tuberculin hypersensitivity of individuals.

These devices have been clinically compared with intradermal administration of 5 TU of PPD-S, the US Reference Standard. Multiple-puncture devices are useful in mass tuberculosis screening programs, to establish priorities for additional testing (eg, intradermal PPD, chest radiographs) and in epidemiological surveys to identify areas with high levels of infection. Multiple-puncture devices aid in the identification of old or recent *Mycobacterium tuberculosis* infection, with or without disease. Multiple-puncture devices are advantageous in persons who may object to

use of needle and syringe, such as young children.

Regular, periodic testing (eg, annual, biennial) of tuberculin-negative persons may be recommended in some populations (eg, healthcare workers). This procedure is especially valuable because the conversion of an individual from negative to positive is highly indicative of recent tuberculosis infection.

Repeated testing of uninfected individuals does not cause sensitization to tuberculin. In persons with waning hypersensitivity to mycobacterial antigens, however, the stimulus of a tuberculin test may "boost" or increase the size of the reaction to a subsequent test given a week to a year later. This may be misinterpreted as recent development of hypersensitivity in some instances.

 Contraindications:
Absolute: None

Relative: Do not administer tuberculin to known tuberculin-positive reactors because of the severity of reactions (eg, vesiculation, ulceration, necrosis) that may occur at the test site in very highly hypersensitive individuals. Rarely, tuberculin testing may activate quiescent lesions in individuals with active tuberculosis.

Elderly: Skin test responsiveness may be delayed or reduced in magnitude among older persons.

Pregnancy: *Category C.* The risk of unrecognized tuberculosis and the close postpartum contact between a mother with active disease and her infant leaves the infant in grave danger of tuberculosis and complications such as tuberculous meningitis. No adverse effects on the fetus recognized as being due to tuberculosis skin testing have been reported.

Lactation: It is not known if tuberculin is excreted in breast milk. Problems in humans have not been documented.

Children: A child known to have been exposed to a tuberculous adult must not be considered free of infection until the child demonstrates a negative tuberculin reaction at least 10 weeks after contact with the tuberculous person(s) has ceased. If tuberculin screening of children is conducted, the American Academy of Pediatrics recommends that skin tests be applied at 12 months, 4 to 6 years, and 14 to 16 years of age.

Adverse Reactions:
In hypersensitive individuals, strongly positive reactions including vesiculation, ulceration or necrosis may occur at the test site. Cold packs or topical corticosteroid preparations may be employed for symptomatic relief of the associated pain, pruritus and discomfort.

Minimal bleeding may occur at the puncture site. This occurs infrequently and does not affect test interpretation.

Pharmacologic & Dosing Characteristics

Dosage: One application, pressed firmly without twisting. Hold the device in place at least 1 second. Exert sufficient pressure to assure that all tines penetrate the skin. If adequate pressure is applied, it will be possible to observe the puncture marks of each tine. Simultaneous application of two or more multipuncture devices is not recommended because such use may alter the patient's response.

Route & Site: Variously described as percutaneous, transcutaneous, intradermal, or topical. The flexor (volar) surface of the forearm, about 4 inches below the elbow, is preferred. Alternately, use the dorsal surface or other sites. Avoid areas without adequate SC tissue, such as above a tendon or bone.

Cleanse application sites with 70% isopropyl alcohol, acetone, ether or soap and water and allow to dry before test application. In persons with severe skin rashes, do not administer the test in areas where the rash occurs. Similarly, avoid hairy areas, scars, pimples, moles and other marks. Grasp the patient's forearm firmly to stretch the skin taut at the test site and to prevent any jerking motion of the arm that could cause scratching with the tines.

Drug Interactions: Reactivity to any tuberculin test may be suppressed in persons receiving corticosteroids or other immunosuppressive drugs, or in persons recently immunized with live virus vaccines (eg, measles, mumps, rubella, poliovirus). If tuberculin skin testing is indicated, perform it either preceding or simultaneous with immunization or 4 to 6 weeks after immunization.

Persons previously immunized with BCG vaccine may test positive to a tuberculin skin test. Tuberculin reactions caused by BCG cannot reliably be distinguished from reactions caused by natural mycobacterial infections. Test conversion rates after vaccination maybe much less than 100%. The mean reaction size among vaccinees is often <10 mm and tuberculin hypersensitivity tends to wane after vaccination. The American Thoracic Society suggests it may be appropriate to consider large reactions to 5 TU of PPD tuberculin in BCG-vaccinated persons as indicating infection with *Mycobacterium tuberculosis*, especially among persons from countries with a high prevalence of tuberculosis. Tuberculin reactivity in BCG vaccinees does not reliably predict protection against *Mycobacterium tuberculosis.*

Several weeks of cimetidine therapy may augment or enhance delayed-hypersensitivity responses to skin-test antigens, although this effect has not been consistently observed. The effect may be mediated through cimetidine binding to suppressor T-lymphocytes (Kumar, 1990). It is presently unknown if other H2-antagonists possess similar activity.

Pharmaceutical Characteristics

Concentration: Standardized by clinical evaluation in human subjects to give reactions equivalent to or more potent than 5 TU of standard PPD administered by intradermal injection.

Packaging:

Connaught: Box of 25 tests. Each package includes patient-oriented induration illustration cards with palpable diagrams of typical reactions.

Wyeth-Lederle: Jar of 25 individual tests, box of 100 individual tests, box of 250 individual tests. Each package includes patient-oriented induration illustration cards with palpable diagrams of typical reactions.

Dose Form: Sterile, single-use, multiple-puncture antigen applicators:

Connaught: Contains old tuberculin in viscous liquid form on points of a white plastic scarifier consisting of 9 plastic tines, each 2 mm long and 4 mm apart. Covered with an airtight seal to maintain sterility.

Wyeth-Lederle: A stainless-steel disc attached to a plastic handle. Projecting from the disc are 4 triangular prongs (tines), each 2mm long and 4 mm apart. The tines are mechanically dipped in a solution of old tuberculin and then dried.

Storage/Stability: Store at room temperature, <30°C (86°F). Contact manufacturer regarding prolonged exposure to elevated or freezing temperatures. Shipped at ambient temperature.

Connaught: Discard if frozen.

Wyeth-Lederle: Discard if refrigerated or frozen.

Tuberculin Purified Protein Derivative Solution
MYCOBACTERIAL ANTIGENS

NAME:
Tubersol Diagnostic Antigen;
Aplisol (Stabilized Solution)

MANUFACTURERS:
Tubersol Diagnostic Antigen, Connaught Laboratories; *Aplisol* (Stabilized Solution), Parke-Davis

Synonyms: PPD, Mantoux test, tuberculin skin test (TST)

Comparison: The various PPD solutions are generically equivalent, but differ from PPD multipuncture devices and from old tuberculin products. Intradermal PPD is more sensitive and more specific than any tuberculin delivered by multipuncture device.

Limited published data suggest that commercial brands of purified protein derivative (PPD) of tuberculin may vary in their false-positive reaction rate. Several published reports suggest that Parke-Davis' *Aplisol* may have a higher false-positive rate than Connaught's *Tubersol*, while *Tubersol* produces somewhat more false-negative results than *Aplisol* (Lifson AR, et al, 1993; Lanphear BP, et al, 1994; Rupp ME, et al, 1994; Johnson JL, et al, 1995). The clinical significance of these data are not clear.

Viability: Inactivated

Antigenic Form: Isolate from culture filtrates

Antigenic Type: Protein. Skin tests assess delayed (type IV) hypersensitivity.

Use Characteristics

Indications: For detection of delayed hypersensitivity to *Mycobacterium tuberculosis*. Tuberculin PPD is used as an aid in the diagnosis of infection with *Mycobac- terium tuberculosis*. The 5 TU/0.1 ml strength is the standard selected for the routine testing of individuals for tuberculosis, for testing of individuals suspected of having contact with active tuberculosis and as a follow-up verification test in individuals who have had reactions to skin tests with tuberculin multiple-puncture devices, which are less sensitive diagnostic tools. Do not use multiple-puncture devices to screen high-risk populations.

Alternate concentrations: Use the 1 TU/0.1 ml concentration only for individuals suspected of being highly sensitized, since larger initial doses may result in severe skin reactions. Reserve PPD preparations containing 250 TU/0.1 ml exclusively for testing individuals who fail to react to a previous injection of 5 TU; it may be given in the opposite forearm. Do not use, under any circumstances, the 250 TU/0.1 ml product for an initial test. Use of 1 TU or 250 TU products is not recommended by ATS or CDC.

The CDC Advisory Council for the Elimination of Tuberculosis recommends that the following groups be screened for tuberculosis and tuberculosis infection:

—Close contacts, those sharing the same household or other enclosed environments, of persons known or suspected to have tuberculosis;

—People infected with HIV;

—People who inject illicit drugs or other locally identified high-risk substance users (eg, crack cocaine users);

—People who have medical risk factors known to increase the risk for disease if infection occurs (eg, diabetes mellitus, conditions requiring prolonged high-dose corticosteroid therapy or other immunosuppressive therapy, chronic renal failure, leukemias, lymphomas, carcinoma of the head or neck, weight loss to ≥10% below ideal body weight, silicosis, gastrectomy, jejunoileal bypass);

—Residents and employees of high-risk congregate settings (eg, correctional institutions, nursing homes, mental institutions, other long-term residential facilities, shelters for the homeless);

—Health-care workers who serve high-risk clients;

—Foreign-born people,including children, who arrived within the last 5 years from countries that have a high tuberculosis incidence or prevalence (eg, most parts of Asia, Africa, Latin America);

—Some medically underserved, low-income populations;

—High-risk racial or ethnic minority populations, defined locally;

—Infants, children and adolescents exposed to adults in high-risk categories above.

High-risk categories will change over time as the epidemiology of tuberculosis infection changes. Screening people not members of high-risk groups is not recommended because it diverts resources from other, more important activities.

The purpose for screening is to identify infected people who are at high risk for disease and who would benefit from preventive therapy or to find people who have clinical disease and need treatment. Screening programs can also provide epidemiologic data for assessing tuberculosis trends in a community, assessing the value of continued screening and compiling baseline data to assess if subsequent exposure occurs (eg, for nursing-home residents and employees in some occupations). Do not undertake screening programs if necessary facilities for patient evaluation and treatment are unavailable or if patients found to be positive are unlikely to complete preventive therapy.

The American Academy of Pediatrics recommends the following criteria for tuberculin skin testing of children:

Children for whom imminent skin testing is indicated:

• Contacts of persons with confirmed or suspected infectious tuberculosis (contact investigation), including children in contact with family members or associates who spent time in jail or prison in the last 5 years.

• Children with radiographic or clinical findings suggesting tuberculosis.

• Children immigrating from endemic countries (eg, Asia, Middle East, Africa, Latin America).

• Children with travel histories to endemic countries or significant contact with indigenous persons from such countries.

Test these children annually for tuberculosis:

• Children infected with HIV.

• Incarcerated adolescents.

Test these children every 2 to 3 years (apply initial test upon diagnosis or circumstance):

• Children exposed to the following people: HIV-infected people, homeless people, residents of nursing homes, institutionalized adolescents or adults, users of illicit drugs, incarcerated adolescents or adults and migrant farm workers. This includes foster children exposed to adults in these high-risk groups.

Consider testing these children at 4, 6 and 11 to 16 years of age:

• Children whose parents immigrated (with unknown tuberculin skin test status) from regions of the world with high prevalence of tuberculosis. Continued potential exposure by travel to the endemic areas or household contact with people from endemic areas (with unknown tuberculin skin test status) is an indication for repeat tuberculin skin testing.

• Children without specific risk factors who reside in high-prevalence areas. In general, a high-risk neighborhood or community does not mean an entire city is at high risk; rates in any city vary by neighborhood, or even from block to block. Be aware of these patterns in determining the likelihood of exposure; public health officials or local tuberculosis experts can help clinicians identify areas that have appreciable tuberculosis rates.

AAP notes the following medical factors increase a child's risk for progression to disease: diabetes mellitus, chronic renal failure, malnutrition and congenital or acquired immunodeficiencies. Without recent exposure, these people are not at increased risk of acquiring tuberculosis infection. Underlying immune deficiencies theoretically enhance the possibility for progression to severe disease. Ask all these patients about potential exposure to tuberculosis. If exposure is possible, consider immediate and periodic tuberculin skin testing. Perform an initial intradermal tuberculin skin test before beginning immunosuppressive therapy in any child.

 Contraindications:

Absolute: None.

Relative: Do not administer tuberculin to known tuberculin-positive reactors because of the severity of reactions (eg, vesiculation, ulceration, necrosis) that may occur at the test site in very highly hypersensitive individuals. Rarely, tuberculin testing may activate quiescent tuberculous lesions in individuals with active tuberculosis.

Elderly: Skin-test responsiveness may be delayed or reduced in magnitude among older persons. Two-step testing is important, especially in persons ≥35 years of age.

Pregnancy: *Category C*. The risk of unrecognized tuberculosis and the close postpartum contact between a mother with active disease and her infant leaves the infant in grave danger of tuberculosis and complications such as tuberculous meningitis. No adverse effects upon the fetus recognized as being due to tuberculosis skin testing have been reported. The state of pregnancy does not interfere with PPD test results. Test women with PPD if they have any substantial risk of disease.

Lactation: It is not likely that tuberculin is excreted in breast milk. Problems in humans have not been documented and are unlikely.

Children: A child known to have been exposed to a tuberculous adult must not be considered free of infection until the child demonstrates a negative tuberculin reaction ≥10 weeks after contact with the tuberculous person(s) has ceased.

Adverse Reactions:

Immediate erythematous or other reactions may occur at the injection site. In hypersensitive individuals, strongly positive reactions including vesiculation, ulceration or necrosis occur at the test site. The reasons for these infrequent occurrences are unknown. Cold packs or topical corticosteroid preparations can be used for symptomatic relief of the associated pain, pruritus and discomfort.

Pharmacologic & Dosing Characteristics

Dosage: 0.1 ml of the appropriate concentration. The 5 TU/0.1 ml strength is the standard concentration.

Alternate concentrations: Use the 1 TU/0.1 ml concentration only for individuals suspected of being highly sensitized. Use PPD preparations con- taining 250 TU/0.1 ml exclusively for the testing of individuals who fail to react to a previous injection of 5 TU. Do not use, under any circumstances, the 250 TU/0.1 ml product for an initial test. Use of these products is not recommended by ATS or CDC.

Route & Site: Intradermal, also described as intracutaneous or the Mantoux method. A $^1/_2$-inch, 26- or 27-gauge needle is recommended. Do not use syringes that have previously been used for another purpose or another person.

Insert the point of the needle into the most superficial layers of the skin with the bevel pointing upward. As the tuberculin solution is injected, a pale bleb 6 to 10 mm in diameter rises over the point of the needle. This is quickly absorbed and no dressing is required. If no bleb forms (suggesting the fluid has been injected SC) or if a significant part of the dose leaks from the injection site, reapply the test at another site >5 cm away from the first site.

Avoid injecting SC. In such cases where no bleb forms, no local reaction develops, but a general febrile reaction or acute inflammation around old tuberculous lesions may occur in highly hypersensitive individuals.

The flexor (volar) or dorsal surface of the forearm about 4 inches below the elbow is preferred, although other sites may be used. Cleanse the site with 70% isopropyl alcohol and allow to dry before test injection. In persons with severe skin rashes, do not administer the test in areas where the rash occurs. Similarly, avoid hairy areas, scars, pimples, moles and other marks.

Drug Interactions: Reactivity to

any tuberculin test may be suppressed in people receiving high doses of corticosteroids or other immuno-suppressive drugs, or in people who were recently immunized with live virus vaccines (eg, measles, mumps, rubella, poliovirus). If tuberculin skin testing is indicated, perform it either preceding or simultaneous with immunization or 4 to 6 weeks after immunization.

Persons previously immunized with BCG vaccine may test positive to a tuberculin skin test. Tuberculin reactions caused by BCG cannot reliably be distinguished from reactions caused by natural mycobacterial infections. Test conversion rates after vaccination may be much less than 100%. The mean reaction size among vaccinees is often <10 mm, and tuberculin hypersensitivity tends to wane after vaccination. The ATS suggests it is appropriate to consider any significant reaction to 5 TU of PPD tuberculin in BCG-vaccinated persons as indicating infection with *Mycobacterium tuberculosis*, especially among persons from countries with a high prevalence of tuberculosis. Tuberculin reactivity in BCG vaccinees does not reliably predict protection against *Mycobacterium tuberculosis*.

Several weeks of cimetidine therapy may augment or enhance delayed-hypersensitivity responses to skin-test antigens, although this effect has not been consistently observed. The effect may be mediated through cimetidine binding to suppressor T-lymphocytes (Kumar, 1990). It is presently unknown if other H_2-antagonists possess similar activity.

Patient Information: Howard & Solomon (1988) reported that only 37.2% of patients with >10 mm induration following 5 TU tuberculin PPD thought any induration was present. Do not rely on patients to read their own tests.

Pharmaceutical Characteristics

Concentration: 1, 5 and 250 tuberculin units (TU) per 0.1 ml, comparable to the US Reference Standard, PPD-S. The 1 TU/0.1 ml concentration has also been referred to as the "first strength" of PPD, 5 TU/0.1 ml as the "intermediate strength," and 250 TU/0.1 ml as the "second strength." In order to avoid misinterpretation and dosage errors, do not use these designations.

Packaging:

Connaught: 1 TU/0.1 ml, 10 tests per 1 ml vial; 5 TU/0.1 ml, 10 tests per 1 ml vial, 50 tests per 5 ml vial; 250 TU/0.1 ml, 10 tests per 1 ml vial

Parke-Davis: 5 TU/0.1 ml, 10 tests per 1 ml vial; 50 tests per 5 ml vial

Dose Form: Solution

Solvent: *Connaught*: 0.28% phenol

Parke-Davis: 0.35% phenol

Storage/Stability: Store at 2° to 8°C (36° to 46°F). Discard if frozen. PPD is light sensitive; expose to light only while measuring doses. Discard vials 1 month after first entry, since air introduced into the vial permits oxidation that reduces potency.

Prefilling Syringes: PPD solution is stable when prefilled into syringes and stored in a refrigerator up to 30 days. Manipulation during prefilling increases the risk of microbial contamination. Aseptic technique in laminar-flow hoods will minimize this risk.

Connaught: Product can tolerate 24 hours at room temperature not exceeding 24°C (75°F). Vials that have not yet been entered can tolerate 24°C (75°F) for 72 hours. Use such products promptly. Shipped in insulated containers with coolant properties.

Parke-Davis: Product can tolerate ≥ 2 to 3 weeks at room temperature or 1 week at elevated temperature. Stability data suggest that frozen *Aplisol* is stable for 24 hours at −16°C (3°F). Shipped at ambient temperature.

Tuberculin Purified Protein Derivative (Multipuncture Device)

MYCOBACTERIAL ANTIGENS

NAME:

Tuberculin, TineTest PPD, Aplitest, SclavoTest-PPD

MANUFACTURERS:

Tuberculin, Wyeth-Lederle Vaccines & Peiatrics; *Aplitest,* Parke-Davis; *SclavoTest-PPD,* Biocine Sclavo

Synonyms: Tine test, tuberculin skin test (TST). *Tine Test* is the registered trademark of Wyeth-Lederle's multiple-puncture device. This device is also used to deliver other immunodiagnostic skin test reagents.

Comparison: The various multiple-puncture PPD devices are generically equivalent, but differ from PPD solution products and from old tuberculin products. Intradermal PPD is more sensitive and more specific than any tuberculin delivered by multipuncture device.

Viability: Inactivated

Antigenic Form: Isolate from culture filtrates

Antigenic Type: Protein. Skin tests assess delayed (type IV) hypersensitivity.

Use Characteristics

Indications: For detection of delayed hypersensitivity to *Mycobacterium tuberculosis*. Multiple-puncture devices are screening tools that aid in determining the tuberculin hypersensitivity of individuals.

These devices have been clinically compared with intradermal administration of 5 TU of PPD-S, the US Reference Standard. These devices are useful in mass tuberculosis screening programs, to establish priorities for additional testing (eg, intradermal PPD, chest radiographs) and in epidemiological surveys to identify areas with high levels of infection. They aid the identification of old or recent *Mycobacterium tuberculosis* infection, with or without disease. Multiple-

puncture devices are advantageous in persons who may object to use of needle and syringe (eg, young children).

Regular, periodic testing (eg, annual or biennial) of tuberculin-negative persons may be recommended in some populations such as health-care workers. This procedure is especially valuable because the conversion of an individual from negative to positive is highly indicative of recent tuberculosis infection.

Repeated testing of uninfected individuals does not sensitize patients to tuberculin. In persons with waning hypersensitivity to mycobacterial antigens, however, the stimulus of a tuberculin test may "boost" or increase the size of the reaction to a subsequent test given a week to a year later. This may be misinterpreted as recent development of hypersensitivity in some instances.

Contraindications:

Absolute: None.

Relative: Do not administer tuberculin to known tuberculin-positive reactors because of the severity of reactions (eg, vesiculation, ulceration, necrosis) that may occur at the test site in very highly hypersensitive individuals. Rarely, tuberculin testing may activate quiescent tuberculous lesions in individuals with active tuberculosis.

Elderly: Skin test responsiveness may be delayed or reduced in magnitude among older persons.

Pregnancy: *Category* C. The risk of unrecognized tuberculosis and the close postpartum contact between a mother with active disease and an infant leaves the infant in grave danger of tuberculosis and complications such as tuberculous meningitis. No adverse effects on the fetus recognized as being due to tuberculosis skin testing have been reported.

Lactation: It is not likely that tuberculin is excreted in breast milk. Problems in humans have not been documented.

Children: A child known to have been exposed to a tuberculous adult must not be considered free of infection until the child demonstrates a negative tuberculin reaction ≥10 weeks after contact with the tuberculous person(s) has ceased. If tuberculin screening of children is conducted, the American Academy of Pediatrics recommends that skin tests be applied at 12 months, 4 to 6 years, and 14 to 16 years of age.

Adverse Reactions:

In highly hypersensitive individuals, strongly positive reactions including vesiculation, ulceration or necrosis may occur at the test site. Cold packs or topical corticosteroid preparations can be used for symptomatic relief of the associated pain, pruritus and discomfort. Minimal bleeding may occur at the puncture site. This occurs infrequently and does not affect the interpretation of the test.

Pharmacologic & Dosing Characteristics

Dosage: One application, applied firmly and without twisting. Hold the device in place at least 1 second. Exert sufficient pressure to assure that all 4 tines have penetrated the skin. If adequate pressure is applied, the puncture marks of each tine will be observed. Do not apply more than one multiple-puncture device since the response of an individual may be altered by the simultaneous administration of several tests.

Route & Site: Variously described as percutaneous, transcutaneous or intradermal. The flexor (volar) surface of the forearm about 4 inches below the elbow is preferred. The dorsal surface or other sites may also be used. Avoid areas without adequate SC tissue, such as above a tendon or bone. Cleanse application sites with 70% isopropyl alcohol, acetone, ether or soap and water and allow to dry before test application. In persons with severe skin rashes, do not administer the test in areas where the rash occurs. Similarly, avoid hairy areas, scars, pimples, moles and other marks. Grasp the patient's forearm firmly to stretch the skin taut at the test site and to prevent any jerking motion of the arm that could cause scratching with the tines.

Drug Interactions: Reactivity to any tuberculin test may be suppressed in persons receiving corticosteroids or other immunosuppressive drugs, or in persons recently immunized with live virus vaccines (eg, measles, mumps, rubella, poliovirus). If tuberculin skin testing is indicated, perform it either preceding or simultaneous with immunization or 4 to 6 weeks after immunization.

Persons previously immunized with BCG vaccine may test positive to a tuberculin skin test. Tuberculin reactions caused by BCG cannot reliably be distinguished from reactions caused by natural mycobacterial infections. Test conversion rates after vaccination may be much less than 100%. The mean reaction size among vaccinees is often <10 mm and tuberculin hypersensitivity tends to wane after vaccination. The American Thoracic Society suggests it is appropriate to consider any significant reaction to 5 TU of PPD tuberculin in BCG-vaccinated persons as indicating infection with *Mycobacterium tuberculosis*, especially among persons from countries with a high prevalence of tuberculosis. Tuberculin reactivity in BCG vaccinees does not reliably predict protection against *Mycobacterium tuberculosis*.

Several weeks of cimetidine therapy may augment or enhance delayed-hypersensitivity responses to skin test antigens, although this effect has not been consistently observed. The effect may be mediated through cimetidine binding to suppressor T-lymphocytes (Kumar, 1990). It is presently unknown if other H_2-antagonists possess similar activity.

Pharmaceutical Characteristics

Concentration: Standardized by clinical evaluation in human subjects to give reactions equivalent to or more potent than 5 TU of standard PPD administered by intradermal injection.

Packaging:

Wyeth-Lederle: Jar of 25 individual tests, box of 100 individual tests. Each package includes patient-oriented induration illustration cards with palpable diagrams of typical reactions.

Parke-Davis: Package of 25 individual tests

Dose Form: Sterile, single-use multiple-puncture antigen applicators

Wyeth-Lederle: Each Tine Test device consists of a stainless-steel disc attached to a light blue plastic handle. Projecting from the disc are 4 triangular steel prongs (tines), each 2 mm long and 4 mm apart. The tines are mechanically dipped into a concentrated solution of PPD.

Parke-Davis: Cylindrical plastic holder bearing 4 equally spaced stainless steel tines at one end, equally spaced around a $\frac{3}{8}$ inch circumference. The tines are coated by dipping in a solution of tuberculin PPD and dried. The tines are covered with a protective cap to maintain sterility.

Storage/Stability: Store at room temperature, at <30°C (86°F). Do not refrigerate or freeze.

Wyeth-Lederle: Discard if refrigerated or frozen. Shipping data not provided.

Parke-Davis: Contact manufacturer regarding prolonged exposure to elevated or freezing temperatures. Shipped at ambient temperature.

Interpretation of Serial Tuberculin Tests

Initial reaction	Subsequent reaction	Time interval	Interpretation
Positive to any multiple-puncture device (OT or PPD)	Positive to intradermal PPD	a few days	Infected
Positive to any multiple-puncture device (OT or PPD)	Negative to any tuberculin test (OT or PPD)	a few days	Not infected (the initial reaction represents a false-positive reaction to the multiple-puncture device)
Negative to any tuberculin test (OT or PPD)	Positive to any tuberculin test (OT or PPD)	a few days, weeks or a month	Infected during the entire period (the second reaction represents a "booster" reaction induced by the first test)
Negative to any tuberculin test (OT or PPD)	Positive to intradermal PPD	months or years	Newly infected (a "converter")
Positive to intradermal PPD (negative history of BCG vaccination)	Negative to intradermal PPD	at any time in the future	Immunosuppressed (anergic, perhaps from tuberculosis itself)
Positive to intradermal PPD (positive history of BCG vaccination)	Negative to intradermal PPD	at any time in the future	Either immuno-suppressed (anergic, perhaps from tuberculosis itself) or waning immunity to BCG
Negative to any tuberculin test (OT or PPD)	Negative to any tuberculin test (OT or PPD)	weeks, months or years	Not infected (assumes anergy is not a factor)

Tuberculin Comparisons			
	Old tuberculin	Purified protein derivative of tuberculin (solution)	Purified protein derivative of tuberculin (multipuncture device)
Abbreviation	OT	PPD	PPD
Synonyms	Tine Test	Mantoux test	Tine Test
Dose Form	Multipuncture device	Solution	Multipuncture device
Proprietary names (manufacturer)	*Old Tuberculin* *Tine Test* (Wyeth-Lederle), *Mono-Vacc OT* (Connaught)	*Aplisol* (Parke-Davis), *Tubersol* (Connaught)	*Tine Test PPD* (Wyeth-Lederle), *Aplitest* (Parke-Davis)
Concentrations available	comparable to 5 TU	1 TU/0.1 ml 5 TU/0.1 ml 250 TU/0.1 ml	comparable to 5 TU
Packaging	25's, 100's, 250's	5th/0.1 ml in 1 and 5 ml vials	25's, 100's
Indications	Screening test	Definitive test	Screening test
Route	Transcutaneous	Intradermal	Transcutaneous
Routine storage	Room temperature	Refrigerate	Room temperature

Coccidioidin

NAME:

Coccidioidin (Mycelial Derivative), *BioCox;* Coccidioidin (Spherule Derivative), *Spherulin*

MANUFACTURERS:

Coccidioidin (Mycelial Derivative), *BioCox,* Iatric Corporation; Coccidioidin (Spherule Derivative), *Spherulin,* ALK Laboratories

Synonyms: *BioCox* is known as CAS # 12622-73-0; *Spherulin* is called *Esferulina* in Spanish. Coccidioidomycosis is also known as San Joaquin valley fever, valley fever, desert fever, desert rheumatism and Posada's disease.

Comparison: The two forms of coccidiodin are generically inequivalent. Coccidioidin derived from spherules is considered more sensitive, although possibly less specific, than coccidioidin derived from mycelia. Either form of coccidioidin may boost the level of existing skin hypersensitivity to coccidioidin. Mycelial coccidioidin may boost titers of complement-fixing antibodies.

Viability: Inactivated

Antigenic Form:

Iatric: Mycelial culture filtrate

ALK: Spherule filtrate

Antigenic Type: Proteins and polysaccharides. Skin tests assess delayed (type IV) hypersensitivity. *BioCox* includes a glycoprotein complex of 31,700 daltons.

Use Characteristics

 Indications: For detection of delayed hypersensitivity to *Coccidioides immitis.* Serves as an aid in the diagnosis of coccidioidomycosis. The skin test is a valuable diagnostic tool to differentiate coccidioidomycosis from the common cold, influenza and other mycotic or bacterial infections (eg, blastomycosis, histoplasmosis, tuberculosis, sarcoidosis).

Unlabeled Uses: In endemic areas (eg, the southwestern US), coccidioidin may be a useful addition to anergy skin-test panels to assess competence of recipients' cell-mediated immunity, but use of mycelial coccidioidin may obscure the results of other fungal assays.

STOP **Contraindications:**

Absolute: None.

Relative: Use with caution in individuals hypersensitive to thimerosal. Such persons may yield false positive reactions. Skin testing during primary coccidioidomycosis may precipitate or produce a recurrence of erythema nodosum. Test such persons, if necessary, with dilutions of the usual-strength reagent.

Elderly: No specific information is available about geriatric use of coccidioidin.

Pregnancy: *Category* C. Use only if clearly needed. It is unlikely that coccidioidin crosses the placenta.

Lactation: It is not likely that coccidioidin is excreted in breast milk. Problems in humans have not been documented.

Children: Safety and efficacy of mycelial coccidioidin have not been specifically established in children; but spherule-derived coccidioidin is safe and effective in children, including those <5 years of age.

Adverse Reactions:

An immediate-type induration and erythema reaction may occur at the injection site. Anaphylaxis develops very rarely following injection. Patients with great hypersensitivity to coccidioidin or with primary coccidioidomycosis rarely develop a systemic reaction consisting of fever or erythema nodosum. There are no reports that skin testing can cause a relapse of the disease. Occasionally, large local reactions develop, leading to vesiculation, tenderness, pruritus, ulceration, regional lymphadenopathy, rash, local tissue necrosis and scar formation at the injection site.

Pharmacologic & Dosing Characteristics

Dosage: 0.1 ml of a 1:100 dilution initially. Use a weaker 1:1000 or 1:10,000 dilution if erythema nodosum is evident. Use the 1:10 dilution only in persons who are negative to the 1:100 dilution.

Route & Site: Intradermal, typically applied to the volar surface of the forearm.

Drug Interactions: Reactivity to any delayed-hypersensitivity test may be suppressed in persons receiving corticosteroids or other immunosuppressive drugs, or in persons who were recently immunized with live virus vaccines (eg, measles, mumps, rubella, poliovirus). If delayed-hypersensitivity skin testing is indicated, perform it either preceding or simultaneous with immunization or 4 to 6 weeks after immunization.

Several weeks of cimetidine therapy may augment or enhance delayed-hypersensitivity responses to skin test antigens, although this effect was not consistently observed. The effect may be mediated through cimetidine binding to suppressor T-lymphocytes (Kumar, 1990). It is presently unknown if other H_2-antagonists possess similar activity.

Laboratory Interferences: A positive reaction to *BioCox* may cause a rise in titers of complement-fixing antibodies against *Emmonsiella capsulata* (formerly *Histoplasma capsulatum*) and coccidioidin. Unlike *BioCox*, *Spherulin* does not induce humoral antibodies nor does it affect complement-fixation titers for either histoplasmosis or coccidioidomycosis. Either coccidioidin may boost existing hypersensitivity in recipients, manifested after a subsequent test.

Pharmaceutical Characteristics

Concentration:

Iatric: 1:10 and 1:100 (ratio is not described as w/v or v/v)

ALK: 1:10 v/v (high strength) and 1:100 v/v (usual strength)

Packaging:

Iatric: 1:100 w/v, 1 ml 10-test multidose vial 1:10 w/v, 1 ml 10-test multidose vial

ALK: 1:100 v/v, 1 ml 10-test multidose vial 1:10 v/v, 0.5 ml 5-test multidose vial

Dose Form: Solution

Solvent: *Iatric*: Bicarbonate-buffered saline

ALK: Isotonic sodium chloride

Diluents:

ALK: 0.9% sodium chloride or buffered saline for test dilutions

Storage/Stability: Store at 2° to 8°C (36° to 46°F). Discard if frozen.

Iatric: Relatively tolerant to elevated temperatures. Contact manufacturer regarding prolonged exposure to room temperature or elevated temperatures.

Shipping data not provided. Stability data for compounded dilutions not provided.

ALK: Product can tolerate 14 days at room temperature. Shipped by second-day courier, without any special insulation or refrigeration. Refrigerate dilutions after compounding and discard within 24 hours.

Coccidioidin Comparisons		
	BioCox	*Spherulin*
Source	Mycelial filtrate	Spherule filtrate
Manufacturer	Iatric	ALK
Concentration	1:10 and 1:100	1:10 and 1:100 v/v
Packaging	1 ml vials	1:10–0.5 ml vial 1:100–1 ml vial
Sensitivity	Not described	Not described
Specificity	Not described	Not described
Related effects	Testing may boost skin hypersensitivity to subsequent tests. Positive reactions may elevate titers of complement-fixing antibodies against *Emmonsiella* (ie, *Histoplasma*) and coccidioidin.	Testing may boost skin hypersensitivity to subsequent test. Positive reactions probably do not elevate titers of complement-fixing antibodies against *Emmonsiella* (ie, *Histoplasma*) and coccidioidin.
Cross-reactivity	*Blastomyces, Emmonsiella* (ie, *Histoplasma*)	No cross reactions when 1:100 v/v strength is used

Histoplasmin

NAME:

Generic Histoplasmin (Mycelial Derivative) (stabilized solution), Histoplasmin (Controlled Yeast Lysate), *Histolyn-CYL*

Synonyms: P-D: CAS # 9008-05-3; ALK: CYL

Comparison: The two forms of histoplasmin are generically inequivalent.

Viability: Inactivated

Antigenic Form:

Parke-Davis: Cell-free culture filtrate from mycelial-phase cultures

ALK: Extract filtrate of whole yeast lysate

Use Characteristics

 Indications: For detection of delayed hypersensitivity to *Emmonsiella capsulata* (ie, *Histoplasma capsulatum*). Histoplasmin serves as an aid in the diagnosis of histoplasmosis and the differentiation of possible histoplasmosis from coccidioidomycosis, tuberculosis, sarcoidosis and other mycotic or bacterial infections, and in the interpretation of radiographic plates showing pulmonary infiltration and calcification. The test may also be useful in epidemiologic studies of groups of persons with exposure to histoplasmosis and other infectious diseases.

Three criteria have been used to distinguish lesions associated with histoplasmin hypersensitivity from those due to other causes:

MANUFACTURERS:

Generic Histoplasmin (Mycelial Derivative) (stabilized solution), Parke-Davis; ✸ Parke-Davis; Histoplasmin (Controlled Yeast Lysate) *Histolyn-CYL,* ALK Laboratories

Mycelial histoplasmin is more likely to boost complement-fixing antibody titers than yeast-lysate histoplasmin.

Antigenic Type: Extract filtrate of whole yeast lysate

Parke-Davis: Mycelial protein and other constituents, such as carbohydrate, lipid and nucleic acid components; two major antigens are known: h and m.

(1) The individual has skin hypersensitivity to histoplasmin but not tuberculin; (2) lesions persist for 2 months, to exclude transient pneumonic lesions; (3) laboratory and clinical examinations to exclude tuberculosis, sarcoidosis or other granulomatous diseases (Furcolow et al, 1947).

Unlabled Uses: In endemic areas (eg, the Ohio and Mississippi River valleys), histoplasmin may be a useful addition to anergy skin test panels to assess competence of recipients' cell-mediated immunity, but use of mycelial histoplasmin may obscure the results of other fungal assays.

STOP **Contraindications:**

Absolute: None.

Relative: Do not administer histoplasmin to known histoplasmin-positive reactors because of the severity of reactions (eg, vesiculation, ulceration, necrosis) that may occur at the test site in very highly hypersensitive individuals.

Elderly: No specific information is available about geriatric use of histoplasmin.

Pregnancy: *Category C.* Use only if clearly needed. It is unlikely that histoplasmin crosses the placenta.

Lactation: It is unlikely that histoplasmin is excreted in breast milk. Problems in humans have not been documented.

Children: Safety and efficacy of mycelial histoplasmin have not been established; but yeast-lysate histoplasmin has been routinely administered to children with no special safety problems noted.

Adverse Reactions: Occasionally a patient may develop an immediate-hypersensitivity skin reaction to either histoplasmin, manifested as induration and erythema. Rarely, urticaria, angioedema, wheezing, excessive perspiration and shortness of breath may occur. Anaphylaxis may follow administration of either histoplasmin.

Doses >0.1 ml increase the frequency of severe local reactions, with large induration, necrosis and ulceration. In highly hypersensitive persons, strongly positive skin-test reactions consisting of vesiculation, necrosis, ulceration and scarring may occur. There is no way to predict the strong reactions, which may occur in as many as 1% of tests. Cold packs and topical corticosteroids may be used for symptomatic relief of discomfort and itching at the site of a large local reaction. Severe erythema and induration followed by necrosis and ulceration may last for several weeks.

Dosage: 0.1 ml of the 1:100 dilution

Route & Site: Intradermal, usually applied to the flexor surface of the forearm. Cleanse skin with 70% isopropyl alcohol and allow to dry. A 26 or 27 gauge, $\frac{3}{8}$ inch to $\frac{1}{2}$ inch needle is recommended. If the test is injected correctly, a small bleb rises within the skin over the point of the needle.

Drug Interactions: Reactivity to any delayed-hypersensitivity test may be suppressed in persons receiving corticosteroids or other immunosuppressive drugs, or in persons who were recently immunized with live virus vaccines (eg, measles, mumps, rubella, poliovirus). If delayed-hypersensitivity skin testing is indicated, perform it either preceding or simultaneous with immunization or 4 to 6 weeks after immunization.

Several weeks of cimetidine therapy may augment or enhance delayed-hypersensitivity responses to skin-test antigens, although this effect was not consistently observed. The effect may be mediated through cimetidine binding to suppressor T-lymphocytes (Kumar, 1990). It is presently unknown if other H2-antagonists possess similar activity.

Laboratory Interference: The mycelial histoplasmin skin test, but generally not the yeast-phase form, may cause elevation of serum complement-fixing antibody titers to histoplasmin. If serological studies are clinically indicated, obtain the blood sample before administering the skin test. If the sample is not drawn before test application, draw it within 48 to 96 hours following test application. After that time, a rise in titer may occur, usually associated with a positive skin test.

Pharmaceutical Characteristics

Concentration:
Parke-Davis: 1:100 w/v
ALK: 1:100 v/v

Packaging:
Parke-Davis: 1 ml, 10-test multidose vial
ALK: 1.3 ml multidose vials

Dose Form: Solution

Storage/Stability: Store at 2° to 8°C (36° to 46°F). Discard if frozen.

Parke-Davis: Stability data suggest the product can tolerate 7 days at 40°C (104°F). Shipping data not provided.

ALK: Contact manufacturer regarding prolonged exposure to room temperature or elevated temperatures. Product can tolerate ambient temperature during mailing for 3 to 4 days.

Histoplasmin Comparisons		
Source	Mycelial filtrate	Yeast lysate
Propietary name	Generic	*Histolyn-CYL*
Manufacturer	Parke-Davis	ALK Laboratories
Concentration	1:100 w/v	1:100 v/v
Packaging	1 ml vial	1.3 ml vial
Sensitivity	96%	83%
Specificity	94%	Very high
Related effects	Positive reactions may elevate titers of complement-fixing antibodies against *Emmonsiella*.	Rarely elevates *Emmonsiella* titers.
Cross-reactivity	*Blastomyces, Coccidioides*	*Blastomyces*

NAME:
MSTA

MANUFACTURERS:
Connaught Laboratories, ⚜ Connaught

Viability: Inactivated

Antigenic Form: Whole virus

Antigenic Type: Protein and other

constituents. S and V major antigens have been isolated. Skin tests assess delayed (type IV) hypersensitivity.

Use Characteristics

Indications: For detection of delayed hypersensitivity to mumps antigens and assessment of cell-mediated immunity. Since most of the population have had contact or infection with mumps virus, they usually demonstrate a delayed-hypersensitivity reaction to mumps skin test antigen if they possess an adequate cellular immune system; 67% to 90% of healthy adults demonstrate a delayed hypersensitivity reaction.

Contraindications:
Absolute: None

Relative: Generally, do not administer this product to anyone with a history of hypersensitivity, especially anaphylactic reactions, to eggs or egg products. Similarly, use it with caution in individuals known to be hypersensitive to thimerosal.

Elderly: Skin test responsiveness may be delayed or reduced in magnitude in older persons.

Pregnancy: *Category* C. Use only if clearly needed. It is unlikely that MSTA crosses the placenta.

Lactation: It is unlikely that MSTA is excreted into breast milk. Problems in humans have not been documented.

Children: Safety and efficacy in children have not been established.

Adverse Reactions:
Local reactions may include tenderness, pruritus, vesiculation and rash. Sloughing, necrosis, abscess formation, or regional lymphadenopathy may be associated with unusually large delayed-hypersensitivity reactions. Adverse reactions may include nausea, anorexia, headache, unsteadiness, drowsiness, sweating, sensation of warmth, and lymphadenopathy.

Pharmacologic & Dosing Characteristics

Dosage: 0.1 ml. Shake vial well before withdrawing each dose.

Route & Site: Intradermal, usually applied to the inner, volar surface of the forearm. Cleanse the skin with 70% isopropyl alcohol and allow to dry. If MSTA is injected SC, no reaction or an unreliable reaction may occur.

Drug Interactions: Reactivity to any delayed-hypersensitivity test may be suppressed in persons receiving corticosteroids or other immunosuppressive drugs, or in persons who were recently immunized with live virus vaccines (eg, measles, mumps, rubella, poliovirus). If delayed-hypersensitivity skin testing is indicated, perform it either preceding or simultaneous with immunization or 4 to 6 weeks after immunization.

Several weeks of cimetidine therapy may augment or enhance delayed-hypersensitivity responses to skin-test antigens, although this effect was not consistently observed. The effect may be mediated through cimetidine binding to suppressor T-lymphocytes (Kumar, 1990). It is presently unknown if other H_2-antagonists possess similar activity.

Pharmaceutical Characteristics

Concentration: 40 complement-fixing units per ml (*USP requirement*: At least 20 CFU per ml)

Packaging: 10 tests per 1 ml multidose vial

Dose Form: Suspension

Solvent: 0.9% sodium chloride

Storage/Stability: Store at 2° to 8°C (36° to 46°F). Discard if frozen. Product can tolerate ≤4 days at ≤37°C (100°F). Shipped in insulated containers with coolant packs.

Candida albicans Skin Test Antigen

NAME:
Candin

MANUFACTURERS:
Manufactured by Allermed Laboratories, distributed by ALK Laboratories

Synonym: An obsolete term is candidin. The *Candida* genus of fungi was formerly called *Oidium* and later *Monilia*.

Comparison: Unlike the now-obsolete oidiomycin and other unstandardized *Candida* albicans allergen extracts, *Candin* is standardized in vivo against an internal reference product to assure potency and reproducibility of cutaneous test results.

In the literature, the incidence of delayed-hypersensitivity reactions to unstandardized *Candida* antigens has been reported to vary from 52% to 89%, depending upon the strength of the antigen and the induration size defined as a positive test. In contrast, when healthy subjects were tested with two reagents, *Candin* and mumps skin test antigen, 92% were positive to at least one antigen, a higher response rate than to either antigen used alone.

Viability: Inactivated

Antigenic Form: Fungal culture filtrate

Antigenic Type: Presumably polysac-charides and proteins, representing fungal cell-wall antigens. Skin tests assess delayed (type IV) hypersensitivity.

Use Characteristics

Indications: For use as a recall antigen for detecting delayed hypersensitivity by intracutaneous (intradermal) testing. The product may be useful in evaluating the cellular immune response in patients suspected of having reduced cell-mediated immunity.

Published studies confirm that antigens of *Candida albicans* are useful in the assessment of diminished cellular immunity in persons infected with human immunodeficiency virus. Responses to delayed-hypersensitivity antigens have been reported to have prognostic value in patients with cancer.

Because HIV infection can modify the delayed-hypersensitivity response to tuberculin, it is advisable to skin test HIV-infected patients at high risk of tuberculosis with antigens in addition to tuberculin, to assess their competency to react to tuberculin.

Contraindications:

Absolute: Patients who had a previous unacceptable adverse reaction to this antigen or to a similar product, (ie, extreme hypersensitivity or allergy). As has been observed with other, unstandardized antigens used for delayed-hypersensitivity skin testing, it is possible that some patients may have exquisite immediate hypersensitivity to *Candin*.

Relative: Patients with bleeding tendency; bruising and non-specific induration may occur due to the trauma of the skin test.

Elderly: No specific information is available about geriatric use of *Candin*. The delayed-hypersensitivity response to *Candin* may be diminished in geriatric patients, since the aging process is known to alter cell-mediated immunity.

Fertility Impairment: Long-term studies in animals have not been conducted with *Candin* to determine its potential for impairing fertility.

Pregnancy: *Category* C. Animal reproduction studies have not been conducted with *Candin*. It is not known whether *Candin* can cause fetal harm when administered to a pregnant woman. Use *Candin* in pregnant women only if clearly needed. Considering the safety record of tuberculin in pregnant women, problems are unlikely.

Lactation: It is not known if *Candin* crosses into human breast milk. Problems in humans have not been documented and are unlikely.

Children: Safety and efficacy of *Candin* in children <18 years old have not been established.

Adverse Reactions:

Systemic: Systemic reactions to *Candin* have not been observed. However, all foreign antigens have the remote possibility of causing anaphylaxis and even death when injected intradermally. Systemic reactions usually occur within 30 minutes after the injection of antigen and may include the following symptoms: Sneezing, coughing, itching, shortness of breath, abdominal cramps, vomiting, diarrhea, tachycardia, hypotension and respiratory failure in severe cases. Progression of the delayed reaction to vesiculation, necrosis and ulceration is possible. Systemic allergic reactions including anaphylaxis must be immediately treated with epinephrine HCl 1:1,000. Additional measures may be required depending upon the severity of the reaction.

Immediate hypersensitivity reactions to *Candin* occur in some individuals. These reactions are characterized by the presence of an edematous hive surrounded by a zone of erythema. They occur approximately 15 to 20 minutes after the intradermal injection of the antigen. The size of the immediate reaction varies depending upon the sensitivity of the individual. Immediate hypersensitivity reactions have been reported in 17% to 22% of patients, with erythema of 10 to 24 mm in diameter, and in another 5% to 13% of patients, with erythema of 5 to 9 mm.

Local: Local reactions to *Candin* can include redness, swelling, pruritus, excoriation and discoloration of the skin. These reactions usually subside within hours or days after administration of the skin test. In some patients, skin discoloration may persist for several weeks. Local reactions may be treated with a cold compress and topical steroids. Severe local reactions may require additional measures as appropriate.

In a published study of 479 HIV positive adults tested with *Candin*, adverse local reactions were observed in six subjects as follows: Pruritus (n=3), swelling at the test site (n=1), vesiculation (n=1) and vesiculation with weeping edema (n=1). Pruritus and swelling cleared within 48 hours; vesiculation with edema required approximately 1 week to resolve. In two studies involving 171 people, one adverse reaction was observed. This reaction consisted of induration 22 x 55 mm at 48 hours, which resolved within 1 week.

Severe local reactions including rash, vesiculation, bullae, dermal exfoliation and cellulitis have been reported to MedWatch for unstandardized allergenic extracts of *Candida albicans* used for anergy testing.

Pharmacologic & Dosing Characteristics

Dosage: The test dose is 0.1 ml.

Route & Site: Inject *Candin* intradermally on the volar surface of the forearm or on the outer aspect of the upper arm. Cleanse the skin with 70% alcohol before applying the skin test. The intradermal injection must be given as superficially as possible, causing a distinct, sharply defined bleb. An unreliable reaction may result if the product is injected subcutaneously. Do not inject into a blood vessel.

Efficacy: In one group of 18 healthy adults, 14 (78%) of the individuals reacted to *Candin* with an induration response of ≥5 mm at 48 hours. In a second study of 35 subjects, 21 (60%) had induration reactions ≥5 mm at 48 hours. In this study, 65% of males tested positive compared with 53% of females; the mean induration in responding males was 12.8 mm and in responding females was 13 mm. When subjects in these studies were tested with two reagents, *Candin* and mumps skin test antigen, 92% were positive to at least one antigen, a higher response rate than to either antigen used alone.

In another study, the skin test responses of adults with HIV infection were compared with those of healthy control subjects. The responses in HIV-infected patients who did not meet the definition of AIDS were less than those in uninfected subjects, but the differences were not statistically significant. A significant difference was found between AIDS patients and uninfected controls in both mean induration (p <0.01) and proportion with ≥5 mm response (p<0.01).

In a related study involving 20 male patients diagnosed with AIDS, one subject responded to *Candin*. In this study, 65% of the male control subjects had delayed-hypersensitivity reactions ≥5 mm to *Candin*. The mean induration response at 48 hours for control subjects was 8.33 mm, compared with 1.78 mm for the AIDS subject. AIDS vs control p-values were <0.01 for mean induration and <0.01 for unduration ≥5 mm.

In a published study of delayed-hypersensitivity anergy, 479 subjects (334 males and 145 females) infected with HIV and being screened for tuberculosis were skin tested with several additional antigens, including *Candin*. Only 12% reacted to tuberculin (≥5 mm), 57% reacted to *Candin* (≥3 mm) and 60% reacted to either tuberculin or *Candin* or both. In this study, a 3 mm induration response to *Candin* was considered positive. The authors concluded that in HIV-infected subjects, testing with other delayed-hypersensitivity antigens increases the accuracy of interpretation of negative tuberculin reactions.

In another study of 18 patients with lung cancer, *Candin* elicited a positive induration response in five patients (28%). In a second series of 20 patients with metastatic cancer, no reactions >5 mm were observed.

Drug Interactions: Pharmacologic doses of corticosteroids may variably suppress the delayed-hypersensitivity skin test response after 2 weeks of therapy. The mechanism of suppression is believed to involve a decrease in monocytes and lymphocytes, particularly T-cells. The skin test response usually returns to the pretreatment level within several weeks after steroid therapy is discontinued.

Pharmaceutical Characteristics

Concentration: *Candin* is not explicitly labeled in potency units.

Packaging: 1 ml multidose vials containing ten 0.1 ml doses

Dose Form: Solution

Solvent: 0.5% sodium chloride, 0.25% sodium bicarbonate

Storage/Stability: Store at 2° to 8°C (36° to 46°F). Discard frozen product. Product can tolerate up to 7 days at 40°C (104°F). Shipped under ambient conditions in uninsulated containers for second-day delivery.

Multiple Skin Test Antigen Device
UBIQUITOUS DELAYED ANTIGENS

NAME:
Multitest CMI

MANUFACTURERS:
Institut Mérieux, distributed by Connaught Laboratories, ✤ Connaught

Viability: Inactivated

Antigenic Form: Toxoids and culture filtrates

Antigenic Type: Multiple, primarily proteins and oligosaccharides. Skin tests assess delayed (type IV) hypersensitivity.

Use Characteristics

⊙ Indications: For detection of delayed hypersensitivity and assessment of cell-mediated immunity. Cutaneous anergy, the lack of responsiveness to delayed-hypersensitivity antigens, may indicate functional impairment of, or abnormalities in, the cellular immune system. Delayed hypersensitivity is a valuable measure of immune response because it involves a complex series of immunologic, cellular, mediator-associated, and vascular effects.

Delayed-hypersensitivity skin testing may be useful in evaluating individuals suspected of having primary or acquired immune deficiency disorders in which cell-mediated immunity is decreased or absent.

A positive correlation exists between defective cell-mediated immunity (as indicated by anergy to multiple skin-test antigens) and disseminated cancer. The occurrence of anergy may be correlated to some extent with advanced stage disease. Demonstration of anergy can be a negative prognostic factor in certain malignant diseases, since diminished cutaneous reactivity has been associated with poor prognosis. In general, patients capable of displaying normal delayed-hypersensitivity skin test reactions may have a better prognosis, whereas those who remain anergic or who exhibit significantly impaired reactivity, tend to have a poor response to therapy, an increased incidence of recurrences and a shortened survival.

Assessment of cellular hypersensitivity reactions may be useful in other conditions. For example, protein calorie malnutrition is often complicated by increasing frequency and severity of infection. Moderate to severe malnutrition (<70% of standard weight for height) is almost invariably associated with impaired immune response. Even marginal malnutrition may be associated with alterations in immunocompetence. Delayed-hypersensitivity tests can serve as a comparative immunocompetence parameter. Deficiencies of certain minerals, trace elements or vitamins (eg, ascorbic acid) have been associated with decreased delayed hypersensitivity. Skin testing at periodic intervals may be useful to determine if a state of immunosuppression persists or if delayed-hypersensitivity responsiveness returns to normal limits. Delayed-hypersensitivity testing has been used to assess nutritional and immunocompetence criteria in pre-

and post-surgical evaluations to detect high-risk groups and adopt improved nutritional support.

 Contraindications:

Absolute: None.

Relative: Although severe systemic reactions to diphtheria or tetanus antigens are rare, perform the test in persons known to have a history of systemic reactions to this product only after removing test heads containing these antigens (#1 and #2).

Elderly: Skin test responsiveness may be delayed or reduced in magnitude in older persons.

Pregnancy: *Category C.* Use only if clearly needed. It is unlikely that the Multitest-CMI antigens cross the placenta.

Lactation: It is unlikely that the Multitest-CMI antigens are excreted in breast milk. Problems in humans have not been documented.

Children: Until data are available for infants and children, skin testing with this product is recommended only for persons ≥17 years of age.

Adverse Reactions: Vesiculation, ulceration or necrosis at the test site occurs in highly hypersensitive subjects. Pain or pruritus at the test site may be relieved with topical corticosteroids or cold packs. Systemic reactions may occur in persons hypersensitive to product constituents.

Pharmacologic & Dosing Characteristics

Dosage: One application. Tap the device on a hard surface, foil side up, to release antigen from the top of the cap. Carefully remove the protective foil and then the plastic caps from each preloaded test head by twisting. Apply once, pointing the T-bar end of the device toward a consistent reference point, such as the elbow or head of the subject being tested, to avoid later identification problems. Keep the skin at the test site taut while applying the device.

Press the device into the skin with sufficient pressure to puncture the skin and allow adequate penetration of all points. Maintain firm contact with the skin for at least 5 seconds. During application, gently rock the device back and forth and from side to side without removing any of the test heads from the skin sites. Bleeding rarely occurs with proper pressure.

If adequate pressure is applied, the puncture marks of the 9 tines on each of the 8 test heads will be observed, an imprint of the circular platform surrounding each test head, and residual antigen and glycerin surrounding each test site. If any of these three criteria are not fulfilled, test results may not be reliable. Identify the area of test sites by drawing a line $\frac{1}{4}$ inch above test sites #1 and #8 and another line below test sites #4 and #5, using an indelible marker. Allow residual antigens and glycerin to remain on the skin surface for 3 minutes, then gently dab with a sterile gauze pad so as not to cross-contaminate test sites with other antigens. Do not smear. Discard applicator safely; do not reuse.

Route & Site: Transcutaneous. Select a test site with sufficient surface area and SC tissue to allow adequate penetration of all points of all 8 test heads. Preferred sites are the volar surfaces of the forearm and the back. Skin of the posterior thighs may be used if necessary. Avoid hairy areas when possible, because test interpretation will be more difficult. Do not apply at sites involving acneiform, infected, or inflamed skin. Cleanse site with 70% isopropyl alcohol, ether or acetone and allow to dry.

If periodic testing is conducted more frequently than every 2 months, rotate test sites so that retesting is not conducted at the same site at <2 month intervals.

Efficacy: See Prevalence of Delayed-Hypersensitivity Responses Among Healthy Adults in the Rational Anergy Test Panels monograph.

Drug Interactions: Reactivity to any delayed-hypersensitivity test may be suppressed in persons receiving corticosteroids or other immunosuppressive drugs, or in persons who were recently immunized with live virus vaccines (eg, measles, mumps, rubella, poliovirus). If delayed-hypersensitivity skin testing is indicated, perform it either preceding or simultaneous with immunization or 4 to 6 weeks after immunization.

Several weeks of cimetidine therapy may augment or enhance delayed-hypersensitivity responses to skin-test antigens, although this effect has not been consistently observed. The effect may be mediated through cimetidine binding to suppressor T-lymphocytes (Kumar, 1990). It is presently unknown if other H_2-antagonists possess similar activity.

Laboratory Interferences: The effect of repeated skin testing on specific antibody levels is not yet known; consequently, conduct in vitro testing only with the understanding that repeated skin testing may alter antibody levels.

Pharmaceutical Characteristics

Concentration:

Test head #1: Tetanus toxoid antigen - 550,000 Mérieux units per ml

Test head #2: Diphtheria toxoid antigen - 1.1 million Mérieux units per ml

Test head #3: Streptococcus Group C antigen - 2000 Mérieux units per ml

Test head #4: Old tuberculin antigen - 300,000 IU per ml

Test head #5: 70% w/v glycerin negative control

Test head #6: Candida albicans antigen - 2000 Mérieux units per ml

Test head #7: Trichophyton mentagrophytes antigen - 150 Mérieux units per ml

Test head #8: Proteus mirabilis antigen - 150 Mérieux units per ml

Packaging: Individual cartons containing 1 single-use, disposable white plastic applicator.

Dose Form: *Multi-Tester,* white acrylic resin applicator, consisting of 8 sterile test heads, numbered clockwise, preloaded with 7 delayed-hypersensitivity antigens and a glycerin negative control. Each head contains approximately 0.3 ml of each antigen in solution, depositing about 0.1% or less of this volume in the skin. Each head consists of 9 tines each and 0.9 mm apart.

Storage/Stability: Store at 2° to 8°C (36° to 46°F). Discard if frozen. Remove from refrigerator 1 hour before use. Stable at room temperature for at least 1 week. Lots produced by the same process for distribution in Europe can tolerate 2° to 25°C (36° to 77°F) for 1 to 2 years. Shipped in insulated containers.

Rational Anergy Test Panels
UBIQUITOUS DELAYED ANTIGENS

Delayed-hypersensitivity skin testing is a tool to diagnose certain infectious diseases (eg, tuberculosis, coccidioidomycosis, histoplasmosis) or to determine patients' general cellular immune competence. If patients have previously been exposed to antigens represented in immunodiagnostic reagents, they normally mount an anamnestic ("memory" or "recall") immune response. Negative responses imply either no previous exposure or anergy, which is a state of immunologic incompetence or deficiency. Numerous factors suppress the immune system and can induce a state of anergy. These factors include such things as infections (eg, bacterial, mycobacterial, viral, fungal, parasitic), congenital immune deficiencies, acquired immune deficiencies (eg, neoplastic, related to medications or radiation) or other. This latter group includes rheumatic diseases, Crohn's disease, alcoholic or biliary cirrhosis, uremia, sarcoidosis, diabetes, anemia, leukocytosis, pregnancy, advancing age, malnutrition, pyridoxine deficiency and recovery from surgery. These factors have been reviewed in detail elsewhere.

To assess immune competence, apply a battery of several immunodiagnostic reagents, which is often called an anergy-test panel. Assemble an assortment of products with a high probability of a positive reaction; multiple positive responses to a skin-test panel are preferred. Most clinicians use a battery of 4 to 6 delayed-hypersensitivity antigens, expecting 2 to 4 positive reactions.

Record results of anergy tests, measured in mm diameter of induration, not simply as a positive or negative response. Tests should be read by medical personnel trained for the intricacies of the task and not by the patient. Timing is critical, since reading reactions too soon can miss a true-positive response. Similarly, reading a test site too late may also pose problems.

A rational anergy-test panel might include a *Candida* antigen (eg, *Candin*), diluted fluid tetanus toxoid, mumps skin test antigen (*MSTA*), and purified protein derivative (PPD) of tuberculin. In endemic areas, a fungal skin test allergen (eg, coccidioidin or histoplasmin) may be added to the panel. In some settings, *Multitest-CMI* may suffice by itself. These settings might involve pediatric patients or settings where personnel familiar with intradermal injection techniques are not available. Any patient who fails to recognize the antigens, testing negative to each of them, is presumed to be immunodeficient with regard to those factors responsible for cell-mediated immunity.

Any patient who fails to recognize the antigens, testing negative to each of them, is presumed to be immunodeficient with regard to those factors responsible for cell-mediated immunity.

Anergy Test Panel, Example 1

Site #	Antigen	Volume and Concentration
1	Mumps Skin Test Antigen	0.1 ml of 40 CFU/ml
2	*Candida* antigen	0.1 ml
3	Fluid Tetanus Toxoid	0.1 ml of either a 1:10 v/v dilution (0.08 to 0.1 Lf u/dose) or a 1.5 to 2 Lf u/ml solution
4	Tuberculin PPD	0.1 ml with 5 TU intradermally

Anergy Test Panel, Example 2

Site #	Antigen	Volume and Concentration
1	Mumps Skin Test Antigen	0.1 ml of 40 CFU/ml
2	*Candida* antigen	0.1 ml
3	Fluid Tetanus Toxoid	0.1 ml of either a 1:10 v/v dilution (0.08 to 0.1 Lf u/dose) or a 1.5 to 2 Lf u/ml solution.
4	Tuberculin PPD	0.1 ml with 5 TU intradermally
5	*Spherulin*	0.1 ml of 1:100 (usual strength) (eg, in the desert southwestern US, or other endemic areas)
–or– 5	*Histolyn-CYL*	0.1 ml of 1:100 concentration (eg, in the Ohio and Mississippi River valleys, or other endemic areas)

Prevalence of Delayed-Hypersensitivity Responses Among Healthy Adults

Antigen	Probability of a positive reaction in healthy adults
Candida albicans allergen extracts	26% to 92%
Mycelial histoplasmin	26% to 80%
Yeast-lysate histoplasmin	up to 80%
Mycelial coccidioidin	10% to 13%
Spherule coccidioidin	Data not provided
Trichophytin allergen extracts	26% to 62%
Mumps skin test antigen	59% to 92%
Purified protein derivative (PPD) of tuberculin	20% to 48%
Tetanus toxoid	28% to 90%

Nonimmunologics

Diluents

Epinephrine

Diluents

NONIMMUNOLOGICS

Diluents are important to the clinician for reconstituting lyophilized drugs and for compounding reagent dilutions for hypersensitivity testing and immunotherapy. Various sterile diluents are available in 1.8, 4, 4.5, 9, 30 ml and 100 ml vials. Manufactuters and resellers include ALK Laboratories, Allergy Laboratories, Allermed, ALO Laboratories, Antigen Laboratories, Center Laboratories, Greer Laboratories, Iatric Corporation, Meridian Division, Miles Pharmaceutical Division, Nelco Laboratories and others.

Preferred Diluents

Human Albumin: Aqueous allergen extracts are commonly diluted with a solution containing 0.03% human serum albumin (HSA) as a protein preservative, 0.9% sodium chloride for isotonicity, and 0.4% phenol as an antimicrobial agent. Dilute Hymenop-tera venoms with HSA diluent.

Glycerin: Dilution in 50% glycerin in sterile water for injection provides a higher degree of protein preservation than human serum albumin (HSA), but glycerin injections may cause local irritation or sterile abscesses. Glycerin is often used as the diluent for prick skin test dilutions, since the viscosity of the glycerin retards the flow of one prick-test reagent into neighboring reagents. Glycerin may increase the incidence of false-positive skin test reactions, especially in the higher dose associated with ID injection. Injections 0.2 ml of a 50% glycerin product may be painful.

Various concentrations of sterile parenteral glycerin, ranging from 10% to 50%, diluted with either sterile water or various combinations of sodium chloride or phosphate or bicarbonate buffers, are available from ALK Laboratories, Allergy Laboratories, Greer Laboratories, Miles Pharmaceutical Division, Meridian Division and other manufacturers. Undiluted sterile parenteral glycerin, with a glycerin content ≥95%, is available from Miles Pharmaceutical Division and perhaps other manufacturers.

Sodium Chloride: Isotonic 0.9% sodium chloride can serve as an effective diluent, although dilutions are not stable for more than several hours to days.

The presence of perservations (eg, thimerosol, phenol) in sodium chloride diluents generally poses no problems, except in the extraordinary patient who may be hypersensitive to the preservative. "Phenol-saline" (0.9% sodium chloride with 0.4% phenol) is the preferred diluent for alum-precipitated allergen extracts (eg, Allpyral, Center-Al).

Inadequate Diluents

Several diluents are sold by allergen-extract manufacturers that provide less than optimal protein stability. Use of suboptimal diluents may cause allergen extracts to lose potency faster and may cause a greater differential in potency when beginning a new treatment formula.

Suboptimal fluids for diluting aqueous allergen extracts and other immunologic drugs include: Phenol-saline (0.9% sodium chloride with 0.4% phenol).

Phosphate-buffered saline (0.5% sodium chloride with 0.08% to 0.11% Na_2HPO_4, 0.036% to 0.04% K_2HPO_4, and 0.4% phenol).

Coca's solution, also called buffered saline (bicarbonate-saline: 0.5% sodium chloride, 0.275% sodium bicarbonate, 0.4% phenol).

Various glycero-saline solutions (eg, 10% glycerin, 0.5% sodium chloride, 0.4% phenol; 25% glycerin, 0.5% sodium chloride, sodium phosphate, potassium phosphate, 0.4% phenol).

Epinephrine Injection

NAMES:

For self administration:

Epinephrine Hydrochloride Injection—1 mg/ml (0.1% or 1:1000 w/v) (Solution), in kits for self-administration: *Ana-Guard,* available separately or as a constituent of the *Ana-Kit* Generic Kit

EpiPen, EpiPen Jr. auto-injectors (1:1000 w/v or 1:2000 w/v), *EpiPen* training device, *EpiE-Z Pen, EpiE-Z Pen Jr.* auto-injectors (1:1000 w/v or 1:2000 w/v), *EpiE-Z Pen* training device

For professional administration:

Epinephrine Injection 1 mg/ml (0.1% or 1:1000 w/v) (Solution) *Adrenalin Chloride Solution* Epinephrine Injection 5 mg/ml (0.5% or 1:200 w/v) (Suspension) *Sus-Phrine.* Generic

MANUFACTURERS:

Wyeth-Ayerst Laboratories, distributed by Bayer Corporation

Wyeth-Ayerst Laboratories, distributed by Derm/Buro Survival Technology, distributed by Center Laboratories

Elkins-Sinn

Parke-Davis Steris Laboratories, distributed by Forest Pharmaceuticals

Various manufacturers

Synonyms: Epi, *Adrenalin*, adrenaline

Comparison: Generically equivalent, adjusting for concentration

Use Characteristics

Indications: Emergency treatment of severe allergic reactions, including anaphylaxis, induced by insect stings or bites, foods, drugs and other allergens. Epinephrine is widely considered the drug of choice for treatment of such emergencies. It can also be used in the treatment of idiopathic or exercise-induced anaphylaxis. Severe immediate hypersensitivity reactions, including ana-

phylaxis, may be induced by the administration of allergen extracts or any biological agent.

Ana-Kit and *EpiPen* products are intended for self-administration by a person with a history of an anaphylactic reaction. Such reactions may occur within minutes after exposure and consist of flushing, apprehension, syncope, tachycardia, or thready or unobtainable pulse associated with a fall in blood pressure, convulsions, vomiting, diarrhea and abdominal cramps, involuntary urination, wheezing, dyspnea due to laryngeal spasm, pruritus, rashes, urticaria or angioedema. Products for self-administration are designed as emergency supportive therapy only and do not substitute for immediate medical or hospital care.

Contraindications

STOP *Absolute*: None in a life-threatening situation.

Relative: Use epinephrine with extreme caution to patients who have heart disease. Use of epinephrine with drugs that may sensitize the heart to dysrhythmias (eg, digitalis, mercurial diuretics, quinidine) ordinarily is not recommended. Anginal pain may be induced by epinephrine in patients with coronary insufficiency, including angina pectoris. The effects of epinephrine may be potentiated by tricyclic antidepressants and monoamine oxidase (MAO) inhibitors. Hyperthyroid persons, persons with cardiovascular disease, hypertension, diabetes, organic brain damage, psychoneurotic disorders. elderly individuals, pregnant women and children weighing <30 kg (for *EpiPen Jr.* or *EpiE-Z Pen Jr.*, children weighing <15 kg) may be theoretically at greater risk of developing adverse reactions after epinephrine administration.

Epinephrine may aggravate narrow-angle (congestive) glaucoma. Despite these concerns, epinephrine is essential for the treatment of anaphylaxis.

Elderly: Elderly persons may theoretically be at greater risk of developing adverse reactions after epinephrine administration.

Pregnancy: Category C. Use only if clearly needed. Pregnant women may be theoretically at greater risk of developing adverse reactions after epinephrine administration. Epinephrine crosses the placenta and may cause anoxia in the fetus. Use only if the potential benefit justifies the potential risk to the fetus.

Lactation: Epinephrine is excreted in breast milk. Use by nursing mothers may cause serious adverse reactions in the infant. Because of this potential, decide whether to discontinue nursing or to withhold epinephrine, taking into account the importance of the drug to the mother.

Children: Children weighing <30 kg (for *EpiPen Jr.* or *EpiE-Z Pen Jr.*, children weighing <15 kg) may theoretically be at greater risk of developing adverse reactions after epinephrine administration. Syncope has occurred following administration of epinephrine in asthmatic children. Epinephrine may be given safely to children at a dosage appropriate to body weight.

Adverse Reactions: Palpitations, tachycardia, sweating, nausea and vomiting, respiratory difficulty, pallor, dizziness, weakness, tremor, headache, apprehension, nervousness and anxiety. These effects are more likely to occur, and in an exaggerated form, in those with hypertension or hyperthyroidism. Cardiac dysrhythmias may follow epinephrine administration. Excessive doses may cause acute hypertension and cardiac dysrhythmia.

Pharmacologic & Dosing Characteristics

Dosage: Usual dosage of epinephrine 1:1000 w/v solution in allergic emergencies:

Adults and children ≥ 12 years: 0.3 to 0.5 mg, 0.3 to 0.5 ml of a 1:1000 w/v solution

Children 6 to 12 years: 0.2 mg, 0.2 ml of a 1:1000 w/v solution

Children 2 to 6 years: 0.15 mg, 0.15 ml of a 1:1000 w/v solution

Infants <2 years: 0.05 mg/0.05 ml to 0.10 mg/0.10 ml of a 1:1000 w/v solution

Give more or less, based on individual assessment of the patient. With severe persistent anaphylaxis, repeat injections if necessary every 5 to 15 minutes according to patient response. The general dose in children is 0.01 mg/kg.

Discard the *Ana-Guard* syringe and obtain a replacement if the second dose is not administered during any given allergic emergency.

Sus-Phrine 1:200 w/v suspension: Give adults 0.5 mg/0.1 ml to 1.5 mg/0.3 ml SC depending 6n patient response. Give children from 1 month to 12 years of age 0.005 ml/kg body weight. The maximum dose for children weighing <30 kg is 0.75 mg/0.15 ml. Give subsequent doses of *Sus-Phrine* only when necessary and not more frequently than every 6 hours.

Route & Site: SC or IM, when given for allergic emergency treatment. Epinephrine may be administered intracardially or IV diluted to <0.1 mg/ml. Inject Sus-Phrine only SC. Instruct patients prescribed epinephrine for self-administration to inject into the anterolateral aspect of the thigh, not the buttock. *EpiPen* products may be administered through a thin layer of clothing, if necessary. Accidental injection of epinephrine into hands or feet may result in loss of blood flow to the affected area and should be avoided. In case of accidental injection into these areas, instruct the patient to go

immediately to the nearest emergency room for treatment. Diluted epinephrine 1:10,000 w/v may be administered through an endotracheal tube, if no other parenteral access is available, directly into the bronchial tree. It is rapidly absorbed there from the capillary bed of the lung.

Additional Doses: In severe persistent anaphylaxis, if symptoms are not noticeably improved, repeat injections if necessary at 10 to 15 minute intervals.

Efficacy: Very high

Onset:

Solutions: Rapid. SC administration produces bronchodilation within 5 to 10 minutes, with maximal effects occurring within 20 minutes.

Suspension: Sus-Phrine provides both rapid and sustained epinephrine activity, due to the dissolved and suspended components, respectively.

Duration:

Solutions: Short. Additional doses may be warranted at 10 to 15 minute intervals.

Suspension: Sus-Phrine effects persist >6 hours.

Drug Interactions: Rapidly acting vasodilators (eg, nitrates, alpha-adrenergic antagonists) can counteract the vasopressor effects of epinephrine. The beta-1- and beta-2-adrenergic-agonist effects of epinephrine are antagonized by beta-adrenergic antagonists (ie, "beta blockers"), while the alpha-adrenergic effects of epinephrine predominate. This may result in increased systolic and diastolic blood pressure and decreased heart rate. Most patients on beta blockers receiving epinephrine to treat anaphylaxis survived the experience, but difficulty in main taining blood pressure and pulse often lasted hours longer than in uncomplicated anaphylactic treatment. Do not use epinephrine to counteract circulatory collapse or hypotension due to phenothiazines (eg, chlorpromazine). Because phenothiazines may reverse the vasopressor effect of epinephrine, such an act could lead to a further lowering of blood pressure. Use of epinephrine with drugs that may sensitize the heart to dysrhythmias (eg, digitalis, mercurial diuretics, quinidine) ordinarily is not recommended. The effects of epinephrine may be potentiated by tricyclic antidepressants, monoamine oxidase (MAO) inhibitors, levothyroxine and certain antihistamines (eg, chlorpheniramine, tripelennamine, diphenhydramine). Because epinephrine may cause hyperglycemia, diabetic patients receiving epinephrine may require an increased dosage of insulin or oral hypoglycemic agents.

If epinephrine and sodium bicarbonate are to be coadministered, inject individually at separate sites. Epinephrine is unstable in alkaline solutions.

Patient Information: Advise patients prescribed epinephrine for self-administration (eg, *Ana-Kit*, *EpiPen*) to read and understand thoroughly the patient instructions before any emergency arises. Counsel patients chronically treated with beta-adrenergic antagonists or other drugs that may potentially interact with epinephrine (eg, monoamine oxidase inhibitors), for whom repeated injections of allergen extracts are indicated, regarding the increased risk of such immunotherapy because of the added difficulty in treating possible anaphylactoid reactions.

Pharmaceutical Characteristics

Concentration: 1:1000 w/v solution (1 mg epinephrine base per ml, 0.1%) or 1:2000 w/v solution (0.5 mg/ml, 0.05%), as the hydrochloride salt

1:200 w/v suspension (5 mg epinephrine base per ml, 0.5%)

Other epinephrine formulations are described at the end of this monograph.

Package Size:

Ana-Guard: 1 multidose 1:1000 syringe with a 25 gauge, 1/8 inch needle housed in a plastic cylinder with clip (NDC #: 00118-9982-01). The syringe plunger is designed for the delivery of two 0.3 mg/0.3 ml doses; smaller doses can also be given.

Ana-Kit: In addition to 1 Ana-Guard syringe, the complete kit includes two 70% isopropyl alcohol sterilizing pads, four chewable 2 mg Chlo-Amine (chlorpheniramine maleate) tablets (colored with FD&C yellow dye #6), a tourniquet and patient instructions in a plastic carrying case with belt clip (00118-9988-01).

Insect Sting Treatment Kit, Derm/ Buro: Comparable contents to Ana-Kit (NDC #: none assigned).

EpiPen: Spring-loaded auto-injector, containing 2 ml of 1:1000 w/v epinephrine, delivering a single dose of 0.3 mg/0.3 ml epinephrine through a 23 gauge, 1/2 inch needle, when activated with 2 to 8 pounds of pressure at the tip, with patient instructions, in a clear plastic tube; 1 syringe (00268- 0301-01).

EpiPen Jr.: Spring-loaded auto-injector, containing 2 ml of 1:2000 w/v epinephrine, delivering a single dose of 0.15 mg/0.3 ml epinephrine through a

23 gauge, 1/2 inch needle, when acti-vated with 2 to 8 pounds of pressure at the tip, with patient instructions. in a plastic tube; 1 syringe (00268-0302-01).

EpiPen Trainer: Spring-loaded simulator that simulates the action of an auto-injector but contains no needle or drug. Includes a resetting device for repeated use (NDC #: none assigned).

EpiE-Z Pen: Spring-loaded auto-injector, containing 2 ml of 1:1000 w/v epineph-rine, delivering a single dose of 0.3 mg/0.3 ml epinephrine through a 22-gauge, 1/8-inch needle, when activated by pressing the gray button at the top of the injector with light pressure, with patient instructions, in a clear plastic package; 1 syringe plus training device (00268-0303-01).

EpiE-Z Pen Jr.: Spring-loaded auto-injec-tor, containing 2 ml of 1:2000 w/v epi-nephrine, delivering a single dose of 0.15 mg/0.3 ml epinephrine through a 22-gauge, Y2-inch needle, when acti-vated by pressing the gray button at the top of the injector with light pressure, with patient instructions, in a clear plastic package; 1 syringe plus training device (00268-0304-01).

EpiE-Z Pen Trainer: Spring-loaded simula-tor that simulates the action of an auto-injector but contains no needle or drug (NDC #: none assigned).

Generic, Elkins Sinn: 1:1000 w/v epineph-rine: 1 mg/1 ml ampules; 25 ampules (00641-1420-35), 100 ampules (00641-1420-36).

Adrenalin: 1:1000 w/v epinephrine: Ten 1 mg/1 ml ampules (00071-4188-03); 30 ml multidose vial (00071-4011-13).

Generic injection, various manufacturers: 1:1000 w/v epinephrine, 1 mg/1 ml ampules; 30 ml multidose vials.

Sus-Phrine: 0.3 ml single-dose ampules and 5 ml multidose vials of 1:200 w/v (5 mg/ml) epinephrine in suspension; 10 ampules (00456-0664-39), 25 ampules (00456-0664-34), 1 vial (00456-0664-05). Approximately 80% of the epi-nephrine is in suspension, with the balance in solution.

Dose Form: Various solutions and one suspension (*Stis-Phrine*)

Solvent: Sterile Water with various excipients added to adjust tonicity and pH

Diluent for Infusion: For direct IV infusion, epinephrine must be diluted to 1 mg per 250 ml. In extreme emer-gencies, epinephrine 0.1 mg/ml (1:10,000) can be administered intrac-ardially or through an endotracheal tube.

Storage/Stability: Epinephrine dete-riorates rapidly on exposure to air or light, turning pink from oxication to adrenochrone and brown from the for-mation of melanin. Protect from light. Protect from excessive heat.

Epinephrine Comparisons, for Self Administration

	Ana-Kit (and similar kits)	EpiPen and EpiE-ZPen	EpiPen Jr. and EpiE-ZPen Jr.
Proprietary Name			
Manufacturer	Bayer and others	Center	Center
Concentration	1:1000, 1 mg/ml	1:1000, 1 mg/ml	1:2000,0.5 mg/ml
Packaging	Manual syringe	Auto-injector	Auto-injector
Number of epinephrine doses per device	2	1	1
Dose delivered	2 doses of 0.3 mg/0.3 ml or other combinations	1 dose of 0.3 mg/0.3 ml	1 dose of 0.15 mg/0.3 ml
Number of chlorpheniramine doses per device	Four tablets of 2 mg each	None	None
Needle	25-gauge, 5/8-inch	original: 23-gauge, 1/2-inch EZ: 22-gauge, 5/8-inch	original: 23-gauge, 1/2-inch EZ: 22 gauge, 1/2-inch
Other components	2 alcohol swabs, tourniquet, case	EZ versions feature an easy trigger	EZ versions feature an easy trigger

Epinephrine Comparisons, for Professional Administration

	Generic, Adrenalin	Stis-Phrine
Manufacturer	Elkins-Sinn, Parke-Davis, others	Forest
Concentration	1:1000 W/V, 1 mg/ml	1:200 w/v, 5 mg/ml
Packaging	1 ml ampules, 30 ml vials	0.3 ml ampules, 5 ml vials
Dose Form	Solution	Suspension
Route	SC or IM	SC
Onset	1 to 5 minutes	30 minutes
Duration of effect	30 to 60 minutes	6 hours

Appendices

Appendix A
VACCINE INDICATIONS BY RISK GROUP

There are many factors to consider when deciding which vaccinations a patient requires. This section deals with such personal factors as age, health and occupation.

Vaccine Indications Based on Age and Other Factors

The following tables summarize authoritative guidelines on immunization. First appears the harmonized schedule for recommended childhood vaccination. Next, Table I summarizes vaccine needs based on the patient's age. Table II reports vaccines indicated (and immunity needed) by the patient's occupation, health status, lifestyle or other factors. Note that recommendations for Haemophilus influenzae type b (Hib) vaccine differ for each formulation licensed in the US.

These summaries condense a large volume of information. Readers must consider all notes carefully and apply their clinical skills in assessing each patient individually. Consult authoritative references for complete information about dosage schedules, booster doses and intervals, contraindications and other use factors. Many of the notes in the tables are mnemonic devices to aid repeated use of the tables. For example, T corresponds to travelers, CC refers to contacts of pathogen carriers or infectious cases and CS refers to close contacts of susceptible patients.

Vaccine recommendations change from time to time and clinicians should stay up-to-date by reading the professional literature (eg, MMWR and summaries in other journals). Subsequent revisions of authoritative guidelines, on which these tables were based, obviously take precedence.

How to Use the Immunization Summary Tables

1. Consider an individual patient known to you.
2. Read the column captions in Table I from left to right.
3. For the caption pertaining to this patient, read down the column looking for indicated vaccines. Read all pertinent footnotes. Compare these recommendations to the patient's actual vaccination and medical history. Consider possible contraindications.
4. Repeat with each appropriate column in Table II.
5. Remember that vaccine recommendations change periodically. Read the professional literature to stay up-to-date.

References:

ACIP. General recommendations on immunization. *MMWR* 1994;43(RR-1):1-38.

ACIP. Recommended childhood immunization schedule--United States, July-December 1996. *MMWR* 1996;45:635-8.

American College of Physicians. Guide for Adult Immunization, 3rd ed. Philadelphia: *American College of Physicians, 1994.*

Canadian National Advisory Committee on Immunizations. *Canadian Immunization Guide, 4th ed.* Ottawa: Ministry of National Health & Welfare, 1993. Updated by fax: 613-941-3900.

CDC. Health Information for International Travel. Washington, DC: Government Printing Office; revised annually and updated biweekly.

Peter G, ed. *1994 Red Book: Report of the Committee on Infectious Diseases, 23rd ed.* Elk Grove Village, IL: American Academy of Pediatrics, 1994.

WHO. International Travel & Health: Vaccination Requirements & Health Advice. Albany, NY: WHO, revised annually.

Recommended childhood vaccination schedule* — United States, January-June 1996

Vaccine	Birth	1 Mo.	2 Mos.	4 Mos.	6 Mos.	12 Mos.	15 Mos.	18 Mos.	4-6 Yrs.	11-12 Yrs.	14-16 Yrs.
Hepatitis B†	Hep B-1	Hep B-2			Hep B-3					Hep B§	
Diphtheria and tetanus toxoids and pertussis vaccine¶			DTP	DTP	DTP	DTP(DTaP at ≥15 mos.)			DTP or DTaP	Td	
Haemophilus influenzae type b**			Hib	Hib	Hib	Hib					
Poliovirus††			OPV	OPV	OPV				OPV		
Measles-mumps-rubella§§						MMR			MMR or MMR		
Varicella zoster virus¶¶						Var				Var***	

☐ Range of Acceptable Ages for Vaccination

▨ "Catch-Up" Vaccination§***

*Vaccines are listed under the routinely recommended ages.

†Infants born to hepatitis B surface antigen (HBsAg)-negative mothers should receive 2.5 mcg of *Recombivax HB* (Merck) or 10 mcg of *Engerix-B* (SmithKline Beecham). The second dose should be administered ≥1 month after the first dose. **Infants born to HBsAg-positive mothers** should receive 0.5 ml hepatitis B immune globulin (HBIG) within 12 hours of birth, and either 5 mcg of *Recombivax HB* or 10 mcg or *Engerix-B* at a separate site. The second dose is recommended at 1-2 months and the third dose at 6 months. **Infants born to mothers whose HBsAg status is unknown** should receive either 5 mcg of *Recombivax HB* or 10 mcg of *Engerix-B* within 12 hours of birth. The second dose of vaccine is recommended at age 1 month and the third dose at 6 months.

Key for Recommended childhood vaccination schedule

§Adolescents who have not received three doses of hepatitis B vaccine should initiate or complete the series at 11 to 12 years of age. Give the second dose at least 1 month after the first dose. Give the third dose at least 4 months after the first dose and at least 2 months after the second dose.

¶The fourth dose of diphtheria and tetanus toxoids and whole-cell pertussis vaccine (DTwP) may be administered at 12 months of age, in ≥6 months have elapsed since the third dose of DTwP. Diphtheria and tetanus toxoids and acellular pertussis vaccine (DTaP) is licensed for the fourth or fifth vaccine dose(s) for children ≥15 months of age and may be preferred for these doses in this age group. Connaught's brand of DTaP (Tripedia) is licensed for use in children 6 weeks to 7 years of age. Tetanus and diphtheria toxoids adsorbed, for adult use (Td), is recommended at 11 to 12 years of age if at least 5 years have elapsed since the last dose of DTwP, DTaP or diphtheria and tetanus toxoids adsorbed, for pediatric use (DT).

**Three Haemophilus influenzae type b (Hib) conjugate vaccines are licensed for infant use. If PedvaxHIB (Merck) is administered at 2 and 4 months of age, a dose at 6 months is not required. After completing the primary series, any Hib conjugate vaccine may be used as a booster at 12 to 15 months of age.

††Oral poliovirus vaccine (OPV) is recommended for routine infant vaccination. Inactivated poliovirus vaccine (IPV) is recommended for persons or household contacts of persons with a congenital or acquired immune deficiency disease or an altered immune status resulting from disease or immuno-suppressive therapy and is an acceptable alternative for other persons. The primary 3-dose series for IPV should be given with a minimum interval of 4 weeks between the first and second doses and 6 months between the second and third doses. Changes in poliomyelitis vaccination policy to favor IPV for initial doses, if approved, are unlikely to be fully implemented before 1997 because of the need for intensive educational efforts and to address logistic and cost issues.

§§The second dose of measles-mumps-rubella vaccine (MMR) is routinely recommended at 4-6 years or 11 to 12 years of age but may be administered at any visit provided at least 1 month has elapsed since receipt of the first dose.

¶¶Varicella-zoster virus vaccine (Var) can be administered to susceptible children any time after 12 months of age.

***Unvaccinated children who lack a reliable history of chicken pox should be vaccinated at 11 to 12 years of age.

Source: Advisory Committee on Immunization Practices, American Academy of Pediatrics and American Academy of Family Physicians.

References: CDC. Recommended childhood immunization schedule-United States, July-December 1996. *MMWR* 1996;45:635-8.

Table I. Standard Immunization Recommendations Based on Age[AG]

Immunologic Drug	Birth	2 months	4 months	6 months	12 months	15 months	18 months	19-47 months	4-6 years	7-10 years	11-12 years	14-16 years	17-34 years	35-64 years	>64 years
Diphtheria Tetanus Pertussis		DTP #1	DTP #2	DTP #3		DTP #4			DTP #5		Td	Td	Td	Td	Td
Measles Mumps Rubella				MO	MMR#1	MMR#1			MMR#2 or MC		MMR#2 MA	AM MU RF	MU RF	RF	
Haemophilus influenzae type b		Hib#1-L or Hib#1-M or Hib#1-S	Hib#2-L Hib#2-M Hib#2-S	Hib#3-L Hib#3-S	Hib#3-M Hib#4-S	Hib#4-L Hib#1-C Hib#4-S									
Hepatitis B child of HBsAg-negative mother	----------#1----------	----------#2----------		----------#3----------					(if unvaccinated)						
Child of HBsAg-positive mother	HepB#1 at birth, HBIG at birth plus HepB#2, day 30			HepB#3											
Influenza A & B Pneumococcal Poliovirus		IPV#1	IPV#2	SI	SI	SI OPV#1	SI	SI SP	SI SP OPV#2	SI SP	SI SP	SI SP	SI SP	SI SP	+ +
Varicella						+					V	VF	VF	VF	

Key for Table 1

+−Immunity needed. Vaccine indicated if patient is susceptible. Prescriber must still consider possible contraindications, as well as vaccination history.

AG−If not immunized at standard recommended time, alternative schedules have been developed.

AM−Two doses of MMR indicated for those born after January 1, 1957, who are attending post-high school educational institutions, beginning employment as a medical personnel or traveling to measles-endemic areas.

B−BCG is indicated in the US for infants and children at high risk of intimate exposure to persistently untreated or ineffectively treated patients with infectious pulmonary tuberculosis (TB) who cannot be placed on long-term preventive therapy, or those continuously exposed to persons with TB who have bacilli resistant to isoniazid and rifampin, or infants and children in groups in which the rate of new infections is 1% per year.

DTaP−New diphtheria and tetanus toxoids with acellular pertussis vaccine.

DTP−Either DTwP or DTaP may be used. See precautions about product interchange.

DTwP−Original diphtheria and tetanus toxoids with whole-cell pertussis vaccine.

HBIG−Hepatitis B immune globulin.

HepB−Routine Hepatitis B vaccine for infants. Give children of HBsAg-negative mothers 3 doses. Give the first dose between birth and 2 months of age, the second dose between 1 and 4 months of age and the third dose between 6 and 18 months of age. At least 30 days must pass between doses. In newborn children of HBsAg-positive mothers, give vaccine and hepatitis B immune globulin (HBIG) within 12 hours of birth, with booster vaccine doses on days 30 and 180.

Hib−Haemophilus influenzae type b conjugate vaccine, dosage schedule depends on vaccine formulation and manufacturer used. Administer Merck's (M) PedvaxHIB at 2, 4 and 12 months of age; Wyeth-Lederele's (L) HibTITER or Pasteur/SKB's Act-HIB at 2, 4, 6 and 15 months of age; or Connaught's (C) ProHIBit at 12 to 18

months of age. Consult references for modifications to these schedules.

ID−Intradermal infant dose of BCG (for high-risk children <30 days old) is one-half the usual dose, with a full dose repeated at 12 months of age.

MA−AAP recommends a routine second dose of MMR at entry into middle or junior high school.

MC−CDC recommends a routine second dose of MMR at entry into kindergarten or first grade.

MMR−Trivalent measles, mumps and rubella vaccine.

MO−Monovalent measles vaccine may be given as early as 6 months of age in outbreak settings; if so, give 2 more doses of MMR, with the first at 15 months of age.

MU−Two doses of MMR are indicated for most persons born after January 1, 1957.

OPV−Live, attenuated, oral poliovirus vaccine.

RF−Rubella component of MMR principally recommended for females of child-bearing potential <45 years of age.

SI−Annual use recommended for selected patients, based on underlying chronic diseases (eg, heart, lung, metabolic, immune diseases; chronic aspirin therapy; renal failure, diabetes, other severe immunocompromise).

SP−Vaccine effective in patients >24 months of age. Indicated in sickle-cell disease, asplenia, nephrotic syndrome, renal failure, diabetes, Hodgkin's disease, HIV infection and other severe immunocompromise.

Td−Adult strength tetanus-diphtheria toxoids (Td) indicated at 10-year intervals. Wound management guidelines are cited elsewhere.

TST−AAP recommends annual testing in high-risk children. Routine testing of low-risk children had been recommended at 12 to 15 months, 4 to 6 years and 14 to 16 years of age. But testing of low-risk people is no longer recommended.

V−Unvaccinated children who lack a reliable history of chicken pox.

VF−Women of child bearing potential if seronegative for varicella.

Table II: Immunization Recommendations Based on Personal Factors

Immunologic Drug	Occupation					Health Status				Life-Style & Other Factors			
	Health-care workers	Day-care workers	Essential workers (police, fire, etc)	Animal & Lab workers	Military personnel	HIV-infected persons	Other immuno-deficiencies	Pregnant women	Persons with chronic illness[c]	Travelers & Immigrants	Nursing home & Institutional residents or staff	Ethnic & Social groups	Other groups
Routine													
Diphtheria & Tetanus	Td	Td	Td	Td	Td	Td	Td	Td	Td	Td	Td	Td	Td
Measles	+	+			+	HC	0	0		T,I		H	
Mumps	+	+			+	HC	0	0		T,I		H	
Rubella	+	+			+	HC	0	0,RT	S	T,I		H	
Haemophilus influenzae type b						+	AS	NC		—			
Hepatitis B	BX		BX	L (BX)	BX,T	+	HD	HP	HD	T,I	BX,MR,PI	AP,H,LS	BX,CC,PE
Influenza A & B	+	+	+		+	+	+	NC	+	T,I	+	H	CS
Pneumococcal						+	+	NC	+	SR	SR	H	CS
Poliovirus[pv]	IPV	IPV		L	OPV	IPV	IPV	PP		T,I			
Unusual													
Adenovirus				L	BT	0	0	0					
Anthrax				A,L				RB					
Cholera	SR	SR		L	T	S	S	RB		T			
Hepatitis A				L	T			NC		T,I	SR	H,SR	PE,SR
Japanese encephalitis				L	BT,T	NC		NC		T			
Meningococcal					T		AS	RB		T			
Plague				A,L	T	0	0	NC		T			
Rabies				A,L	BT	SQ	SQ	0		T			PE
Smallpox				L	T	0	SV	SQ,RB					
Typhoid				L	SV	0	0	0		T,I			CC
Varicella	SV	SV			T	0	0	RB	0	T		H	
Yellow fever				L		0	0	0		T			
BCG						TST	SR	NC		T,I		B,H	ADU
Tuberculin skin test	TST				TST				SR		TST	H,SR	CC

Key for Table II

+–Immunity needed. Vaccine indicated if patient is susceptible. Prescriber must still consider possible contraindications, as well as vaccination history.

O–Vaccine generally contraindicated. Certain isolated individuals may benefit from this vaccine. Consult detailed references.

A–Animal workers, including veterinarians and their assistants.

ADU–Alcoholics, IV drug abusers and medically under-served low-income populations.

AP–Alaskan natives, Pacific Islanders, immigrants and refugees from hepatitis B endemic areas (particularly Haiti, Africa and eastern Asia).

AS–Asplenic patients.

B–BCG is indicated in the US for infants and children at high risk of intimate exposure to persistently untreated or ineffectively treated patients with infectious pulmonary tuberculosis (TB) who cannot be placed on long-term preventative therapy, or those continuously exposed to persons with TB who have bacilli resistant to isoniazid and rifampin, or infants and children in groups in which the rate of new infections is 1% per year.

BT–Military recruits at basic training.

BX–If exposed to blood or other contaminated body fluids.

C–Chronic illnesses include: Hemodynamically significant cardiovascular disease, pulmonary disease (eg, asthma, active tuberculosis, myasthenia gravis, cystic fibrosis, chronic obstructive pulmonary disease), diabetes mellitus, renal or hepatic dysfunction, sickle-cell and chronic hemolytic anemia, chronic alcoholism or cirrhosis and others.

CC–Close contacts of pathogen carriers or close contacts of infectious cases.

CS–Close contacts of susceptible patients.

H–When assessing the homeless, review status for all routine vaccines.

HA–For treatment of hepatitis A or measles exposure.

HC–HIV-infected children.

HD–Haemophilia, thalassemia, dialysis and renal failure patients.

HIV–Human immunodeficiency virus.

HP–Screen all pregnant women for HBsAg; vaccinate the newborn infants of mothers who are HBsAg positive.

I–Selected immigrants based on origin, age and health; includes refugees, guest workers, foreign students and internationally adopted children.

IPV–Enhanced-potency inactivated poliovirus vaccine (e-IPV), if not vaccinated as a child.

L–Laboratory workers potentially exposed to the corresponding pathogen.

LS–Homosexual and bisexual men, intravenous drug abusers, prostitutes, heterosexually active persons with multiple sexual partners or recently acquired sexually transmitted disease.

MR–Clients and staff of institutions for the mentally or developmentally retarded.

NC–Not contraindicated.

OPV–Oral, attenuated poliovirus vaccine.

P–Includes women planning to become pregnant within 3 months.

PE–Used for post-exposure prophylaxis.

PI–Prison inmates.

PP–Vaccinate pregnant women only if at high risk of exposure to poliovirus. OPV is acceptable if immediate protection is needed. Alternately, 2 doses of e-IPV may be used. Use c-IPV to boost women who previously received a complete primary series.

PV–When choosing between e-IPV and OPV, consult detailed references.

RB–Consider the risk-benefit ratio; vaccinate only if clearly needed.

RT–Screen all pregnant women for rubella antibody titer. If vaccine needed, administer after delivery, but before patient's discharge. Rho(D) immune globulin does not interfere with rubella vaccine.

S–Vaccine indicated for selected individuals in this category. See diagnosis and drug tables on following pages.

SC–Live, oral typhoid-vaccine capsules are contraindicated. Inactivated, subcutaneous vaccine may be acceptable. Consider risk-benefit ratio.

SR—Many in this category warrant vaccinations, based on other risk factors. See diagnosis and drug tables on following pages.

SV—Women of childbearing potential if seronegative for varicella.

T—Selected travelers, depending on destinations and itinerary. For further information,

telephone CDC's international health requirements and recommendations 24-hour hotline: 404-332-4559.

Td—Adult strength tetanus-diphtheria toxoids (Td) indicated at 10-year intervals. Wound-management guidelines are cited elsewhere.

TST—Many in this category warrant testing.

Vaccine Recommendations for Persons Infected with HIV

Special immunization recommendations are appropriate for persons infected with the human immunodeficiency virus (HIV):

Live Bacterial or Viral Vaccines

Persons infected with HIV and persons who have developed the acquired immunodeficiency syndrome (AIDS) are theoretically at risk of disseminated infection following immunization with a live, albeit attenuated, bacterial or viral vaccine. Specific recommendations follow:

BCG (injection or instillation)—Disseminated mycobacterial infection may result from exposure to this drug. Do not expose HIV-infected persons in the US to BCG (Braun & Cauthen, 1992).

BCG vaccination of children who are born to HIV-infected mothers in developing nations and who are vaccinated shortly after birth appears to be relatively safe but questionably effective. WHO recommends that only HIV-infected infants who are asymptomatic and live in areas with high tuberculosis risk receive BCG (Braun & Cauthen, 1992). Waiting to immunize children at 1 year of age has also been suggested for developing countries (Athale et al, 1992).

Measles, mumps & rubella (MMR)—Vaccinate both symptomatic and asymptomatic children and adults according to routine schedules; consider the possibility of less than optimal immunogenicity.

Poliovirus (oral form, OPV)—Do not administer live, oral poliovirus vaccine to any HIV-infected child or adult in the US, nor to their household contacts. Give inactivated poliovirus vaccine (e-IPV) injection instead. WHO continues to recommend routine use of OPV, a rational approach in developing nations with a substantial risk of endemic poliomyelitis.

Typhoid (capsule form)—Do not administer live, oral typhoid vaccine to any HIV-infected child or adult. Inactivated typhoid vaccine injection may be used if needed.

Vaccinia (smallpox—Do not administer live vaccinia (smallpox) vaccine to any HIV-infected child or adult.

Varicella (chicken pox)—Do not administer live varicella vaccine to any HIV-infected child or adult, until results of ongoing studies are published. Consider the value of VZIG for immunocompromised people.

Yellow fever—Base decisions to administer live yellow fever vaccine to an HIV-infected child or adult on an assessment of the patient's state of immunosuppression and the risk of exposure to the yellow fever virus. Offer the option of immunization to asymptomatic persons infected with HIV who cannot avoid potential exposure to yellow fever virus.

Inactivated Vaccines or Toxoids

In general, immunization with an inactivated vaccine or toxoid poses no additional risk to persons infected with HIV and persons who have developed AIDS. But these persons may be less likely to develop an adequate immune response to vaccination and may remain susceptible to the disease at issue. While HIV-infected persons and AIDS patients may develop less than optimal immunity, compared with uninfected persons, immunization is often still recommended to confer at least partial protection. Optimally, complete the immunization of HIV-infected persons before they meet the criteria for AIDS. Specific recommendations follow:

Cholera—Observe standard recommendations; consider the possibility of less than optimal immunogenicity. Encourage standard food and water precautions.

Diphtheria & tetanus toxoids with pertussis vaccine (DTP)—Observe routine pediatric DTP vaccination schedules among HIV-infected children; consider the possibility of less than optimal immunogenicity.

Diphtheria & tetanus toxoids (pediatric)—Observe routine pediatric DT vaccination schedules among HIV-infected children; consider the possibility of less than optimal immunogenicity. DTP is the preferred drug for most children.

Haemophilus influenzae type b (Hib)—Observe routine pediatric Hib vaccination schedules among HIV-infected children; consider the possibility of less than optimal immunogenicity. Routine Hib vaccination of all HIV-infected adults is generally recommended to decrease susceptibility to Hib infections. Optimally, complete immunization of HIV-infected persons before they meet the criteria for AIDS.

Hepatitis A—Observe standard recommendations; consider the possibility of less than optimal immunogenicity.

Hepatitis B—Observe routine pediatric hepatitis B vaccination schedules among HIV-infected children; consider the possibility of less than optimal immunogenicity. Routine hepatitis B vaccination of all HIV-infected adults (unless known to already be infected with hepatitis B) is generally recommended to decrease susceptibility to hepatitis B infections. Optimally, complete immunization of HIV-infected persons before they meet the criteria for AIDS.

Influenza—Routine influenza vaccination of all HIV-infected persons is generally recommended to decrease susceptibility to influenza infections; consider the possibility of less than optimal immunogenicity. Chemical antiviral prophylaxis (eg, amantadine) may be appropriate during periods of increased influenza A activity in a community.

Meningococcal A/C/Y/W-135—Observe standard recommendations; consider the possibility of less than optimal immunogenicity.

Plague—Observe standard recommendations; consider the possibility of less than optimal immunogenicity.

Pneumococcal—Routine pneumococcal vaccination of all HIV-infected persons is generally recommended to decrease susceptibility to pneumococcal infections; consider the possibility of less than optimal immunogenicity. Optimally, complete immunization of HIV-infected persons before they meet the criteria for AIDS.

Poliovirus (injection, e-IPV)—Observe standard recommendations; consider the possibility of less than optimal immunogenicity. Use of e-IPV is preferred over the oral, attenuated poliovirus vaccine.

Rabies—Observe standard recommendations; consider the possibility of less than optimal immunogenicity.

Tetanus & diphtheria (Td adult)—Routine Td vaccination of all HIV-infected adults is recommended to decrease susceptibility to tetanus and diphtheria infections; consider the possibility of less than optimal immunogenicity. Furste has suggested a lower threshold for deciding to use TIG in wounded HIV-infected persons, under the assumption that their circulating antitetanus antitoxin level may be lower than among uninfected persons (Furste, 1986).

Typhoid (injection)—Observe standard recommendations; consider the possibility of less than optimal immunogenicity. Encourage standard food and water precautions.

Summary Recommendations for Routine Immunization of HIV-Infected Persons in the US

Drug	Known asymptomatic	Symptomatic
DTP/Td	yes	yes
OPV	no	no
e-IPV[1]	yes	yes
MMR	yes	yes[2]
Hib[3]	yes	yes
Pneumococcal	yes	yes
Influenza	yes[2]	yes

[1]For adults ≥18 years of age, use only if indicated
[2]Consider risk and benefit
[3]Consider for HIV-infected adults also

Safety of Immunizing HIV-Infected Persons

In vitro studies show that proliferating CD4 cells are more susceptible to infection with HIV than nonproliferating cells, raising the possibility that immunization may be a cofactor in exacerbating the progression of HIV infection to AIDS. Recent reports show temporary increases in plasma HIV viremia after injection of tetanus toxoid or influenza or hepatitis B vaccines. These increases lasted up to 6 weeks. Is this clinically important? No clinical data have substantiated the concern about antigenic stimulation causing deterioration of clinical status. We encounter natural antigenic stimulation innumerable times during our lives. Actual infections may be riskier than an immunization, due to more prolonged antigenic stimulus. The risk to an HIV-infected person from a vaccine is probably outweighed by the value of induction of specific antibodies. CDC and WHO continue to recommend immunization of HIV-infected persons as described above, when the benefits of immunization outweigh the risks of infection.

References:

CDC. Update on adult immunization: Recommendations of the Immunization Practices Advisory Committee (ACIP). *MMWR* 1991;40(RR-12):1-94.

Hibberd PL, Rubin RH. Approach to immunization in the immunosuppressed host. *Infect Dis Clin N Amer* 1990;4:123-42.

Onorato IM, Markowitz LE, Oxtoby MJ. Childhood immunization, vaccine-preventable diseases and infection with human immunodeficiency virus. Pediatr Infect Dis J 1988;7:588-95.

Jewett JF, Hecht FM. Preventive healthcare for adults with HIV infection. JAMA 1993;269:1144-53.

Pav AK, McNicholl IR, Pursell KJ. Active immunization with HIV-infected patients. Pharmacotherapy 1996;16:163-70.

Patients with other Immune Deficiencies

People with immune deficiencies include those with antibody or thymus disorders, leukemia, lymphoma or other cancers. Also included are people with lowered resistance to infection after getting corticosteroids, alkylating drugs, antimetabolites or radiation. Patients taking drugs that weaken the immune system or who have other immune deficiencies may not produce enough antibodies after vaccination. They can be vulnerable despite the vaccine.

Most people with a deficiency of their immune system should avoid live vaccines. These include measles-mumps-rubella, oral poliovirus, oral typhoid, yellow fever and BCG vaccines. Some exceptions to this rule exist, including routine vaccines for children. For poliovirus and typhoid, use the inactivated vaccines.

People whose spleens have been removed or do not work properly need vaccines against *Haemophilus influenzae* type b and meningococcal bacteria.

People with hemophilia, thalassemic or renal failure need hepatitis B vaccine. People on hemodialysis also need the hepatitis B vaccine.

People with an immune deficiency of any kind need an influenza vaccine every year. They also need at least one dose of the pneumococcal vaccine. Influenza and pneumococcal disease are contagious infections of the lungs. They can kill older people and people with chronic diseases. These vaccines may not completely protect people with immune system problems, but they can expect at least partial immunity. Side effects from these vaccines are no different than in healthy people.

Weakened Immune Systems: Medications and Diseases

This section lists immune suppressive drugs and reviews some of their characteristics.

1. Alkylating Agents
   a. Nitrogen Mustards
      - Chlorambucil (*Leukeran*)
      - Cyclophosphamide (*Cytoxan, Neosar*)
      - Ifosfamide (*Ifex*)
      - Mechlorethamine (*Mustargen*)
      - Melphalan (*Alkeran*)
      - Uracil Mustard
   b. Nitrosoureas
      - Carmustine (BCNU, BiCNU)
      - Lomustine (CCNU, *CeeNu*)
      - Streptozocin (*Zanosar*)
   c. Busulfan (*Myleran*)
   d. Cisplatin (*Platinol*)
   e. Pipobroman (*Vercyte*)
   f. Thiotepa
   g. Carboplatin (*Paraplatin*)
2. Antimetabolites
   a. Azathioprine (*Imuran*)
   b. Cytarabine (*ARA-C, Cytosar-U*)
   c. Floxuridine (*FUDR*)
   d. Fludarabine (*Fludara*)
   e. Fluorouracil (*Adrucil*)
   f. Mercaptopurine (*6-MP, Purinethol*)
   g. Methotrexate (amethopterin, *MTX, Folex, Mexate*)
   h. Thioguanine
3. Cyclosporine (*Sandimmune*)
4. Glucocorticosteroids
   a. Corticotropin (ACTH, *Acthar, Cortrophin Gel*)
   b. Cortisone acetate
   c. Betamethasone (*Celestone*)
   d. Dexamethasone (*Decadron, Dexone, Hexadrol*)
   e. Hydrocortisone (*Cortisol, A-hydroCort, Cortef, Solu-Cortef, Cortenema, Hydrocortone*)
   f. Methylprednisolone (*A-methaPred, Medrol, Depo-Medrol, Solu-Medrol*)
   g. Paramethasone (*Haldrone*)
   h. Prednisolone, various salts (*Delta-Cortef, Hydeltrasol*)
   i. Prednisone (*Deltasone, Liquid Pred, Meticorten, Orasone*)
   j. Triamcinolone (*Aristocort, Aristospan, Kenacort, Kenaject, Kenalog*)
5. Mitotic Inhibitors
   a. Etoposide (*VP-16, VePesid*)
   b. Vinblastine (*Velban*)

c. Vincristine (*Oncovin*)
6. Radiopharmaceuticals
   a. Chromic Phosphate 32-P
      (*Phosphocol P32*)
   b. Sodium Iodide 131-I (*Iodotope*)
   c. Sodium Phosphate 32-P
7. Other immunosuppressants
   a. Altretamine (*Hexalen*)
   b. Dacarbazine (*DTIC-Dome*)
   c. Gold Compounds
      Auranofin (*Ridaura*)
      Aurothioglucose (*Solganal*)
      Gold sodium thiomalate
      (*Myochrysine*)
   d. Hydroxyurea (*Hydrea*)
   e. Procarbazine (*Matulane*)

Other drugs that suppress the bone marrow at high doses include:
   a. Amphotericin B (*Fungizone*)
   b. antibiotic antineoplastic drugs
      dactinomycin (*Cosmegen*)
      daunorubicin (*Cerubidine*)
      doxorubicin (*Adriamycin*)
      mitomycin (*Mutamycin*)
      Plicamycin (*Mithracin*)
   c. Antithyroid Drugs
      Propylthiouracil
      Methimazole (*Tapazole*)
   d. Chloramphenicol
      (*Chloromycetin*)
   e. Aminoquinolone Compounds
      Chloroquine (*Aralen*)
      Hydroxychloroquine (*Plaquenil*)
   f. Colchicine
   g. Flucytosine (*Ancobon*)
   h. Interferons
      (*Intron-A*, *Roferon-A*)
   i. Mitoxantrone (*Novantrone*)
   j. Penicillamine (*Cuprimine*)
   k. Pentamidine (*NebuPent*,
      Pentam 300)
   l. Zidovudine (*Retrovir*)

Immune suppression is often related to the dose of drug given. Large cumulative doses can produce reversible bone-marrow damage. Immune suppression can increase the risk of bacterial, viral, fungal, or other infections. Infections are more likely to occur when steroid and other immune sup-

pressive therapies are used together. Infections may require changing or stopping the dose.

Use of some immunosuppressive drugs (such as cyclophosphamide) can increase the risk of secondary tumors. Some immune suppressants are carcinogenic (such as azathioprine).

People with Chronic Illness

Patients with any of the following disorders need an influenza vaccine every year. They also need at least one dose of the pneumococcal vaccine. This applies equally to adults and children with the listed diseases.

- Alcoholism
- Anemia
- Asthma
- Chronic heart, lung, liver or kidney disease
- Cirrhosis
- Diabetes
- Problems of the spleen

Adults with any of the following diseases need *Haemophilus influenzae* type b vaccine:

- Sickle-cell disease
- Hodgkin's disease or other cancers of the blood
- Weakened spleen or other immune disorders

Pregnant Women

To protect the unborn child, pregnant women should avoid some live vaccines. These include measles-mumps-rubella, oral typhoid, yellow fever and BCG vaccines. Some exceptions to this rule exist, including oral poliovirus vaccine. For typhoid, use the inactivated vaccine.

Pregnant women who are not immune to rubella need rubella vaccine shortly after giving birth, which will protect future children from the terrible effects of rubella.

All pregnant women need to be tested for the hepatitis B virus. If positive, their children need hepatitis B vaccine plus a special dose of hepatitis B antibodies.

Healthcare Workers

People who work in hospitals, clinics, nursing homes, physicians' offices and other health care settings have two kinds of vaccine needs. They need to protect themselves from on-the-job infection risks, and they have a duty to not transmit infections to the patients they serve.

Workers likely to be exposed to blood or blood products need hepatitis B vaccine. In fact, the Occupational Safety & Health Administration (OSHA) requires that these workers be offered hepatitis B vaccine.

Health workers need to be immune to measles, mumps, rubella, varicella, poliovirus, and influenza so they don't pass these diseases to sick patients. This is especially important if they work with vulnerable patients with weak immune systems. For this reason health care workers need to get a skin test to detect tuberculosis from time to time.

Day Care Workers

Vaccine needs of child-care givers are similar to those of healthcare workers. Day care workers need to be immune to measles, mumps, rubella, varicella, poliovirus and influenza. This is especially important when working with vulnerable children with weak immune systems.

Essential Community Workers

This group includes police, fire, ambulance and similar workers. It is a good idea to vaccinate these workers against influenza. If an influenza epidemic strikes a community, these workers would be protected and able to remain on the job.

Workers likely to be exposed to blood or blood products need hepatitis B vaccine. OSHA requires that these workers be offered hepatitis B vaccine.

Animal Workers:

Veterinarians, their assistants and others who handle a lot of animals need rabies vaccine. In unusual cases, these workers might need anthrax or plague vaccine.

Laboratory Workers:

Workers likely to be exposed to blood or blood products need hepatitis B vaccine. OSHA requires that these workers be offered hepatitis B vaccine.

Military Personnel:

Soldiers, sailors, marines, and airmen need adenovirus and meningococcal vaccines during basic training to prevent lung diseases. They also get booster doses of measles-mumps-rubella and poliovirus vaccines. Military troops are vaccinated against vaccinia (smallpox) during basic training to protect against the biological warfare threat of smallpox.

These workers get influenza vaccines each year to keep them on the job during an influenza outbreak. Military healthcare workers get a hepatitis B vaccine.

Depending on chance of travel and destination, military people can get several vaccines. Most often, this includes typhoid, meningococca, and hepatitis A. National Guard and military reserve troops need a variety of vaccines to meet standards of military readiness.

Travelers

Vaccine guidelines for international travel vary with the route, lodging plans, eating habits and other factors. At least 6 weeks before a major trip, refer to the information in the section "Vaccines for Travelers."

Immigrants

People who move to the U.S. may come from places where they received inadequate health care and vaccines. Do a complete work-up of these people to see what vaccines are needed. They may even need routine childhood vaccines.

Nursing Home & Other Institutional Workers
Residents and Staff

Like healthcare workers, people who live or work in nursing homes and other organized homes have two kinds of vaccine needs. They need to protect themselves from infection risks around them; and they have a duty to not transmit infections to people around them.

Residents need influenza vaccines each year to stop out breaks in their homes. This is especially important for older individuals or those with chronic illnesses. They are most vulnerable to the sometimes fatal effects of influenza. Many of these elderly and ill patients need at least one dose of pneumococcal vaccine. Prison inmates often need protection against hepatitis B.

Clients and workers at homes for the mentally or developmentally retarded need hepatitis B vaccine.

Workers likely to be exposed to blood or blood products need hepatitis B vaccine. In fact, OSHA requires that these workers be offered hepatitis B vaccine.

A tuberculin skin test may be recommended from time to time to control the spread of tuberculosis.

Homeless People

Our nation's homeless rarely have access to healthcare, including vaccines. A complete work-up of these individuals is required to determine what vaccines they need.

Ethnic and Social Groups

Certain ethnic and social groups are at increased risk of hepatitis B. These groups include Alaskan natives, Pacific Islanders and immigrants and refugees from areas where hepatitis B is common. These areas include Haiti, Africa, and eastern Asia.

Other people who need the protection of hepatitis B vaccine include:

- homosexual and bisexual men
- intravenous drug users
- prostitutes
- people with multiple sexual partners
- people with a recent sexually transmitted disease (eg, syphilis, gonorrhea)

Close Contacts of People with Infection

Individuals who have close contact with people who are infected with hepatitis B virus or typhoid bacteria need to be vaccinated.

Drug Interactions

Live Vaccines: Live viral or bacterial vaccines given to patients getting immune suppressive therapy may not produce the expected antibody response. These patients may remain vulnerable and get infected despite immunization. They may get infected despite vaccination. In immune suppressed patients, the risk of widespread infection resulting from vaccination can increase. If both live and killed vaccines are made (such as poliovirus or typhoid), use the killed vaccine. For example, never give live oral poliovirus vaccine (OPV) to immune compromised patients or members of their family. Rather, use the parenteral inactivated poliovirus vaccine (IPV).

Inactivated Vaccines: Inactivated viral and bacterial vaccines and toxoids given to patients getting immune suppressive therapy may not produce the expected antibody response. These patients may remain vulnerable and get an infection despite immunization. They may get infected despite vaccination. Response to the vaccine may be best if given 10 to 14 days before chemotherapy or radiation; or give the vaccine 3 to 12 months after stopping immune suppressive therapy.

Interviewing & Counseling About Immunizations

Through effective interviewing and counseling, clinicians can increase vaccine acceptance. Interviewing comes first. The only way to determine a patient's needs is to question and evaluate that patient's health risks. In a good interview, which might last just 1 to 5 minutes, the clinician solicits pertinent information regarding medical and immunization history. This information is used in subsequent decisions about vaccines or immunologic tests needed by the patient.

Counseling is the second step in educating patients to change their immunization behavior. Effective counseling of any type requires that the healthcare professional provide information individualized to the patient's needs. Conduct educational counseling in an understandable manner that enables the patient to accept and carry out immunization recommendations. In this regard, counseling about vaccines is very similar to counseling patients about other medications.

Behavioral experts report that there are four primary factors involved in patients' decisions whether or not to be vaccinated:

a. Perceived barriers to vaccination (eg, expense, ease of access, knowledge),

b. Belief in the effectiveness of the vaccine,

c. Perceptions of susceptibility to disease and

d. Perceptions of severity of disease if they contract it.

Counseling patients about vaccination should center around these four issues. The simple act of advising patients of their susceptibility and informing them where vaccine is available can dramatically increase vaccine-acceptance rates.

The patient's perceptions of disease susceptibility and vaccine efficacy may not correspond with scientifically accepted fact. In such cases, education can serve a real need. Barriers to vaccination include factors such as fear, anxiety, inconvenience, pain and expense. If the person considers barriers to be relatively weak and their readiness to be vaccinated is great, then he or she is likely to be immunized. Conversely, if the person's readiness is low and the perceived barriers are strong, then the desired behavior is less likely to occur.

In many cases, the clinician will counsel not the patient, but the patient's agent. For example, parents make immunization decisions for their children and many adults assist with immunization decisions for their aging parents. Viewing the immunization decision through the eyes of the decision maker is important. The key elements in a patient's immunization decision are perceptions of disease susceptibility, disease severity, barriers and vaccine effi-

cacy. Knowing this, clinicians can target their counsel to improve the probability of influencing the decision-making process regarding immunization.

Minimize suggestive or leading inquiries when interviewing and counseling. Such questions tend to include the desired response within the question itself and often reflect the opinions of the person asking the questions. For example, asking "You've had all your shots, haven't you?" is likely to prejudice the response. One exception to this rule might be in taking a patient's history of prior tetanus immunization. "Have you been treated in an emergency room in the last few years, where you may have received a tetanus booster?" can be helpful in interviewing. Leading questions can be useful to test how closely the counselor and patient agree but, overall, this type of question tends to bias answers.

An important role of the immunization counselor is to dispel misconceptions and misinformation about particular vaccines. For example, be prepared to counter common misconceptions about influenza vaccine with facts regarding its safety and low incidence of side effects. Similarly, the risks of encephalopathy following pertussis vaccine are now recognized to be much lower than earlier thought, if there is any causal link at all (Cherry, 1990) and fears of human immunodeficiency virus (HIV) transmission from hepatitis B vaccine have been conclusively put to rest. The key issue whenever confronted with side-effect disputes is to ask if the risk of side effects does or does not outweigh the risk of the disease to be prevented.

Before the counseling phase, gather enough data to identify diseases to which the patient is susceptible. Clinicians can then suggest a set of immunizations to protect the patient against potential infections. The goal is to inform the patient of his or her immunization needs and convince the individual to accept these vaccines, in light of the risks and benefits involved.

Diseases & Diagnoses Warranting Immunization

Disease/Diagnosis	Vaccine(s) indicated
Age >64 years, even if healthy	Influenza, pneumonia
Alcoholism, chronic	Pneumonia
Antibiotic allergies, multiple (especially penicillin and erythromycin)	Influenza, pneumonia
Anemia, chronic, severe, including sickle-cell and chronic hemolytic	Influenza, pneumonia
Artificial heart valve	Influenza, pneumonia
Aspirin therapy, long-term, in children	Influenza
Asplenia	Influenza, pneumonia
Asthma	Influenza, pneumonia
Atherosclerosis	Influenza, pneumonia
Azotemia	Influenza
Bedridden, chronically	Influenza, pneumonia
Cancer	Influenza, pneumonia
Cardiovascular disease ("altered circulatory dynamics")	Influenza, pneumonia
Cerebrospinal fluid leaks	Pneumonia
Cirrhosis	Pneumonia
Claudication, intermittent	Influenza, pneumonia
Congestive heart failure	Influenza, pneumonia
Cystic fibrosis	Influenza, pneumonia
Diabetes mellitus	Influenza, pneumonia
Dialysis, kidney	Influenza, hepatitis B, pneumonia
Hemophilia	Hepatitis A, hepatitis B
Hepatitis B, chronic carriers of	Hepatitis A
HIV infection	Influenza, pneumonia
Immunodeficiency, natural or induced	Influenza, pneumonia
Kidney disease, chronic	Influenza, pneumonia
Liver failure	Hepatitis A, influenza
Mitral stenosis	Influenza, pneumonia
Myesthenia gravis	Influenza, pneumonia
Nephrotic syndrome	Infleunza, pneumonia
Panacinar emphysema (with use of alpha$_1$-proteinase inhibitor)	Hepatitis B
Pulmonary disease	Influenza, pneumonia
Renal failure	Influenza, pneumonia
Septral defect	Influenza pneumonia
Sexually transmitted diseases, repeated	Hepatitis A, hepatitis B
Splenic dysfunction, asplenia	Influenza, pneumonia
Thalassemia	Hepatitis B
Transplantation, organ	Influenza, pneumonia
Tuberculosis, active	Influenza, pneumonia

In developing an immunization plan, consider the individual's age, occupation, place of residence, travel plans, life-style, underlying disease states and other individual factors. Then, in consultation with detailed immunization references, construct a specific list and schedule of needed vaccines. The immunization advice may be communicated verbally if it is simple, but written recommendations may make it easier for the patient to follow complex schedules. Providing written handouts or appointment cards can remind patients of important data or dates after they leave the counseling session. Handouts are available from the CDC (404-639-1836), many vaccine manufacturers and other sources. Be prepared to explain specifically when and where immunizations are available and what costs to expect.

The final part of the counseling process is the evaluation phase. By asking the patient to summarize the material communicated, the counselor can determine if the patient understands the ideas discussed. The ultimate success of immunization counseling is determined by whether or not the patient actually is immunized. Immunization is favored if convenience can be enhanced: Suggest the patient get influenzae vaccine along with a friend who also needs it. Ask for the promise of a parent to obtain a child's immunizations by a certain date. Ask the patient to report back to you how he or she found the vaccination experience to be. Remind the patient that the small inconvenience involved in getting immunized is an investment in health that pays dividends for years to come. Congratulate vaccinees on their wise decision and suggest that they encourage family or friends with similar vaccine needs to be vaccinated as well.

Reference: Kirk JK, Grabenstein JD. Interviewing and counseling patients about immunizations. Hosp Pharm 1991;26:1006-10.

Activities for Immunization Advocacy

The Need for Advocacy

Advocacy of immunizations is needed because as many as 80,000 Americans die of vaccine-preventable infections every year, primarily from influenza, pneumococcal pneumonia, hepatitis B and measles. The vast majority of these persons visited healthcare providers in the year preceding their death, either as inpatients or outpatients, but were not vaccinated.

Tens of millions of Americans are susceptible to these infections, despite the availability of effective vaccines. About 30% to 40% of American children from 2 to 6 years old are inadequately immunized with routine vaccines, although over 95% of children are vaccinated in compliance with regulations before entry into kindergarten or elementary school (the so-called school-entry gate). The majority of American adults are inadequately vaccinated, especially against influenza, pneumococcal pneumonia, hepatitis B, tetanus and diphtheria.

Influenza and pneumonia combined are the eighth leading cause of premature mortality in the US: 172,000 excess hospitalizations due to pneumonia or influenza occur with each moderate influenza epidemic, costing over millions of dollars. Patients 64 years of age account for 80% of pneumonia or influenza deaths.

Remarkably, 40% to 55% of patients who die following influenza receive medical care at a hospital during the year preceding their death; 75% of those who will die visit an outpatient clinic in the year before their death. Despite this access to healthcare, 30% of high-risk groups are immunized. Although influenza vaccine has been recommended for all members of high-risk groups since 1960, a third of a century, many clinicians fail to offer vaccine to those most at risk. More than 40 million Americans should receive influenza vaccine each year because of their increased susceptibility. Increased use of influenza vaccine, assuming 70% efficacy and 70% coverage, could prevent 20,000 deaths and 80,000 hospitalizations each year in the US. Canadians appear to be more successful at delivering influenza vaccine to high-risk groups than their southern neighbors.

Similarly, for pneumococcal pneumonia, only 10% to 20% of a likely 48 million vaccine candidates have been immunized. The mortality rate from this infection (5% for pneumonia, 15% to 40% for bacteremia, 30% to 50% for pneumococcal meningitis) has not changed substantially since the 1950s, despite advances in antibiotic therapy. At least two-thirds of patients with serious pneumococcal infections had been hospitalized at least once within 3 to 5 years before the illness, but had not been vaccinated.

Specific Advocacy Activities

Methods for Determining Immunization Needs

Methods of screening for immunization needs may be organized in several ways and model screening forms have been included in the Immunization Documents Appendix. Clinicians can be involved in some or all of the following forms of immunization surveillance:

a. Occurrence screening identifies vaccine needs at the time of particular events, such as hospital or nursing home admission or discharge, an ambulatory or emergency-room visit, mid-decade birthdays (years 25, 35, 45 and so forth) and any contact with the healthcare delivery system for any patient 8 years or 64 years.

b. Diagnosis screening reviews vaccine needs among patients with conditions that

place them at increased risk of preventable infections. Diagnoses such as hemophilia, thalassemia, most types of cancer, sickle-cell anemia, chronic alcoholism, cirrhosis, cerebrospinal fluid leaks, human immunodeficiency virus (HIV) infection, multiple antibiotic allergies and other disorders should prompt specific attention to the patients' vaccine needs.

c. Procedure screening identifies vaccine needs on the basis of medical or surgical procedures. These include splenectomy, heart or lung surgery, organ transplant, chemotherapy, radiation therapy, immunosuppression of other types, dialysis and prescription of certain medications.

d. Periodic mass screening can be conducted during autumn influenza programs and during programs to control outbreaks (eg, local measles epidemics). Schools and other institutions can perform such screening when registering new cohorts of students, residents or other groups. Mass screening may also be appropriate where no comprehensive immunization program has been conducted in the past few years. Mass screenings help improve vaccine-coverage rates acutely, but long-term benefits are much greater when such intermittent programs are combined with ongoing, comprehensive screening efforts.

Once patients in need of immunization have been identified, they must be advised of their infection risk and encouraged to accept the immunizations they need. If appropriate, also remind the patients' physician(s) of the patients' need for vaccination. Do not reschedule patients needing immunization to a future appointment that may be missed. Rather, vaccinate them during the current healthcare contact unless valid contraindications exist. In general, mild fevers or mild diarrheal illness do not contraindicate immunization, nor do current antimicrobial therapy, con valescence, prematurity, pregnancy, recent exposure to an infectious disease, breast-feeding, history of nonspecific allergies, or family histories of allergies, convulsions, sudden infant death syndrome or adverse events following vaccinations.

Advising patients of their need for immunization can take several forms. In the ambulatory setting, individualized or form letters or postcards can be mailed to patients, patients can be telephoned, or an insert can be included with prescriptions informing patients of their infection risk and the availability and efficacy of vaccines.

Adhesive warning labels can also be affixed to prescription containers for drugs that indicate need for vaccination against influenza and pneumonia (eg, digoxin, warfarin, theophylline, insulin). These labels would be analogous to labels currently in wide-spread use (eg, "shake well," "take with food or milk"). Such labels might read "You May Need Flu or Pneumonia Vaccine: Ask Your Doctor or Pharmacist." For inpatients and institutional residents, chart notes, consultations, messages to patients and similar means can be used.

While most of the screening criteria described above are specific for indications of influenza or pneumococcal vaccines, conduct comprehensive screening on the patients thus identified. In other words, interest in a patient might be initiated because of his or her need for pneumococcal vaccine. But while assessing that patient, take the opportunity to check for needs for any vaccine: Influenza, pneumococcal, or hepatitis B vaccine, tetanus-diphtheria boosters, etc.

Drugs Indicative of Diseases Warranting Immunization

Category title	Representatative drugs	Immunization-Indicating disease states
ANTI-INFECTIVE DRUGS		
Antifungal antibiotics	Ketoconazole	Hyperadrenocorticism
Anti-influenza agents	Amantadine	Influenzae A prophylaxis
Antimalarial agents	Chloroquine, hydroxychloroquine	Rheumatoid arthritis, travel to hepatitis-B endemic area
Antitubercular agents	Rifampin, pyrazinamide	Tuberculosis treatment
Antivirals	Zidovudine, didanosine	HIV infection
Sulfonamides	Sulfasalazine	Crohn's disease
ANTINEOPLASTIC DRUGS		
Alkylating agents	Cyclophosphamide	Cancer, various
Antimetabolites	Azathioprine	Glomerulonephritis, immunosuppression, nephrotic syndrome, cirrhosis
Interferons	Interferon-alfa	Cancer, hepatitis, various
Mitotic inhibitors	Etoposide	Cancer, various
BLOOD MODIFIERS		
Anticoagulants	Heparin, warfarin	Cardiovascular disease
Folic-acid products	Leucovorin	Antagonist rescue, anemia
Hemorrheologic agents	Pentoxifylline	Cardiovascular disease
Hemostatics	Coagulation factors VIII, IX	Hemophilia
Thrombolytic agents	Alteplase, streptokinase	Cardiovascular disease
CARDIOVASCULAR DRUGS		
Cardiac drugs	Digoxin, disopyramide	Cardiovascular disease
Diuretics	Furosemide	Congestive heart failure
Vasodilating agents	Dipyridamole, isosorbide nitroglycerin	Cardiovascular disease
CNS DRUGS		
Gold compounds	Auranofin	Rheumatoid arthritis
Heavy metal antagonists	Penicillamine	Rheumatoid arthritis
GI DRUGS		
Digestants	Pancreatin, pancrelipase	Cystic fibrosis
Miscellaneous GI drugs	Mesalamine	Crohn's disease
	Colchicine	Cirrhosis
HORMONES		
Adrenal hormones	Corticosteroids	Asthma, certain anemias, immunosuppression
Adrenal steroid inhibitors	Aminoglutethimide, Trilostane	Hyperadrenocorticism
Insulins	Insulins	Diabetes mellitus
Sulfonylureas	Glyburide	Diabetes mellitus

Table continued

Drugs Indicative of Diseases Warranting Immunization (cont.)

Category title	Representatative drugs	Immunization-Indicating disease states
IMMUNOLOGIC DRUGS		
Immune globulins	IV immune globulin	Immunodeficiency
	Anti-thymocyte globulin	Organ transplant
	Muromab-CD3	Organ transplant
Immunosuppressants	Cyclosporine	Organ transplant
RADIOISOTOPES		
Therapeutic isotopes	NaI-131, NaP-32	Certain cancers
RENAL DRUGS		
Agents for gout	Allopurinal	Renal calculi
Ammonia detoxicants	Potassium acid phosphate	Renal calculi
RESPIRATORY DRUGS		
Anticholinergic agents	Ipratropium	Pulmonary disease
Parasympathomimetics	Pyridostigmine bromide	Myasthenia gravis
Respiratory smooth muscle relaxants	Aminophylline, theophylline	Pulmonary disease
Sympathomimetic agents	Albuterol	Pulmonary disease
Enzyme replacements	Alpha₁-proteinase inhibitor	Congenital panacinar emphysema

Administrative Matters

Infection-control committees can prevent infections among staff and patients by encouraging sound institutional policies on:

a. Hepatitis B pre-exposure prophylaxis, to provide immunity to healthcare workers exposed to blood products and other contaminated items.

b. Hepatitis B post-exposure (eg, needle-stick) prophylaxis, to protect previously unvaccinated patients from infection.

c. Rabies pre- and post-exposure prophylaxis, to protect individuals at occupational risk of rabies or following exposures to potentially rabid animals. Rabies vaccine is the only overused immunization in the US; sound policies can minimize unneeded vaccinations.

d. Wound-management guidelines, to prevent tetanus and diphtheria in patients with trauma.

e. Pertussis contraindications, to minimize inappropriate exclusions from vaccination and to maximize the number of people protected.

f. Employee immunization requirements (against measles, rubella, influenza, hepatitis B and other diseases), to reduce disease transmission from patient to employee and from employee to patient.

g. Tuberculosis screening of patients and staff, to conduct rational surveillance of high-risk populations served by the institution and to preclude nosocomial infection.

Adopt quality indicators and monitoring systems to ensure that all patients are assessed for immunization adequacy prior to leaving the facility. In some settings, standing orders to this effect may be helpful. Drug-use evaluation (DUE) criteria for drugs that indicate need for influenzae and pneumococcal vaccine should include immunization of these patients. For example, immunize all patients on digoxin, war farin, insulin or chronic theophylline therapy against influenza and pneumococcal pneumonia.

Institutional policies on the administration of immunizations should include immediate availability of epinephrine and other products used to treat adverse events. Similarly, have Advanced Cardiac Life Support (ACLS) providers readily available when immunizations are offered.

Planning Influenza Vaccination Programs

1. Ensure that adequate vaccine supplies have been ordered.

2. Name one or two primary vaccine advocates on the staff to coordinate department activities. Charge these people with developing an outreach program to identify patients at risk of influenza and pneumococcal pneumonia.

3. Work with the employee health department to encourage vaccination of the staff of the whole institution, since nosocomial transmission of influenza from staff to immunosuppressed patients can be fatal.

4. Prepare for ill-founded excuses. Explain to the unwilling that modern influenza vaccines cause far fewer side effects than vaccines produced in the 1960s and 1970s and are far more effective at preventing disease and death. A recent double-blind, placebo-controlled study demonstrated no difference between modern influenza vaccine and saline placebo in terms of disability or systemic symptoms (Margolis et al, 1990).

5. Fight the myth that influenza vaccine can cause influenza. The malaise some persons experience following vaccination is common to many vaccines and is not an infectious process. People who develop true influenza within a few days after being vaccinated were certainly incubating the virus at the time of injection and would have got-

ten sick whether they were vaccinated or not. In the American vernacular, "flu" is casually used as a generic term for a wide class of viral illnesses, including "stomach flu," that have nothing to do with influenzae. Avoid using the term "flu," favoring the specific term influenza instead.

Take advantage of existing resources, such as CDC's manual, Managing an Influenza Vaccination Program in the Nursing Home (1987, revision in progress).

Model Activities for National Adult Immunization Awareness Week

1. Lead your infection-control committee in declaring a local observation of National Adult Immunization Awareness Week. Invite the print, radio and television media to a ceremony marking the week to see what a good job you do protecting the public health. Vaccinate a local celebrity in front of their cameras.

2. Lead your Pharmacy and Therapeutics (P&T) committee in recommending influenza and pneumococcal vaccine for patients receiving appropriate medications.

3. Devote an issue of the pharmacy or hospital newsletter to explaining the need to protect adults against preventable infections. Or review a vaccine-preventable disease every issue or two.

4. For every admission with a vaccine-indicating diagnosis, recommend influenza and pneumococcal vaccination just prior to discharge. Use any medium that communicates: Sticky notes, index cards, letters, chart notes, preprinted forms.

5. Start screening for vaccine needs by medication use; send an individualized, preprinted message to the physician recommending vaccination.

6. As you take medication histories, start taking immunization histories as well. Add this information to computerized patient profiles, so that dates for booster doses can be generated.

7. Encourage good documentation of immunizations (eg, state form, PHS Form 731), computerized immunization profiles, inpatient and outpatient chart entries.

8. Codify your vaccine-use policies, following national guidelines: Hepatitis B (preexposure and needle-stick), rabies prophylaxis (to preclude unneeded vaccination), DTP to DT conversion in pediatrics (strict criteria, to maximize pertussis prophylaxis) and wound management.

9. Order immunization references for your drug-information center and libraries.

10. Conduct educational programs for pharmacy staff, nurses, physicians, patients and other groups. Incorporate immunization routines into diabetic, asthmatic and heart disease clinics. Give talks at local civic and retirement centers and to other groups.

11. Encourage your own parents and older relatives to be vaccinated.

12. Obtain pamphlets, videotapes and additional information from the National Foundation for Infectious Diseases (301-656-0003) or from Technical Information Services, Centers for Disease Control and Prevention (404-639-1836).

13. Encourage recognition that buying vaccines saves total costs to the healthcare system by reducing the number of hospital admissions and the number of deaths.

Drug-Product Selection

1. Delete tetanus toxoid from formularies in favor of combined tetanus-diphtheria toxoids for wound prophylaxis, in order to sustain diphtheria immunity in the population. If this decision is not accepted, purchase adsorbed tetanus toxoid in place of fluid tetanus toxoid.

2. Favor trivalent measles-mumps-rubella (MMR) vaccine over single- or double-antigen formulations, in order to boost immunity against each of the three diseases. Change requests for single- or dou-

ble-antigen vaccines to trivalent MMR, in consultation with the prescriber, as frequently as possible.

3. Stock inactivated poliovirus vaccine (e-IPV), in addition to attenuated, oral poliovirus vaccine (OPV), to immunize adults and certain high-risk patients and families of patients with immunodeficiencies.

4. Favor oral typhoid vaccine capsules over the subcutaneous vaccine, because of the lesser incidence of adverse reactions. Do emphasize the need for compliance with all four doses of the capsules.

5. Generally favor tuberculin PPD over old tuberculin (OT), since PPD is both more sensitive and more specific than OT, producing fewer false-negative and fewer false-positive reactions.

6. Favor the spherule-derived form of coccidioidin, since it is more sensitive than cocidiodidin, USP, and does not boost antibody titers that interfere with complement-fixation tests.

7. Favor the controlled yeast lysate (CYL) form of histoplasmin, since it is more sensitive than histoplasmin, USP, and does not boost anti-Histoplasma antibody titers that interfere with complement-fixation tests.

8. Reassess agents and doses used in anergy skin-test batteries (refer to Rational Anergy Test Batteries in the Hypersensitivity Agents section).

9. Ensure sufficient vials of crotalid antivenin are stocked to treat the entire course of severe envenomation in a pit viper snakebite victim (8 to 15 vials).

Ten Things To Do First In Immunization Advocacy

1. Increase use of influenza and pneumococcal vaccines by staff and patients.

2. Start screening for vaccine needs on admission, on discharge, by drug use, etc. Use any medium that communicates: Sticky

notes, index cards, letters, chart notes, preprinted forms.

3. Codify vaccine use policies: Hepatitis B (preexposure and needle-stick), rabies (to preclude unneeded immunization), DTP to DT switch (to maximize pertussis vaccination), wound management (Td, rather than TT).

4. Delete tetanus toxoid, in favor of Td.

5. Favor PPD over old tuberculin.

6. Conduct educational programs for pharmacy, nursing, physicians, patients and other groups (eg, classes, newsletters). Conduct an educational program (eg, grand rounds, in-service) on patient immunization or occupational immunization; publish a newsletter on immunizations.

7. Start keeping vaccine profiles and taking vaccine histories.

8. Build immunization advocacy into continuous quality-improvement (CQI) activities or drug-use evaluation (DUE) programs.

9. Encourage your own parents and older relatives to be vaccinated against influenzae and pneumococcal pneumonia.

10. Do something special for the next National Adult Immunization Awareness Week, the last full week of each October.

Inappropriate Contraindications

Conditions often inappropriately regarded as contraindications are printed below. Do NOT routinely withhold immunization in the following instances:

1. Reaction to a previous dose of diphtheria and tetanus toxoids with pertussis vaccine (DTP) that involved only soreness, redness or swelling in the immediate vicinity of the vaccination site or temperature 40.5·C (105·F).

2. Mild acute illness with low-grade fever or mild diarrheal illness in an otherwise well child.

3. Current antimicrobial therapy or the convalescent phase of an illness.

4. Prematurity. The appropriate age to initiate immunization of the prematurely born infant is the usual chronologic age from birth. Do not reduce vaccine doses for preterm infants.

5. Pregnancy in the patient or a household contact.

6. Recent exposure to an infectious disease.

7. Breastfeeding. The only vaccine virus that has been isolated from breast milk is rubella vaccine virus. There is no good evidence that breast milk from women immunized against rubella is harmful to infants.

8. A history of nonspecific allergies or relatives with allergies.

9. Allergies to penicillin or any other antibiotic, except anaphylactic reactions to neomycin (pertinent for MMR-containing vaccines) or streptomycin (pertinent for oral poliovirus vaccine). No vaccine licensed in the US or Canada contains penicillin.

10. Allergies to duck meat or duck feathers. No vaccine available in the US or Canada is produced in substrates containing duck antigens.

11. A family history of convulsions in persons considered for pertussis or measles vaccination.

12. A family history of sudden infant death syndrome (SIDS) in children considered for DTP vaccination.

13. A family history of an adverse event, unrelated to immunosuppression, following vaccination.

14. History of an adverse reaction to one of the older influenza vaccines prior to the zonal centrifuge (1960s) and improved purification (1970s).

Adapted from: ACIP. General recommendations on immunization. MMWR 1989;38:205-14,219-27.

True Contraindications & Precautions	Not True (Vaccines May Be Administered)
General For all Pediatric Vaccines *(DTwP, DTaP, OPV, IPV, MMR, Hib, HBV)*	
Contraindications	
Anaphylactic reactions to a vaccine contraindicate further doses to that vaccine Anaphylactic reaction to a vaccine constituent contraindicates the use of vaccines containing that substance Moderate or severe illnesses with or without fever	Mild to moderate local reaction (soreness, redness, swelling) after a dose of an injectable antigen Mild acute illness with or without low-grade fever Current antimicrobial therapy Convalescent phase of illnesses Prematurity (use same dose and indications as for normal, full-term infants) Recent exposure to an infectious disease History of penicillin or other nonspecific allergies or family history of such allergies
DTwP or DTaP	
Contraindications	
Encephalopathy within 7 days of administration of previous dose of DTP	Temperature of <40.5°C (105°F) following a prior dose of DTP Family history of convulsions
Precautions[1]	
Fever ≥40.5° (105°F) within 48 hours after vaccination with a prior dose of DTP Collapse of shock-like state (hypotonic-hyporesponsive episode) within 48 hours of receiving a prior dose of DTP Seizures within 3 days of receiving a prior dose of DTP Persistent, inconsolable crying lasting ≥3 hours within 48 hours of receiving a prior dose of DTP	Family history of sudden infant death syndrome (SIDS) Family history of an adverse event following DTP administration
OPV	
Contraindications	
Infection with HIV or a household contact with HIV Known altered immunodeficiency (hematologic and solid tumors; congenital immunodeficiency; long-term immunosuppressive therapy) Immunodeficient household contact	Breastfeeding Current antimicrobial therapy Diarrhea
Precautions[1]	
Pregnancy	
IPV	
Contraindications	
Anaphylactic reaction to neomycin or streptomycin	Infection with HIV
Precautions[1]	
Pregnancy	

Table continued

True Contraindications & Precautions	Not True (Vaccines May Be Administered)
MMR	
Contraindications	
Anaphylactic reaction to egg ingestion or to neomycin Pregnancy Known altered immunodeficiency (hematologic and solid tumors; congenital immunodeficiency; long-term immunosuppressive therapy)	Tuberculosis or positive skin test Simultaneous tuberculin skin testing Pregnancy of mother of recipient Immunodeficient family member or household contact Infection with HIV
Precautions[1]	
Receipt of an immune globulin product within preceeding 3 months	Nonanaphylactic reaction to egg or neomycin
Hib	
None identified	
HBV	
None identified	

[1]Events or conditions listed as precautions, although not contraindications to immunization, should be carefully reviewed, considering the benefits and risks of giving a specific vaccine to that individual.

Adapted from: CDC. Standards for pediatric immunization practices. *MMWR* 1993;42(RR-5):1-13.

Standards for Pediatric Immunization Practices

1. Immunization services are readily available.

2. There are no barriers or unnecessary prerequisites to the receipt of vaccines.

3. Immunization services are available free or for a minimal fee.

4. Providers utilize all clinical encounters to screen and, when indicated, immunize children.

5. Providers educate parents and guardians about immunization in general terms.

6. Providers question parents or guardians about contraindications and, before immunizing a child, inform them in specific terms about the risks and benefits of the immunizations their child is to receive.

7. Providers follow only true contraindications.

8. Providers administer simultaneously all vaccine doses for which a child is eligible at the time of each visit.

9. Providers use accurate and complete recording procedures.

10. Providers co-schedule immunization appointments in conjunction with appointments for other child health services.

11. Providers report adverse events following immunization promptly, accurately and completely.

12. Providers operate a tracking system.

13. Providers adhere to appropriate procedures for vaccine management.

14. Providers conduct semiannual audits to assess immunization coverage levels and to review immunization records in the patient populations they serve.

15. Providers maintain up-to-date, easily retrievable medical protocols at all locations where vaccines are administered.

16. Providers operate with patient-oriented and community-based approaches.

17. Vaccines are administered by properly trained individuals.

18. Providers receive ongoing education and training on current immunization recommendations.

Reference: CDC. Standards for pediatric immunization practices. MMWR 1993;42(RR-5):1-13 and JAMA 1993;269:1817-22.

Standards for Adult Immunization Practices

National Coalition for Adult Immunization

The National Coalition for Adult Immunization, recognizing that many adults become victims of vaccine-preventable diseases; and

Recognizing that influenza, pneumococcal and hepatitis B infections account for the majority of adult vaccine-preventable morbidity and death; and

Recognizing that influenza and pneumococcal infections may account for up to 60,000 deaths annually among adults; and

Recognizing that more than 300,000 cases of hepatitis B and more than 5,000 hepatitis B-related deaths occur annually; and

Recognizing that persons 15 years and older accounted for 43% of reported cases of measles and 39% of reported cases of mumps in 1987; and

Recognizing that approximately 11 million young women are unprotected against rubella; and

Recognizing that over 90% of reported cases of tetanus and over 80% of reported cases of diphtheria during 1985-1987 occurred in persons over 20 years of age, most of whom were inadequately immunized; and

Acknowledging that safe, effective vaccines that could reduce disease incidence, morbidity, mortality and healthcare costs from these illnesses are available but are underutilized; and

Noting that healthcare providers often miss opportunities to provide vaccines to adults for whom they are recommended; and

Noting that 40% to 50% or more of persons at high risk for, or who die from, influenza and pneumonia had received medical attention in healthcare institutions during the previous year and at least 70% attended outpatient clinics but failed to receive influenza vaccine; and

Noting that two-thirds or more of patients with serious pneumococcal infections have been hospitalized at least once within the previous three to five years but have not received pneumococcal vaccine; therefore the National Coalition for Adult Immunization

1. Encourages that promotion of appropriate vaccine use through information campaigns for healthcare practitioners and trainees, employers and the public about the benefits of immunizations; and

2. Encourages physicians and other healthcare personnel (in practice and in training) to protect themselves and prevent transmission to patients by assuring that they themselves are completely immunized; and

3. Recommends that all healthcare providers routinely determine the immunization status of their patients, offer vaccines to those for whom they are indicated and maintain complete immunization records; and

4. Recommends that all healthcare providers identify high-risk patients in need of influenza vaccine and develop a system to recall them for annual immunization each autumn; and

5. Recommends that all healthcare providers and institutions identify high-risk adult patients in hospitals and other treatment centers and assure that appropriate vaccination is considered either prior to discharge or as a part of discharge planning; and

6. Recommends that all licensing/accrediting agencies support the development by healthcare institutions of compre

hensive immunization programs for staff, trainees, volunteer workers, inpatients and outpatients; and

7. Encourages states to establish pre-enrollment immunization requirements for colleges and other institutions of higher education; and

8. Recommends that institutions that train healthcare professionals, deliver healthcare or provide laboratory or other medical support services require appropriate immunizations for persons at risk of contracting or transmitting vaccine-preventable illnesses; and

9. Encourages healthcare benefit programs, third party payers and governmental healthcare programs to provide coverage for adult immunization services; and

10. Encourages the adoption of a standard personal and institutional immunization record as a means of verifying the immunization status of patients and staff.

Source:

National Coalition for Adult Immunization (NCAI), 4733 Bethesda Avenue, Bethesda, MD 20832; 301-656-0003

National Foundation for Infectious Diseases (NFID), 4733 Bethesda Avenue, Bethesda, MD 20832; 301-656-0003

Appendix B

Health departments, travel clinics and the Centers for Disease Control and Prevention (CDC) offer expert travel-health advice. Information from the CDC can be obtained by calling one of the following numbers:

- International travel hotline: 404-332-4559.
- Voice-information system: 404-332-4555.
- Fax information service: 404-332-4656.
- Malaria hotline: 404-639-1610.
- On the Internet: www.cdc.gov and follow the prompts.

These telephone lines can help both travelers and healthcare specialists. Use a touch-tone telephone. Rotary calls go to an operator during normal business hours. Have a pen and paper handy to write down drug and vaccine names and other advice.

Vaccine recommendations for international travel change frequently. A review of the patient's health needs should be conducted about 6 weeks before the departure date.

Risk Factors of Preventable Diseases

This section covers major risk factors affecting the health of international travelers. These are only the risks that vaccination or malaria prevention can reduce. It does not include infections that vaccines cannot prevent. Nor are environmental and other hazards discussed, such as heat injury.

Health risks vary within a country. Medical threats vary with the destination and with the type of business and recreation conducted while there. Risk also depends on season, altitude, method of travel and other factors.

- **Food.** Cholera, typhoid and hepatitis are spread in contaminated food, which can be tainted before or during preparation. Proper storage is important as well. Dairy products may not be pasteurized or handled properly.

- **Water.** Water should be purified or bottled (ensuring that the source for the bottled water is safe). Water can be purified by boiling or by adding of household bleach or 2% tincture of iodine. (The use of iodine should be avoided during pregnancy.) There are also water purification tablets that can be purchased commercially. Canned or bottled carbonated beverages, hot coffee or tea from boiled water, and unopened containers of beer or wine are generally safe.

- **Insect control.** Malaria, which is transmitted by mosquitoes, is one of the most widespread and destructive infections in the world. Malaria infects about 270 million people each year, of which approximately 1 million die. To reduce exposure risk, stay indoors during early morning and early evening hours. Wear long-sleeved shirts and long pants and sleep in a screened area. Insect repellents containing DEET (N, N-diethyl-methatolumide) work well. Repellents using a high concentration of DEET should be used sparingly, if at all, on young children. Tick repellents (eg, permethrin, *Permanone*) should only be applied to clothing, never to skin.

- **Medical access.** Observe several general medical precautions. Take along a list of both generic and brand name medications packed, as well as an adequate supply. Plan ahead for special needs by bringing.
  - Insect-sting kits.
  - Medical-alert bracelets.
  - Extra eyeglasses and eyeglass prescriptions.
  - Storage needs for heat-sensitive items.

Carry critical items with you; do not stow them in luggage.

Rabies is common in animals in Latin America, India, the Far East and Africa.

Cleanse any animal bite promptly and thoroughly. Get protection immediately after a bite or mucous contact if the animal is likely to harbor rabies.

In general, early treatment is better than prevention of travelers' diarrhea. The most common cause of such diarrhea is enterotoxigenic *Escherichia coli. Campylobacter, Shigella, Salmonella*, viruses and parasites are also major causes of diarrhea. Many of these infections cannot be prevented with vaccines.

Loperamide *(Imodium)* or bismuth subsalicylate *(Pepto-Bismol)* are often used in mild cases of 2 to 3 loose stools per day. For severe cases, antibiotics such as doxycycline *(Vibramycin)*, sulfamethoxazole-trimethoprim *(Septra, Bactrim)*, and cipro-floxacin *(Cipro)* have been used. When prescribed, antibiotics are often used twice daily for just 3 days. Blood or mucus in the stool or fever suggests the need for more aggressive evaluation. Oral rehydration solutions help in treating severe diarrhea.

Immunization Needs

The patient should be informed that some vaccines require several doses for complete immunity. Medical needs should be reviewed at least 6 weeks before departure date. While most travelers usually focus on protection from exotic diseases, it is also important to ensure that vaccinations for "domestic" diseases are current. These include:

- Tetanus
- Measles
- Rubella
- Varicella
- Influenza
- Hepatitis B
- Poliovirus

Other vaccines to consider for patients traveling abroad are:

- **Hepatitis A or intramuscular immune globulin** (IGIM or "gamma globulin"). This is particularly important when traveling to where hygiene is poor and for those traveling away from standard tourist routes. Hepatitis A vaccine provides more long-lasting protection than IGIM. IGIM may be cheaper if the traveler will make only one visit and stays less than 2 months.

- **Typhoid and cholera vaccines.** Risk is high for travelers staying more than 1 week in rural areas where these diseases are common. Vaccination is also useful for travelers with some stomach disorders. This includes long-time users of antacids, cimetidine *(Tagamet)*, ranitidine *(Zantac)*, omeprazole *(Prilosec)*, and similar medications.

- **Yellow fever.** This vaccine should be given according to specific instructions provided by individual countries.

- **Meningococcal vaccination.** Meningococcal meningitis is a risk in savanna regions of sub-Saharan Africa during the dry season from December to June. Outbreaks can extend up the Nile Valley into northern Egypt. In recent years, Kenya, Tanzania, Nepal and India also reported epidemics. Saudi Arabia may require meningococcal vaccination before admitting Islamic pilgrims to Hajj.

- **Pre-travel and post-travel tuberculin skin test.** This should be done for travel to most developing countries.

- **Plague vaccine.** This should be given for travel to rural areas of Viet Nam and some other Southeast Asian countries.

- **Japanese encephalitis vaccine.** Vaccination should be considered for visitors who are staying a month or longer in rice-growing areas of rural Asia with extensive mosquito exposure.

Vaccination Certificate Requirements

International Health Regulations are adopted by the World Health Organization (WHO). A country can require an International Certificate of Vaccination for certain diseases before allowing a traveler to enter. Americans use Public Health Service (PHS) Form

731, International Certificates of Vaccination, to record these immunizations. This form is commonly called the "yellow shot record." It also can serve as a personal vaccine record.

- **Yellow Fever.** Some countries require travelers to present an "International Certificate of Vaccination Against Yellow Fever." The certificate is valid for 10 years, beginning 10 days after the first vaccination or on the date of revaccination, if within 10 years of an earlier injection. Yellow fever is a viral infection that leads to swelling of the brain.

- **Cholera.** A certificate of cholera immunization is no longer required by any country or territory. Some earlier government requirements exceeded International Health Regulations. The certificate is valid for 6 months, beginning 6 days after the first vaccination or on the date of revaccination, if within 6 months of an earlier injection. Cholera vaccination will not prevent the introduction of the disease into any country. Cholera is a serious infection of the stomach and intestines.

- **Smallpox.** Smallpox was dropped from diseases subject to International Health Regulations, effective January 1, 1982.

Quarantine. Under International Health Regulations, people with suspected infections can be quarantined as follows:

- Cholera—5 days.
- Plague—6 days.
- Yellow Fever—6 days.

For direct travel from the U.S., the following countries require an International Certificate of Vaccination.

- Cholera: None.
- Yellow Fever: Benin, Burkino Faso, Cameroon, Central African Republic, Congo, Côte d'Ivoire, French Guiana, Gabon, Ghana, Liberia, Mali, Mauritania (if staying more than two weeks),

Senegal, Togo and Zaire.

For travel to and between other countries, check individual country requirements. Call CDC's 24-hour international travel information hotline at 404-332-4559 or their Fax Information Service at 404-332-4565. The Fax Information Service system answers 24 hours a day, 7 days a week. Up to five documents may be requested during each call.

No vaccinations are required to enter or return to the U.S.

Advances in vaccine science over the last 50 years have been nothing short of remarkable. Diseases once feared have all but disappeared, tamed by vaccines.

The general public wants more than ever to be involved in its health care. Prevention is no different from therapy in this regard. In the last five years, countless grass-roots coalitions have sprung up around the country to advocate childhood immunizations. Similar efforts for adult immunizations are beginning.

Public service announcements via the mass media reinforce to millions of people to the health benefits of immunization. Medicare reimbursement of influenza and pneumococcal vaccines and the Vaccines For Children program enable more extensive immunization delivery today than at any time in our nation's history. Detailed cost-effectiveness studies repeatedly reveal the magnitude of the benefit of immunizations, both for society and for the individual.

These general forces mean that more and more people will be vaccinated each year. More people than ever expect high-quality immunization services. They expect courtesy, convenience, efficiency and value. Do you meet their expectations?

Are you new at running your immunization clinic? Maybe you're looking for ways to improve the quality of your operation? If so, this section will help you consider obvious and not-so-obvious issues in delivering immunizations in your community, safely, efficiently and courteously. We'll start with the traditional aspects of who, what, when, where and how.

Baseline Considerations

Think about your vaccine clinic the way your clients think about you. Look at the operation as they see you. What do your other senses tell you? Consider sound, touch and smell. Business gurus talk about "management by walking around." Check out your waiting room for sights and sounds and temperature. Test the seats.

Who?

Who will your primary clients be? If they are children, you will want to make your waiting area comfortable and inviting in ways different than you would use to welcome adults. Sit in the waiting area yourself to appreciate the view and atmosphere. Be sure to assess the waiting area during both quiet times and busy ones.

Who are your fellow staff members? Do they know all they need to know to handle unusual cases? What are their educational needs? What would it take to help them develop into top-notch vaccine givers? Be sure everyone has current certification in cardiopulmonary resuscitation (CPR, also called Basic Cardiac Life Support, BCLS). To make learning fun, have each person present the vaccine-of-the-week or make up a trivia game about vaccine and disease characteristics. Don't forget to know the diseases we vaccinate against, even the ones that are in the process of disappearing thanks to vaccines.

What?

What records will you keep? Consider an immunization registry; automated ones are best for retrieving data. Do you have a responsibility to report to a state immunization registry? Don't forget to fill out Vaccine Adverse Event Reporting System (VAERS) forms whenever patients have unusual reactions. Remind patients to report these events to you even if they occur after they leave your clinic. Also remind them to carry their personal immunization records to every health visit. National experts recommend that everyone carry immunization records in their wallets.

What will you say to patients? Once you consider a patient's immunization needs, think globally. Figure out all the vaccines that person needs. Offer pneumococcal as well as influenza vaccine to the elderly and those with chronic disease. Be a good detective: ask the questions that will help you uncover the patient's needs.

When?

When are vaccines needed? Do your patients and their family members know? Post enlarged schedules around the clinic and give copies so people know when they should return for the next immunization. One Hawaiian health department official had the pediatric immunization schedule printed on the back of his business cards.

What hours will you operate? Will these hours meet the needs of your clients? Can you rearrange your staffing so that your present staff is spread out, allowing longer hours of availability? Young parents especially appreciate the ability to have their children vaccinated early in the morning or late in the day. Convenience contributes directly to return visits.

When will you release patients after they have been vaccinated? After 15 minutes, 20 minutes, 30 minutes? Do you have a system for assuring that patients don't leave too early?

Where?

Is your clinic well known? How do your patients most often travel to your clinic? Would they appreciate maps or help with bus connections or parking?

Where will you give the vaccines? Do you have a separate area where you can interview patients calmly and do your record-keeping?

Where will your patients wait? Determine the number of patients you expect to serve on an average day and on a peak day. Inflate that number by the number of family members likely to accompany the patient: parents, siblings, others. If you have no influence over the size of your waiting area, can you suggest good alternative space, like a nearby snack bar or lobby?

Where will you store your vaccines and related supplies? Do your refrigerators and freezers have adequate storage space?

What is you backup plan if the power fails? Does everyone know prudent measures to prevent vaccine wastage? Remind everyone periodically about rotating stock, putting vials with the most distant expiration dates in the back and the shortest dated ones up front. Does the staff know how important it is to recognize vaccines that have been exposed to degrading temperatures and may no longer be potent?

Where will you dispose of used needles and syringes? Be sure to use rigid containers for needles, to protect your staff. Do not recap or clip used needles. Gloves are not generally recommended when injecting vaccines, although this policy may vary from place to place. Nevertheless, observe universal precautions in handling anything contaminated with blood or body fluids. Everyone should wash their hands between patients.

Where will you dispose of vials containing live viruses? It is best to send them off in a manner of disposal that will include autoclaving.

How?

How do you explain informed-consent documents? Do you use it as a chance to teach the patients and parents about the value of vaccines, as well as their unintended (and usually rare) side effects? Be sure to answer patient questions before and after the consent forms are signed. Help the patient keep the benefits of avoiding disease in perspective, compared to the risks of vaccination itself.

How do you respond to questions? Do your receptionist and your staff have ready access to answers to frequently asked questions about hours of access, cost, appropriate reasons to defer immunization, and the like?

How will you handle emergencies? Do you have the necessary equipment and training to respond to anaphylaxis? ...to vasovagal reactions? When was the last time you practiced your emergency drill? How will you access additional support (eg, elsewhere in the building, via 911)?

More and more vaccine combinations

are available. How will you reduce the risk of someone selecting the wrong vaccine from your refrigerator shelf? Consider special labeling, physical separation, individual bins. Don't forget, these measures are not fool-proof. There is no substitute for reading the vial label.

How will you manage your inventory, to ensure an adequate supply while avoiding waste? Do you have a system for checking expiration dates? Who is your principal product-quality checker?

How do you tell patients that you want them to return? Do you make appointment scheduling easy? Are records promptly updated? Do you convey the fact that this patient is important?

How will you keep your staff up-to-date on recent changes in national vaccine policies and schedules? These changes seem to be coming faster and faster, so it may be appropriate to name one person the coordinator for "vaccine news and gossip." Facts about the latest changes should be widely discussed at staff meetings and dedicated educational sessions.

Especially for Kids

Remember that children are not little adults. They often do not have the power to reason or comprehend the value of immunizations. Reward their bravery. It is usually best not to draw up a vaccine dose in front of children, because they may become frightened from viewing the needle and syringe too long. Selecting and preparing doses in a quiet, well-lit setting also reduces the risk of a medication error.

If the parent brings two or more children for immunization, see if the other children can stay in the waiting area temporarily. If this is not possible, immunize the older child first, because they set an example for the others. It is important not to compare children's responses to injections. Instead, praise them all for protecting themselves from nasty germs.

If a child is old enough, explain what vaccines do in simple terms. Do not say that injections will not hurt. Instead, say that the injection will be like a pin prick. Other techniques to minimize pain recog-

nition by children have been proposed by Kachoyeanos & Friedhoff, based on the child's age:

- for infants: a pacifier, music, swaddling, caressing
- for toddlers: blowing bubbles, playing with pop-up toys, looking through a kaleidoscope
- for preschoolers: imagining a superhero, blowing away the pain, gradual desensitization, rehearsing the procedure, using a "magic" glove or blanket, finding Waldo in a "Where's Waldo" poster, looking through a kaleidoscope
- for school-age children: a "magic" glove, using a "pain switch," blowing bubbles, rehearsing

Young children tend to fidget and jump around. Calmly and quietly ask a parent to hold a child's extremities (both arms and legs) while the injection is being administered. Involving the parent helps in tangible cases, like this, as well as in other ways. Colorful adhesive bandages are appreciated by both children and parents alike. Remind parents that children bruise more easily than adults.

For a pediatric waiting area, offer furniture and diversions appropriate for age. If your budget won't allow for such niceties, ask parents to donate them.

Consider a television and videocassette recorder. Rather than connecting the television to the local broadcast stations, play educational videos appropriate to the audience.

Especially for Adults

Remember that adults will appreciate a private area for immunization. This is especially true for women, if tight upper clothing needs to be removed to expose the deltoid area.

Especially for Seniors

Remember that the skin of an older person tends to be drier, less elastic, and more of a challenge when injecting a vaccine. Take special care to dry the skin thoroughly and avoid rubbing it after injection so that it will not bruise.

Think Globally

Remember, when you are preparing to vaccinate a person, to check for all the vaccines that this person might need. Once you begin assessing a person's vaccine needs, think comprehensively. For example, a person might ask for influenza vaccine or a tetanus booster. Be sure to consider pneumococcal vaccine, hepatitis B vaccine and all others appropriate by age, health state, occupation and risk factors.

Immunizations are some of the most powerful tools available to medical science today. They have saved literally billions of lives over the years and made the lives of billions more so much happier. You can be justifiably proud of your work to protect your patients.

Reference: Kachoyeanos MK, Friedhoff M. Cognitive and behavioral strategies to reduce children's pain. *Maternal/Child Nursing 1993*;18;14-9.

Bibliography

Abrutyn E, Berlin JA. Intrathecal therapy in tetanus: A meta-analysis. *JAMA* 1991;266:2262–7.

ACOG. Technical Bulletin #160: Immunization during pregnancy. Washington, DC: ACOG, October 1991.

Adams WG, Deaver KA, Cochi SL, et al. Decline of childhood *Haemophilus influenzae* type b (Hib) disease in the Hib vaccine era. *JAMA* 1993;269:221–6.

Andrew M, Blanchette VS, Adams M, et al. A multicenter study of the treatment of childhood chronic idiopathic thrombocytopenia purpura with anti-D. *J Pediatr* 1992;120:522–7.

Antonelli G, Currenti M, Turriziani O. et al. Neutralizing antibodies to interferon-alfa: Relative frequency in patients treated with different preparations. *J Infect Dis* 1991;163:882–5.

Arbeter AM, Baker L, Starr SE, et al. Combination measles, mumps, rubella, and varicella vaccine. *Pediatrics* 1986;76(Suppl):742–7.

Archer JD. The FDA does not approve uses of drugs. *JAMA* 1984;252:1054–5.

Arthurs B, Flanders M, Codere F, et al. Treatment of blepharospasm with medication, surgery, and type A botulinum toxin. *Can J Ophthalmol* 1987;22:24–8.

Athale UH, Luo-Mutti C, Chintu C. How safe is BCG vaccination in children born to HIV-positive mothers? *Lancet* 1992;340:434–5.

Badaro R, Falcoff E, Badaro FS, et al. Treatment of visceral leishmaniasis with pentavalent antimony and interferon gamma. *N Engl J Med* 1990;322:16–21.

Baker CJ, Melish ME, Hall RT, et al. Intravenous immune globulin for the prevention of nosocomial infection in low-birth-weight neonates. *N Engl J Med* 1992;327:213–9.

Benenson AS. Immunization and military medicine. *Rev Infect Dis* 1984;6:1–12.

Bernard KW, Fishbein DB, Miller KD, et al. Pre-exposure rabies immunization with human diploid-cell vaccine: Decreased antibody responses in persons immunized in developing countries. *Am J Trop Med Hyg* 1985;34:633–47.

Bielory L, Wright R, Nienhuis AW, et al. Antithymocyte globulin hypersensitivity in bone marrow failure patients. *JAMA* 1988;260:3164–7.

Blumhardt R, Pappano JE Jr., Moyer DG. Depression of poison ivy skin tests by measles vaccine. *JAMA* 1968;206:2739–41.

Bolaños R, Cerdas L, Abalos JW. Venoms of coral snakes (*Micrurus* spp): Report on a multivalent antivenin for the Americas. *Bull PAHO* 1978;12:23–7.

Braun MM, Cauthen G. Relationship of the human immunodeficiency virus epidemic to pediatric tuberculosis and *Bacillus Calmette-Guérin* immunization. *Pediatr Infect Dis J* 1992;11:220–7.

Bryan JP, Sjogren MH, Macarthy P, et al. Dosing schedule for recombinant hepatitis B vaccine. *J Infect Dis* 1991;163:1384−5.

CDC. Hepatitis B associated with jet gun injection-California. *MMWR* 1986;35:272−6.

CDC. Inadequate immune response among public safety workers receiving intradermal vaccination against hepatitis B-United States, 1990-1991. *MMWR* 1991;40:569−72.

Crawford J, Ozer H, Stoller R, et al. Reduction by granulocyte colony-stimulating factor of fever and neutropenia induced by chemotherapy in patients with small-cell lung cancer. *N Engl J Med* 1991;325:164−70.

Cupit GC, Self TH, Bekemeyer WB. The effect of pneumococcal vaccine on the disposition of theophylline. *Eur J Clin Pharmacol* 1988;34:505−7.

Decker MD, Edwards KM, Bradley R, et al. Comparative trial in infants of four conjugate *Haemophilus influenzae* type b vaccines. *J Pediatr* 1992;120:184−9.

Diaz W, Salamone FR, Muller RJ. Aplastic anemia-Focus on treatment with anti-thymocyte globulin. *Hosp Pharm* 1989;24:737−41,754.

Edsall G. Specific prophylaxis of tetanus. *JAMA* 1959;171:417−27.

Edwards KM. Diphtheria, tetanus, and pertussis immunizations in adults. *Infect Dis Clin N Amer* 1990;4:85−103.

Edwards KM, Decker MD, Graham BS, et al. Adult immunization with acellular pertussis vaccine. *JAMA* 1993;269:53−6.

Edwards KM, Decker MD, Halsey NA, et al. Differences in antibody responses to whole-cell pertussis vaccines. *Pediatrics* 1991;88:1019-23.

Eibl MM, Wolf HM, Furnkranz H. et al. Prophylaxis of necrotizing enterocolitis by oral IgA-IgG: Review of a clinical study in low birth weight infants and discussion of the pathogenic role of infection. *J Clin Immunol* 1990;10(Suppl):72-9.

English PC. Therapeutic strategies to combat pneumococcal disease: Repeated failure of physicians to adopt pneumococcal vaccine, 1900-1945. *Perspect Biol Med* 1987;30:170−85.

Fedson DS. Pneumococcal vaccination: When in doubt, go ahead. *JAMA* 1991;265:211−2.

Fine PEM, Rodrigues LC. Mycobacterial diseases. *Lancet* 1990;335:1016−20.

Fisher AA. *Contact Dermatitis*, 3rd ed. Philadelphia: Lea and Febiger, 1986.

Furcolow ML, Mantz HL, Lewis I. The roentgenographic appearance of persistent pulmonary infiltrates associated with sensitivity to histoplasmin. *Pub Health Rep* 1947;62:1711−8.

Furste W. The potential development of tetanus in wounded patients with AIDS: Tetanus toxoid and tetanus immune globulin. *Arch Surg* 1986;121:367.

Gaillat J, Zmirou D, Mallaret MR, et al. Essai clinique du vaccin in antipneumococcique chez des personnes agees vivant en institution. *Rev Epidémiol Santé Publique* 1985;33:437−44.

Gheorghiu M. The present and future role of BCG vaccine in tuberculosis control. *Biologicals* 1990;18: 135−41.

Giammanco G, DeGrandi V, Lupo L, et al. Interference of oral poliovirus vaccine on RIT 4237 oral rotavirus vaccine. *Eur J Epidemiol* 1988;4:121−3.

Grabenstein JD. Comment on anaphylactic shock. *Drug Intell Clin Pharm* 1984;18:646−7.

Grabenstein JD. Drug-interactions involving immunologic agents: Part I. Vaccine-vaccine, vaccine-immunoglobulin, and vaccine-drug interactions. *DICP-Ann Pharmacother* 1990;24:67−81

Grabenstein JD. Drug-interactions involving immunologic agents: Part II. Immunodiagnostic and other immunologic drug interactions. *DICP-Ann Pharmacother* 1990;24:186−93.

Grabenstein JD, Baker JR Jr. Comment on cyclosporine and vaccination. *Drug Intell Clinical Pharm* 1985;19:679−80.

Grabenstein JD, Smith LJ, Summers RJ. Incidence of epinephrine self-administration in an outpatient population. *Ann Allergy* 1989;63:184−8.

Greenberg MA, Birx DL. Safe administration of mumps-measles-rubella vaccine in egg-allergic children. *J Pediatr* 1988;113:504−6.

Greenberg PD, Lax KG, Schechter CB. Tuberculosis in house staff: A decision analysis comparing the tuberculin screening strategy with the BCG vaccination. *Am Rev Respir Dis* 1991;143:490−5.

Gross PA, Ennis FA. Influenza vaccine: Split-product versus whole-virus types-How do they differ? *N Engl J Med* 1977;296:567−8.

Halsey NA, Klein D. Maternal immunization. *Pediatr Infect Dis J* 1990;9:574.

Hardy IRB, Gershon AA. Prospects for use of a varicella vaccine in adults. *Infect Dis Clin N Amer* 1990;4: 159−73.

Herman JJ, Radin R, Schneiderman R. Allergic reactions to measles (rubeola) vaccine in patients hypersensitive to egg protein. *J Pediatr* 1983;102:196−9.

Herwaldt LA. Pertussis and pertussis vaccines in adults. *JAMA* 1993;269:93−4.

Hibberd PL, Rubin RH. Approach to immunization in the immunocompromised host. *Infect Dis Clin N Amer* 1990;4:123−42.

Howard PA, Haley C. Duration of immunity from hepatitis B vaccine. *Drug Intell Clin Pharm* 1988;22:985−7.

Howard TP, Solomon DA. Reading the tuberculin skin test: Who, when, and how? *Arch Intern Med* 1988; 148:2457−9.

Insel RA. Maternal immunization to prevent neonatal infections. *N Engl J Med* 1988;319:1219−20.

Ippoliti C, Williams L, Huber S. Toxicity of rapidly infused concentrated intravenous immune globulin. *Clin Pharm* 1992;11:1022−6.

Janeway CA, Merler E, Rosen FS, et al. Intravenous gamma globulin: Metabolism of gamma globulin fragments in normal and agammaglobulinemic persons. *N Engl J. Med* 1968;278:919−23.

Jilg W, Schmidt M, Deinhardt F. Vaccination against hepatitis B: Comparison of three different vaccination schedules. *J Infect Dis* 1989;160:766–9.

Juntunen-Backman K, Peltola H, Backman A, et al. Safe immunization of allergic children against measles, mumps, and rubella. *Am J Dis Child* 1987;141:1103–5.

Kaplan JE, Nelson DB, Schonberger LB, et al. The effect of immune globulin on the response to trivalent oral poliovirus and yellow fever vaccinations. *Bull WHO* 1984;62:585–90.

Karzon DT, Edwards KM. Diphtheria outbreaks in immunized populations. *N Engl J Med* 1988;318:41–3.

Kasperek M, Wetmore R. Considerations in the use of intravenous immune globulin products. *Clin Pharm* 1990;9:909.

Kletz MR, Holland CL, Mendelson JS, et al. Administration of egg-derived vaccines in patients with history of egg sensitivity. *Ann Allergy* 1990;64:527–9.

Krotoski WA, Mroczkowski TF, Rea TH, et al. Lepromin skin testing in the classification of Hansen's disease in the USA. *Am J Med Sci* 1993;305:18–24.

Kumar A. Cimetidine: An immunomodulator. *DICP-Ann Pharmacother* 1990;24:289–95.

Lavi S, Zimmerman B, Koren G, et al. Administration of measles, mumps, and rubella virus vaccine (live) to egg-allergic children. *JAMA* 1990;263:269–71.

Leavengood DC, Renard RL, Martin BG, et al. Cross allergenicity among grasses determined by tissue threshold changes. *J Allergy Clin Immunol* 1985;76:789–94.

Levin MJ, Murray M, Rotbart HA, et al. Immune response of elderly individuals to a live attenuated varicella vaccine. *J Infect Dis* 1992;166:253–9.

Levine HB, Scalarone GM, Campbell GD, et al. Histoplasmin-CYL, a yeast-phase reagent in skin test studies with humans. *Am Rev Respir Dis* 1979;119:629–36.

Livengood JR, Mullen JR, White JW, et al. Family history of convulsions and use of pertussis vaccine. *J Pediatr* 1989;115:527–31.

Losonsky GA, Fishaut JM, Strussenberg J, et al. Effect of immunization against rubella on lactation products. I. Development and characterization of specific immunologic reactivity in breast milk. *J Infect Dis* 1982;145:654–60.

Losonsky GA, Fishaut JM, Strussenberg J, et al. Effect of immunization against rubella on lactation products. II. Maternal-neonatal interactions. *J Infect Dis* 1982;145:661–6.

Losonsky GA, Johnson JP, Winkelstein JA, et al. Oral administration of human serum immunoglobulin in immunodeficient patients with viral gastroenteritis: A pharmacokinetic and functional analysis. *J Clin Invest* 1985;76:2362–7.

Lucas GS, Jobbins K, Bloom AL. Intravenous immunoglobulin and blood-group antibodies. *Lancet* 1987;2:742.

MacKenzie WR, Davis JP, Peterson DE, et al. Multiple false-positive serologic tests for HIV, HTLV-1, and hepatitis C following influenza vaccination, 1991. *JAMA* 1992;268: 1015−7.

Margolis KL, Nichol KL, Poland GA, et al. Frequency of adverse reactions to influenza vaccine in the elderly: A randomized, placebo-controlled trial. *JAMA* 1990;264:1139−41.

Marsh DG, Goodfriend L, King TP, et al. Allergen nomenclature. *J Allergy Clin Immunol* 1987;80:639−45.

McCluskey DR, Boyd NAM. Anaphylaxis with intravenous gammaglobulin. *Lancet* 1990;2:874.

McCollough NC, Gennaro JF. Diagnosis, symptoms, treatment, and sequelae of envenomation by *Crotalus adamanteus and genus Ancistrodon. J Fla Med Assoc* 1968;55:327−9.

Mertin J, Rudge P, Kremer M, et al. Double-blind controlled trial of immunosuppression in the treatment of multiple sclerosis: Final report. *Lancet* 1982;2:351−4.

Meuer SC, Dumann H, Meyer zum Bueschenfelde KH, et al. Low-dose interleukin-2 induces systemic immune responses against HBsAg in immunodeficient non-responders to hepatitis B vaccination. *Lancet* 1989;1:15−8.

Miller JR, Orgel HA, Meltzer EO. The safety of egg-containing vaccines for egg-allergic patients. *J Allergy Clin Immunol* 1983;77:568−73.

Moore DA, Hopkins RS. Assessment of a school exclusion policy during a chickenpox outbreak. *Am J Epidemiol* 1991;133:1161−7.

Mueller JH, Miller PA. Factors influencing the production of tetanal toxin. *J Immunol* 1947;56:143−7.

Murphy KR, Strunk RC. Safe administration of influenza vaccine in asthmatic children hypersensitive to egg proteins. *J Pediatrics* 1985;106:931−3.

Nelson BK. Snake envenomation: Incidence, clinical presentation, and management. *Med Toxicol* 1989;4: 17−31.

Nesbit GH. Canine allergic inhalant dermatitis: A review of 230 cases. *J Am Vet Med Assoc* 1978;172:55.

Nightengale SL. The FDA and drug uses: Reprise. *JAMA* 1985;253:632.

Noble GR, Bernier RH, Esber EC, et al. Acellular and whole-cell pertussis vaccines in Japan: Report of a visit by US scientists. *JAMA* 1987;257:1351−6.

Oren I, Hershow MD, Ben-Porath E, et al. A common-source outbreak of fulminant hepatitis B in a hospital. *Ann Intern Med* 1989;110:691−8.

Ozawa N, Shimizu M, Imai M, et al. Selective absence of immunoglobulin A1 or A2 among blood donors and hospital patients. *Transfusion* 1986;26:73−6.

Pabst HF, Godel J, Grace M, et al. Effect of breast feeding on immune response to BCG vaccination. *Lancet* 1989;1:295−7.

Parrish HM, Hayes R. Hospital management of pit viper envenomations. *Clin Toxicol* 1970;3:501.

Parrish HM, Khan MS. Bites by coral snakes: Report of 11 representative cases. *Am J Med Sci* 1967;253:561–8.

Pillemer L, Grossberg DB, Wittler RG. The immunochemistry of toxins and toxoids. II. The preparation and immunological evaluation of purified tetanal toxoid. *J Immunol* 1946;54:213–24.

Pirofsky B, Reid RH, Bardana EJ Jr., et al. Myasthenia gravis treated with purified antithymocyte antiserum. *Neurology* 1979;29:112–6.

Pollack W. Rh hemolytic disease of the newborn: Its cause and prevention. *Prog Clin Biol Res* 1981;70: 185–203.

Polmar SH, Smith TF, Pirofsky B, et al. Rapid infusion of intravenous immunoglobulin in patients with primary immunodeficiency disease. *J Allergy Clin Immunol* 1992;89:86A.

Prince HE, Morrow MB, Meyer GH, et al. Molds and bacteria in the etiology of respiratory allergic diseases: Studies with mold extracts produced from cultures grown in modified synthetic media: A preliminary report. *Ann Allergy* 1961;19:259–67.

Radosevich CA, Gordon LI, Weil SC, et al. Complete resolution of pure red cell aplasia in a patient with chronic lymphocytic leukemia following antithymocyte globulin therapy. *JAMA* 1988;259:723–9.

Redfield RR, Wright DC, James WD, et al. Disseminated vaccinia in a military recruit with human immunodeficiency virus (HIV) disease. *N Engl J Med* 1987;316:673–6.

Reisman RE. Venom immunotherapy: When is it reasonable to stop? *J Allergy Clin Immunol* 1991;87:618-20.

Robbins JB, Schneerson R. Polysaccharide-protein conjugates: A new generation of vaccines. *J Infect Dis* 1990;161:821–32.

Rodney WM, Chapivsky P, Quan M. Adult immunization: The medical record design as a facilitator for physician compliance. *J Med Educ* 1983;58:576–80.

Rodwell JD, Alvarez VL, Lee C, et al. Site-specific covalent modification of monoclonal antibodies: In-vitro and in-vivo evaluations. *Proc Natl Acad Sci USA* 1986;86:2632–6.

Rose RM, Rey-Martinez J, Croteau C, et al. Failure of recombinant interleukin-2 to augment the primary humoral response to a recombinant hepatitis B vaccine in healthy adults. *J Infect Dis* 1992;165:775–7.

Russell RF, Carlson RW, Wainschel J, et al. Snake venom poisoning in the United States: Experiences with 550 cases. *JAMA* 1975;233:341.

Schiff RI, Sedlak D, Buckley RH. Rapid infusion of Sandoglobulin in patients with primary humoral immunodeficiency. *J Allergy Clin Immunol* 1991;88:61–7.

Schmidt JO. Allergy to *Hymenoptera* venoms. In: Piek T, ed. Venoms of the *Hymenoptera*. London: Academic Press, 1986:50949.

Schmidt JO. Chemistry, pharmacology, and chemical ecology of ant venoms. In: Piek T, ed. Venoms of the *Hymenoptera*. London: Academic Press, 1986:425–508.

Schwarz JA, Koch W, Buehler V, et al. Pharmacokinetics of low molecular (monovalent) dextran (Dx 1) in volunteers. *Int J Clin Pharmacol Ther Toxicol* 1981;19:358–67.

Seeff LB, Zimmerman HJ, Wright EC, et al. Efficacy of hepatitis B immune serum globulin after accidental exposure. *Lancet* 1975;2:939–41.

Seibert FB. The isolation and properties of the purified protein derivative of tuberculin. *Am Rev Tuberc* 1934;30:713–20.

Shapiro GG, Anderson JA. Controversial techniques in allergy. *Pediatrics* 1988;82:935–7.

Shaw FE Jr., Guess HA, Roets JM, et al. Effect of anatomic site, age and smoking on the immune response to hepatitis B vaccination. *Vaccines* 1989;7:425–30.

Shirk MB, Hale KN. Obtaining drugs from foreign markets. *Am J Hosp Pharm* 1992;49:2731–9.

Siber GR. Immune globulin to prevent nosocomial infections. *N Engl J Med* 1992;327:269–71.

Slade HB, Schwartz SA. Mucosal immunity: The immunology of breast milk. *J Allergy Clin Immunol* 1987;80:346–56.

Smith TA II, Figge HL. Treatment of snakebite poisoning. *Am J Hosp Pharm* 1991;48:2190–6.

Spaite DW, Dart RC, Hurlbut K, et al. Skin testing: Implications in the managment of pit-viper envenomation. *Ann Emerg Med* 1988;17:389.

Steinhart R, Reingold AL, Taylor F, et al. Invasive *Haemophilus influenzae* infections in men with HIV infection. *JAMA* 1992;268:3350–2.

Steinhoff MC, Auerbach BS, Nelson KE, et al. Antibody responses to Haemophilus influenzae type b vaccines in men with human immunodeficiency virus infection. *N Engl J Med* 1991;325:1837–42.

Stevens DA, Levine HB, Deresinski SC, et al. Spherulin in clinical coccidioidomycosis: Comparison with coccidioidin. *Chest* 1975;68:697–702.

Stiehm ER. Skin testing prior to measles vaccination for egg-sensitive patients. *Am J Dis Child* 1990;144:32.

Tacket CO, Shandera WX, Mann JM, et al. Equine antitoxin use and other factors that predict outcome in type A foodborne botulism. *Am J Med* 1984;76:794–8.

Todd PA, Brogden RN. Muromonab CD3: A review of its pharmacology and therapeutic potential. *Drugs* 1989;37:871–99.

Trissel LA, Martinez JF. Sargramostim incompatibility. *Hosp Pharm* 1992;27:929.

Ujhelyi MR, Colucci RD, Cummings DM, et al. Monitoring serum digoxin concentrations during digoxin immune Fab therapy. *DICP Ann Pharrnacother* 1991;25:1047–9.

Ujhelyi MR, Green PJ, Cummings DM, et al. Determination of free serum digoxin concentration in digoxin toxic patients after administration of digoxin fab antibodies. *Ther Drug Monit* 1992;14:147–54.

Wainwright RB, McMahon BJ, Bulkow LR, et al. Duration of immunogenicity and efficacy of hepatitis B vaccine in a Yupik Eskimo population. *JAMA* 1989;261:2362–6.

Watt C, Gennaro J. Pit viper bites in south Georgia and north Florida. *Tr South Surg Assoc* 1966;77:378.

Weber RW, Nelson HS. Pollen allergens and their interrelationships. *Clin Rev Allergy* 1985;3:291–318.

Weiss ME, Adkinson NF. Immediate hypersensitivity reactions to penicillin and related antibiotics. *Clin Allergy* 1988;18:515–40.

Wingert WA, Wainschel J. Diagnosis and management of envenomation by poisonous snakes. *South Med J* 1975;68:1015–26.

ADDITIONAL SOURCES

GENERAL REFERENCES

American Academy of Pediatrics (AAP). *Report of the Committee on Infectious Diseases*, 22nd ed. Elk Grove Village, IL: American Academy of Pediatrics, 1991.

American Cancer Society. Cancer *Facts and Figures-1992*. Atlanta: American Cancer Society, 1992.

American College of Physicians (ACP). *Guide for Adult Immunizations*, 2nd ed. Philadelphia: American College of Physicians, 1990.

Australia National Health and Medical Research Council (NHMRC). *Immunisation Procedures*, 4th ed. Canberra: Australian Government Publishing Service, 1991.

Bellanti JA. Basic immunologic principles underlying vaccination procedures. *Pediatr Clin N Amer* 1990; 37:513–30.

Benenson AS, ed. *Control of Communicable Diseases in Man*, 15th ed. Washington, DC: American Public Health Association, 1990.

British Joint Committee on Vaccination and Immunisation. *Immunisation Against Infectious Disease*. London: Her Majesty's Stationary Office, 1988.

Canadian National Advisory Committee on Immunizations. *Canadian Immunization Guide*, 3rd ed. Ottawa: Ministry of National Health and Welfare, 1989.

Centers for Disease Control and Prevention (CDC). *Health Information for International Travel 1992*. Washington, DC: Government Printing Office, 1992; revised annually and updated biweekly.

CDC. Update on adult immunization: Recommendations of the Immunization Practices Advisory Committee (ACIP). *MMWR* 1991;40(RR-12):1–94.

Cryz SJ Jr., ed. *Vaccines and Immunotherapy*. New York: McGraw-Hill, 1991.

deShazo RD, Smith DL, eds. JAMA primer on allergic and immunologic diseases. *JAMA* 1992;268:2789–996.

Immunization Practices Advisory Committee (ACIP). General recommendations on immunization. *MMWR* 1989;38:205-14,219-27 and *Clin Pharm* 1989;8:839–50.

Joklik WK, Willett HP, Amos DB, et al, eds. *Zinsser Microbiology*, 20th ed. Norwalk, CT: Appleton and Lange, 1992.

Koeller J, Tami J, eds. *Concepts in Immunology and Immunotherapeutics*, 2nd ed. Bethesda, MD: American Society of Hospital Pharmacists, 1992.

LaForce FM. Immunizations, immunoprophylaxis, and chemoprophylaxis to prevent selected infections. *JAMA* 1987;257:2464–70.

National Coalition for Adult Immunization (NCAI). Standards for adult immunization practice. *Am J Hosp Pharm* 1990;47:2348.

Plotkin SA, Mortimer EA Jr., eds. *Vaccines*. Philadelphia: WB Saunders, 1988.

Public Health Service (PHS), US Department of Health and Human Services. Immunization and Infectious Disease. In: *Healthy People 2000: National Health Promotion and Disease Prevention Objectives*. Washington, DC: Government Printing Office, 1991:511–28.

Russell FE. *Snake Venom Poisoning*. Great Neck, NY: Scholium International, 1983.

World Health Organization (WHO). *Vaccination Certificate Requirements for International Travel and Health Advice to Travelers*. Albany, NY: World Health Organization, 1992; and revised annually.

VACCINE ADVOCACY & DELIVERY METHODS

Fedson DS. Improving the use of pneumococcal vaccine through a strategy of hospital-based immunization: A review of its rationale and implications. *J Am Geriatr Soc* 1985;33:142–50.

Fedson DS. Influenza and pneumococcal immunization strategies for physicians. *Chest* 1987;91:436–43.

Grabenstein JD, Hayton BD. Pharmacoepidemiologic program for identifying patients in need of vaccination. *Am J Hosp Pharm* 1990;47:1774–81.

Grabenstein JD. Pneumococcal pneumonia: Don't wait, vaccinate. *Hosp Pharm* 1990;25:866–69.

Williams WW, Hickson MA, Kane MA, et al. Immunization policies and vaccine coverage among adults: The risk for missed opportunities. *Ann Intern Med* 1988;108:616–25.

PREGNANCY, BREASTFEEDING & IMMUNIZATIONS

American College of Obstetricians and Gynecologists. Technical Bulletin #160: Immunization during pregnancy. Washington, DC: ACOG, October 1991.

ACOG. Technical Bulletin #147: Prevention of D isoimmunization. Washington, DC: ACOG, October 1990.

ACOG. Technical Bulletin #148: Management of isoimmunization in pregnancy. Washington, DC: ACOG, October 1990.

Barry M, Bia F. Pregnancy and travel. *JAMA* 1989;261:728–31.

CDC. *Health Information for International Travel.* Washington, DC: GPO, 1992 [revised annually].

Halsey NA, Klein D. Maternal immunization. *Pediatr Infect Dis J* 1990;9: 574–81.

Insel RA. Maternal immunization to prevent neonatal infections. *N Engl J Med* 1988;319:1219–20.

Slade HB, Schwartz SA. Mucosal immunity: The immunology of breast milk. *J Allergy Clin Immunol* 1987;80:346–56.

IMMUNOCOMPROMISED HOSTS & IMMUNIZATIONS

CDC. Purified protein derivative (PPD)-tuberculin anergy and HIV infection: Guidelines for anergy testing and management of anergic persons at risk of tuberculosis. *MMWR* 1991;40(RR-5):27–33.

Hibberd PL, Rubin RH. Approach to immunization in the immunosuppressed host. *Infect Dis Clin N Amer* 1990;4:123–42.

Kafidi KT, Rotschafer JC. Bacterial vaccines for splenectomized patients. *Drug Intell Clin Pharm* 1988;22: 192–7.

Onorato IM, Markowitz LE, Oxtoby MJ. Childhood immunization, vaccine-preventable diseases, and infection with human immunodeficiency virus. *Pediatr Infect Dis J* 1988;6:588–95.

HISTORICAL SUMMARYS

Chase A. *Magic Shots.* New York: William Morrow, 1982.

Coombs RRA, Gell PGH. The classification of allergic reactions underlying disease. In: Gell GPH, Coombs RRA, eds. *Clinical Aspects of Immunology.* Philadelphia: FA Davis, 1963:317–37.

Gregg CT. *Plague: An Ancient Disease in the Twentieth Century,* revised edition. Albuquerque: University of New Mexico Press, 1985.

Neustadt RE, Fineberg HV. *The Epidemic That Never Was: Policy-Making and The Swine Flu Affair.* New York: Vintage Books, 1983.

Parish HJ. *A History of Immunizations*. Baltimore: Williams and Wilkins, 1965.

Rosenberg CE. *The Cholera Years: The United States in 1832, 1849, and 1866*. Chicago: University of Chicago Press, 1987.

Silverstein AM. *Pure Politics and Impure Science: The Swine Flu Affair*. Baltimore: Johns Hopkins University Press, 1981.

Smith, Jane S. *Patenting the Sun: Polio and the Salk Vaccine*. New York: William Morrow and Co., 1990.

Starzl TE. *The Puzzle People: Memoirs of a Transplant Surgeon*. Pittsburgh: University of Pittsburgh Press, 1992.

FDA ADVISORY REVIEW PANEL REPORTS

FDA. Biological products; blood and blood derivatives; implementation of efficacy review. *Fed Reg* 1985 Dec 24;50:52602–723.

FDA. Biological products; bacterial vaccines and toxoids; implementation of efficacy review; proposed rule. *Fed Reg* 1985 Dec 13;50:51002–117.

FDA. Biological products; allergenic extracts; opportunity for hearing. *Fed Reg* 1985 Aug 9;50:32314–8.

FDA. Biological products; allergenic extracts; implementation of efficacy review; proposed rule. *Fed Reg* 1985 Jan 23;50:3082–287.

FDA. Viral and rickettsial vaccines; proposed implementation of efficacy review. *Fed Reg* 1980 Apr 15;45:25652–758.

FDA. Skin test antigens; implementation of efficacy review. *Fed Reg* 1979 Jul 10;44:40284–90,45617.

FDA. Skin test antigens; proposed implementation of efficacy review. *Fed Reg* 1977 Sep 30;42:52674–723,61613.

Other detailed references are available from the editor upon request.

Personal Vaccine Profile

Date Prepared: _____ Updated: ____ , ____ , ____

Name	Male / Female	Birth Date / /	Age: ____ Years	ID #
Occupation	Address			Daytime Telephone #

Allergies: eggs, mercury/thimerosal, neomycin, other:	Describe reaction: When?	Primary Physician:

use pencil...

☐ I am now or I might be pregnant.

☐ I take steroids or get other drugs or radiation that might suppress my immune system.

☐ I had a serious reaction to a vaccine in the past. Describe:

☐ My spleen does not work properly.

☐ I have some other problem with my immune system.

☐ Someone with a weak immune system lives in my home.

☐ Medications I take regularly include:

☐ List any other serious medical problems:

☐ I had a positive tuberculin skin test (Tine, PPD) in the past. When?

● My childhood vaccines are probably up-to-date.
Yes / No / Maybe

use pen...

		Dose, Product	Date Given	Comment	Date Next Dose Due	
Diphtheria,	1.	_____	_____	_____	_____	Children need 5 DTP doses.
Tetanus,	2.	_____	_____	_____	_____	
Pertussis	3.	_____	_____	_____	_____	
(DTP, DT, Td)	4.	_____	_____	_____	_____	
	5.	_____	_____	_____	_____	Adults need Td every 10 years.
	6.	_____	_____	_____	_____	
Hepatitis B	1.	_____	_____	_____	_____	Children need 3 hepatitis B doses. Some adults need them too.
	2.	_____	_____	_____	_____	
	3.	_____	_____	_____	_____	
Haemophilus	1.	_____	_____	_____	_____	Children need 3 or 4 Hib doses, depending on brand.
influenzae	2.	_____	_____	_____	_____	
type b (Hib)	3.	_____	_____	_____	_____	
	4.	_____	_____	_____	_____	
Polio-	1.	_____	_____	_____	_____	People need 4 polio doses, any type.
Virus	2.	_____	_____	_____	_____	
(OPV/IPV)	3.	_____	_____	_____	_____	
	4.	_____	_____	_____	_____	

(Continue on other side. List vaccine needs at bottom of other side.)

46

Name:				
	Dose, Product	Date Given	Comment	Date Next Dose Due

(continued from other side)

Measles, 1. _____ _____ _____ _____ — 2 MMR doses needed by everyone born since 1957.

Mumps, 2. _____ _____ _____ _____

Rubella _____ _____ _____ _____

Chickenpox _____ _____ _____ _____ — List disease or vaccine.

Pneumococcal _____ _____ _____ _____ — Needed by all people 65 years and older, plus others.

   Pneumonia _____ _____ _____ _____

Influenza _____ _____ _____ _____ — Needed by all people 65 years and older, plus others.

_____ _____ _____ _____

_____ _____ _____ _____

Tuberculin _____ _____ _____ _____ — If you have a confirmed positive test, do not get tested again.

Skin Tests _____ _____ _____ _____

(PPD, Tine, etc.) _____ _____ _____ _____

Other Vaccines: _____ _____ _____ _____

_____ _____ _____ _____ _____

_____ _____ _____ _____ _____

_____ _____ _____ _____ _____

_____ _____ _____ _____ _____

Vaccines Needed Soon:	Vaccines Needed In Next Few Months:	Vaccines Needed Next Year:

Where to get vaccinated: telephone:

address:

Hours offered: _____ to _____ ; _____ to _____

Conditions: Notes:

Days offered (circle):
Sun Mon Tue Wed Thu Fri Sat

If you have questions, read The Family Vaccine Book or ask your physician, pharmacist, or nurse.

This form may be freely copied for individuals, if you credit The Family Vaccine Book.

Animal Vaccine Profile: DOGS														

Pet Name: | **Owner's Name:** | **Birth Date or Age:** | **Male / Female**

Is this dog outside....? ☐ a little (house dogs)   ☐ sometimes (in between)   ☐ a lot (hunting dogs)

Is the dog with other dogs....? ☐ a little (neighbor dogs)   ☐ sometimes in kennel   ☐ a lot (show dog, stud dog)

Is Lyme disease common in your area?   Yes   Don't know   No   Ask your veterinarian if unsure.

Vaccines to Consider:
- ☐ Rabies
- ☐ Distemper
- ☐ Measles
- ☐ Bordetella bronchiseptica
- ☐ Parvovirus
- ☐ Coronavirus
- ☐ Adenovirus (CAV-1 or CAV-2)
- ☐ Parainfluenza-3 (PI-3)
- ☐ Leptospirosis
- ☐ Lyme disease

Vaccines Given	Dose, Product	Date Given	Comment	Date Next	Rabies	Distemp	Measles	Parvo	Coron a	CAV1/a2	Borde tint f	Paratinsp	Lep to sp	Lyme

Vaccines Needed Soon: | **Vaccines Needed In Next Few Months:** | **Vaccines Needed Next Year:**

Where to get vaccinated: telephone:

address:

hours offered: _____ to _____ ; _____ to _____

Conditions: **Notes:**

days offered (circle):

Sun Mon Tue Wed Thu Fri Sat

If you have questions, ask your veterinarian.

This form may be freely copied for individuals, if you credit The Family Vaccine Book.

Animal Vaccine Profile: CATS			

Pet Name:	Owner's Name:	Birth Date or Age:	Male / Female

Is this cat outside....?	☐ a little (house cats)	☐ sometimes (in between)	☐ a lot (outdoor cats)
Is the cat with other cats....?	☐ a little (neighbor cats) ☐ sometimes in kennel		☐ a lot (show cat, breeder)

Vaccines to Consider:
- ☐ Rabies
- ☐ Chlamydia
- ☐ Calicivirus
- ☐ Rhinotracheitis
- ☐ Feline leukemia
- ☐ Infectious peritonitis
- ☐ Panleukopenia (distemper)

Vaccines Given	Dose, Product	Date Given	Comment	Date Next	Rabies	Chlamydia	Panleuk/Dr	Calicivir	Rhinotrac	Leukemia	Peritonit			

Vaccines Needed Soon:	Vaccines Needed in Next Few Months:	Vaccines Needed Next Year:	

Where to get vaccinated: telephone:

address:

hours offered: _____ to _____; _____ to _____

Conditions: Notes:

days offered (circle):

Sun Mon Tue Wed Thu Fri Sat

If you have questions, ask your veterinarian.

This form may be freely copied for individuals, if you credit The Family Vaccine Book.

VACCINE ADVERSE EVENT REPORTING SYSTEM

VAERS

24 Hour Toll-free information line 1-800-822-7967
P.O. Box 1100, Rockville, MD 20849-1100
PATIENT IDENTITY KEPT CONFIDENTIAL

For CDC/FDA Use Only

VAERS Number _____

Date Received _____

Patient Name:	Vaccine administered by (Name):	Form completed by (Name):
Last First M.I.	Responsible Physician _____	Relation ☐ Vaccine Provider ☐ Patient/Parent to Patient ☐ Manufacturer ☐ Other
Address	Facility Name/Address	Address *(if different from patient or provider)*
City State Zip	City State Zip	City State Zip
Telephone no. (_____) _____	Telephone no. (_____) _____	Telephone no. (_____) _____

1. State	2. County where administered	3. Date of birth ___/___/___ mm dd yy	4. Patient age	5. Sex ☐ M ☐ F	6. Date form completed ___/___/___ mm dd yy

7. Describe adverse event(s) (symptoms, signs, time course) and treatment, if any

8. Check all appropriate:
☐ Patient died   (date ___/___/___ mm dd yy)
☐ Life threatening illness
☐ Required emergency room/doctor visit
☐ Required hospitalization (_____days)
☐ Resulted in prolongation of hospitalization
☐ Resulted in permanent disability
☐ None of the above

9. Patient recovered ☐ YES ☐ NO ☐ UNKNOWN	10. Date of vaccination ___/___/___ mm dd yy Time _____ AM PM	11. Adverse event onset ___/___/___ mm dd yy Time _____ AM PM

12. Relevant diagnostic tests/laboratory data

13. Enter all vaccines given on date listed in no. 10

	Vaccine (type)	Manufacturer	Lot number	Route/Site	No. Previous doses
a.	_____	_____	_____	_____	_____
b.	_____	_____	_____	_____	_____
c.	_____	_____	_____	_____	_____
d.	_____	_____	_____	_____	_____

14. Any other vaccinations within 4 weeks prior to the date listed in no. 10

	Vaccine (type)	Manufacturer	Lot number	Route/Site	No. Previous doses	Date given
a.	_____	_____	_____	_____	_____	_____
b.	_____	_____	_____	_____	_____	_____

15. Vaccinated at: ☐ Private doctor's office/hospital ☐ Military clinic/hospital ☐ Public health clinic/hospital ☐ Other/unknown	16. Vaccine purchased with: ☐ Private funds ☐ Military funds ☐ Public funds ☐ Other /unknown	17. Other medications

18. Illness at time of vaccination (specify)	19. Pre-existing physician-diagnosed allergies, birth defects, medical conditions (specify)

20. Have you reported this adverse event previously? ☐ No ☐ To doctor ☐ To health department ☐ To manufacturer	***Only for children 5 and under***
	22. Birth weight _____ lb. _____ oz.	23. No. of brothers and sisters

21. Adverse event following prior vaccination (check all applicable. specify)	***Only for reports submitted by manufacturer/immunization project***

	Adverse Event	Onset Age	Type Vaccine	Dose no. in series	24. Mfr. / imm. proj. report no.	25. Date received by mfr. / imm. proj.
In patient	_____	_____	_____	_____		
In brother	_____	_____	_____	_____	26. 15 day report?	27. Report type
or sister	_____	_____	_____	_____	☐ Yes ☐ No	☐ Initial ☐ Follow-Up

Health care providers and manufacturers are required by law (42 USC 300aa-25) to report reactions to vaccines listed in the Table of Reportable Events Following Immunization. Reports for reactions to other vaccines are voluntary except when required as a condition of immunization grant awards.

Form VAERS -1

"Fold in thirds, tape & mail - DO NOT STAPLE FORM"

NO POSTAGE
NECESSARY
IF MAILED
IN THE
UNITED STATES
OR APO/FPO

BUSINESS REPLY MAIL
FIRST-CLASS MAIL   PERMIT NO. 1895   ROCKVILLE, MD

POSTAGE WILL BE PAID BY ADDRESSEE

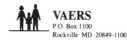 **VAERS**
P.O. Box 1100
Rockville MD 20849-1100

lıılıllııılıılıılılılıımıllıılllıılıımlılıl

DIRECTIONS FOR COMPLETING FORM
(Additional pages may be attached if more space is needed.)

GENERAL

- Use a separate form for each patient. Complete the form to the best of your abilities. Items 3, 4, 7, 8, 10, 11, and 13 are considered essential and should be completed whenever possible. Parents/Guardians may need to consult the facility where the vaccine was administered for some of the information (such as manufacturer, lot number or laboratory data.)

- Refer to the Reportable Events Table (RET) for events mandated for reporting by law. Reporting for other serious events felt to be related but not on the RET is encouraged.

- Health care providers other than the vaccine administrator (VA) treating a patient for a suspected adverse event should notify the VA and provide the information about the adverse event to allow the VA to complete the form to meet the VA's legal responsibility.

- These data will be used to increase understanding of adverse events following vaccination and will become part of CDC Privacy Act System 09-20-0136, "Epidemiologic Studies and Surveillance of Disease Problems". Information identifying the person who received the vaccine or that person's legal representative will not be made available to the public, but may be available to the vaccinee or legal representative.

- Postage will be paid by addressee. Forms may be photocopied (must be front & back on same sheet).

SPECIFIC INSTRUCTIONS

Form Completed By: To be used by parents/guardians, vaccine manufacturers/distributors, vaccine administrators, and/or the person completing the form on behalf of the patient or the health professional who administered the vaccine.

Item 7:   Describe the suspected adverse event. Such things as temperature, local and general signs and symptoms, time course, duration of symptoms diagnosis, treatment and recovery should be noted.

Item 9:   Check "YES" if the patient's health condition is the same as it was prior to the vaccine, "NO" if the patient has not returned to the pre-vaccination state of health, or "UNKNOWN" if the patient's condition is not known.

Item 10:   Give dates and times as specifically as you can remember. If you do not know the exact time, please
and 11:   indicate "AM" or "PM" when possible if this information is known. If more than one adverse event, give the onset date and time for the most serious event.

Item 12:   Include "negative" or "normal" results of any relevant tests performed as well as abnormal findings.

Item 13:   List ONLY those vaccines given on the day listed in Item 10.

Item 14:   List any other vaccines that the patient received within 4 weeks prior to the date listed in Item 10.

Item 16:   This section refers to how the person who gave the vaccine purchased it, not to the patient's insurance.

Item 17:   List any prescription or non-prescription medications the patient was taking when the vaccine(s) was given.

Item 18:   List any short term illnesses the patient had on the date the vaccine(s) was given (i.e., cold, flu, ear infection).

Item 19:   List any pre-existing physician-diagnosed allergies, birth defects, medical conditions (including developmental and/or neurologic disorders) for the patient.

Item 21:   List any suspected adverse events the patient, or the patient's brothers or sisters, may have had to previous vaccinations. If more than one brother or sister, or if the patient has reacted to more than one prior vaccine, use additional pages to explain completely. For the onset age of a patient, provide the age in months if less than two years old.

Item 26:   This space is for manufacturers' use only.

Index